A Computer Model of Human Respiration

A Computer Model of Human Respiration

**Ventilation—blood gas transport
and exchange—hydrogen ion regulation**

*For teaching, research and
clinical use—'MacPuf'*

by

C. J. Dickinson, D.M.

Professor of Medicine in the
University of London
at
St. Bartholomew's Hospital
Medical College

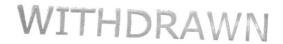

University Park Press
Baltimore

Published in USA and Canada by

University Park Press
Chamber of Commerce Building
Baltimore, Maryland 21202

Published in UK by

MTP Press Limited,
St Leonard's House,
Lancaster, England.

Library of Congress Cataloging in Publication Data

Dickinson, Christopher John.
  A computer model of human respiration.

  Includes bibliographical references and index.
  1. Respiration—Data processing. 2. Respiration—
Mathematical models. I. Title.
QP121.D5   612'.2'0184   77-5853
ISBN 0-8391-1144-4

Printed in Great Britain

To

ARTHUR GUYTON

with admiration and affection

A living organism cannot be correctly studied piece by piece separately, as the parts of a machine can be studied, the working of the whole machine being deduced synthetically from the separate study of each of the parts. A living organism is constantly showing itself to be a self-maintaining whole, and each part must therefore always be behaving as a part of such a self-maintaining whole.

J. S. HALDANE (1922)
Respiration (Oxford; University Press)

Contents

Preface

By trying to make my title both accurate and comprehensive I seem to have finished with one of those trendy mouthfuls like Peter Weiss's play *The Persecution and Assassination of Marat as performed by the Inmates of the Asylum of Charenton under the Direction of the Marquis de Sade*. My purpose, though, is to claim for this book a bit more than a technical description of a well-tested and reasonably accurate model of respiration and gas transport. I hope that some of the devices used in this particular model may be useful to people designing instructional computer models in other fields, and may exemplify some general design principles. There is at present a glut of computer simulations of vital processes, and a dearth of detailed description of such simulations and of the ways in which they can be used. Most present models are only of ephemeral value. No-one except the author can operate his model effectively. This book is to some extent an exercise in public relations, and an attempt to show that models really do have something to offer the scientific community of researchers, instructors and students.

Acknowledgements

I should first acknowledge McMaster University Medical School, Ontario, which appointed me R. Samuel McLaughlin Visiting Professor of Medicine during the exciting year that the first students arrived. There were no facilities for the students to carry out animal or human experiments, but they had the use of a digital computer in the Department of Epidemiology and Bio-statistics. Dr. E. J. Moran Campbell, Chairman of the Department of Medicine, was concerned at our initial lack of laboratory facilities, and asked me to design a physical model of blood circulation which might form the basis of class experiments in haemodynamics during the first year curriculum. I thought it might be interesting to take advantage of the computer resources, to draw on some previous experience in modelling biological systems, and to design an interactive computer model of systemic haemodynamics which could be used in the same way as animals are used in the traditional curriculum. Thanks to the enthusiastic co-operation of Dr. D. L. Sackett and Dr. C. H. Goldsmith the project was brought to a successful conclusion. A simple model has been available as a learning resource to four annual entries of students. This model—christened 'MacMan' as a convenient term for quick reference (Dickinson, Sackett and Goldsmith, 1973)—has been popular, insofar that it has been used by about half the students in most years. Subsequently this and other models have been transferred to time-sharing systems, and I am grateful to Dr. E. M. Chance and Dr. E. P. Shephard at University College, London, for helping me to become familiar with this powerful technique.

The father of 'MacPuf'—the respiratory model which is the subject of this book—is Moran Campbell. He introduced me to respiratory physiology when we were both working on the Medical Unit at the Middlesex Hospital in London, and also suggested to me, when we were both at McMaster, that I might do for respiration and blood gas transport the same as I had already done for systemic haemodynamics. The result pleasantly surprised us. The model has been gradually improved over the last six years, and has now become accurate enough to have some value in clinical work and in research as well as in the purely educational role for which it was conceived. Its progressive improvement has been largely due to the help I have had from Dr. Campbell and his associates, Dr. N. L. Jones and Dr. A. S. Rebuck. During return visits to McMaster they have progressively taught me the respiratory physiology which I have subsequently embedded in the model. Indeed, the discipline has proved an unusual but stimulating way of entering a field about which I was very ignorant. Dr. Gerald Partridge was largely responsible for the description used of bulk lactic acid metabolism. In the last few years Dr. Khursheed Ahmed, Software Supervisor at McMaster, and Dr. David Ingram, Lecturer in Medical Computing and Physics at St. Bartholomew's Hospital Medical College, have helped a lot with programming aspects, and in interfacing the model into the undergraduate teaching programme. During this time many in the Computation Services Unit at McMaster, especially its former Director, Dr. G. D. Anderson and the Computer Manager, Mr. Don Gilchrist, have tolerated gracefully my frequent traumatic dislocations of their other activities. The staffs of the Departments of Computer Science at Imperial College and Queen Mary College, London, especially Mr. Paul Verrier at Q.M.C., have also given unstinted help. Financial support has been generously provided by the Departments of Medicine and of Medical Education at McMaster, by the American Lung Association and by the Hewlett-Packard Corporation.

Dr. Campbell, Dr. Ingram, Dr. Jones and Dr. Rebuck have read and criticised the manuscript at different stages and I am very grateful for all their suggestions. The well-drawn diagrams are by Mr. V. K. Asta: I did the others myself. Dr. D. Ingram and Dr. A. Olszowka have very kindly read the proofs.

I am delighted and honoured that Dr. Arthur C. Guyton, the doyen of physiologists analysing integrated systems, has allowed me to dedicate this book to him. Finally, I must acknowledge the kind help and encouragement of my wife during the lengthy processes of gestation and revision of the book.

C. J. Dickinson,
St. Bartholomew's Hospital Medical College,
West Smithfield,
London, EC1A 7BE.

Part I
Principles of Physiological Design

1
Introduction

A model is a representation of a structure or in more general terms something which resembles, or behaves the same as, something else. The objects of model building are multifarious, but generally involve an attempt to simplify and thereby understand something better, to change the scale, and sometimes to test hypotheses. Watson and Crick's physical model of DNA was a beautiful example of model building. It allowed their proposed structure to be tested for internal consistency. The test was useful, indeed crucial, because their model, though enormous in relation to the size of the DNA molecule, was accurate. *Accuracy is the most essential attribute of any useful scientific model.*

I shall describe in this book a model which is half-way between a physical structure and a conceptual description. It is a computer programme which describes the main structures and functions involved in human respiration, and which has been used successfully in teaching, research, and clinical practice. The model began as a self-instructional device for students, but thanks to the enthusiastic collaboration of many skilful friends it has now, I hope, become accurate enough and economical enough (in terms of storage space and computer resources) to be of wider use, and perhaps worth publishing on that account alone. It has been previously described only in a brief abstract (Dickinson, 1972). The programme was developed over 6 years at McMaster University, University College Hospital Medical School, and St. Bartholomew's Hospital Medical College. It has been available at different stages of development to other medical schools in North America and Europe. However, the needs of one instructor or researcher are not necessarily the same as those of his colleagues elsewhere, and it is obviously desirable to make a complex model explicit, so that it may be adapted, changed or extended by others. For example, 'MacPuf'* could easily be extended into the field of anaesthetics, both for educational and research purposes. Unfortunately, as anyone with experience knows, it is extremely difficult to make sense of a computer programme even in a high level language (in this case Fortran) unless one has written the programme oneself—and it is often difficult even then!—or unless very complete documentation is available. One of my principal aims in this book is to supply that documentation.

---

* I hope readers will forgive the twee name for the model. It was christened one day in a light-hearted moment. The name stuck; and has since proved a useful shorthand term of reference.

All over the world people are building models of physiological systems, and thereby clarifying their thoughts; but it is exceptionally rare to see one group building on the foundations laid by another. The reason seems to be either that the models themselves are banal and not accurate enough to be interesting, or that, if good, they are too complex to be easily understood or used by others.

I might as well come clean at the start and confess that I am no mathematician, and that my understanding of the mathematical formulation and solution of differential equations is intuitive and inexact. I came to this field simply as a clinician and teacher of medical students, and found out for myself, as many others have done, that computers as tools have one transcending merit: the expenditure of a small amount of computer time can substitute not only for mathematical flair but also for native intelligence.

I can best explain what I mean by a simple example. It is related that a mathematician was set a problem. Two cyclists are 40 miles apart. They travel towards each other at 10 miles per hour, while a fly, travelling at 20 miles per hour, flits to and fro between the noses of each, until it is crushed as they meet in the middle. The problem is to find how far the fly has travelled.

According to legend the mathematician expressed the distance travelled as an infinite geometrical series, and summed this to obtain the answer (40 miles). A schoolboy, also according to legend, solved it by native intelligence, realising that the cyclists would each travel 20 miles, taking two hours in doing so, and that the fly (travelling twice as fast) would cover 40 miles in the same time. I will now expand the legend. The stupid non-mathematician,

```
C INITIALISE CUMULATIVE DISTANCE TRAVELLED(DISTAN) AND DISTANCE
C SEPARATING CYCLISTS(SEPAR)
        DISTAN=0.
        SEPAR=40.
C ITERATE UNTIL DISTANCE IS LESS THAN .001 MILES
        DO 1 I=1,100
C FROM SIMULTANEOUS EQUATIONS RELATING RELATIVE SPEEDS COMPUTE
C DISTANCE TRAVELLED BY FLY AT EACH LEG OF ITS JOURNEY
        RUN=SEPAR*2./3.
        DISTAN=DISTAN+RUN
        SEPAR=SEPAR-2.*(SEPAR-RUN)
        IF (RUN.LT..001) GO TO 2
1       CONTINUE
2       WRITE (6,3) DISTAN
3       FORMAT (' TOTAL DISTANCE TRAVELLED BY FLY=', F7.3,' MILES')
        WRITE(6,4) I
4       FORMAT(' NUMBER OF JOURNEYS=',I3,/,' END OF PROGRAMME')
        STOP
        END
        FINISH
14.33.21_ (FORL TEST,CONS,CONS)
STARTED

LOADED .
14.34.54_ (SRUN)

TOTAL DISTANCE TRAVELLED BY FLY= 40.000 MILES
NUMBER OF JOURNEYS= 11
END OF PROGRAMME

DELETED 00
14.35.05_
```

Figure 1.1   Computer programme written in Fortran IV, with execution of the same—see text (compile and run instructions encircled)

perhaps a clinician, lacked both mathematical skill and native intelligence, but was able to solve the problem by using a few milliseconds of time on a computer. It took him only a few minutes to write and run the computer programme in Figure 1.1 which involved no sophisticated mathematics, but gave the same answer by simple iterative additions. Incidentally, it also computed a value not obtainable by the other two methods, i.e. the number of journeys greater than 0.001 mile travelled by the fly.

The point I want to make by this example is that if one has the easily mastered ability to formulate solutions of this sort, difficult problems needing higher mathematics or exceptional intelligence melt away. Indeed, mathematicians nowadays make frequent use of iterative numerical methods to solve tedious problems.

The growing field of biological computer models, however, is not really

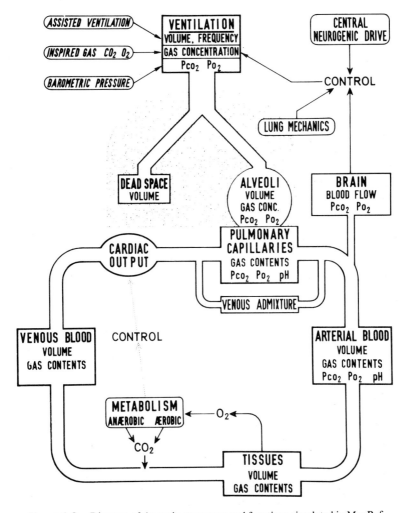

Figure 1.2   Diagram of the main structures and functions simulated in MacPuf

short on mathematical expertise. That is there in abundance. It is quite often short on accuracy and clinical relevance. On these grounds I would justify any attempts by clinicians and physiologists, however lacking they may be in mathematical or programming skill, to construct their own models. The pilot of an aircraft does not have to understand how a jet engine works, but he has to know how to control the plane and react appropriately in emergencies. Just as experienced pilots are needed to design flight simulators, physiologists and clinicians are needed to design analogous instructional models for student training.

The main structures and functions simulated by MacPuf are shown in Figure 1.2, which is a schematic representation of the blood circulation, the gas exchanging system, the control of ventilation, and the metabolism of the tissues. The model is given functional characteristics appropriate for a human being rather than for a lower animal, and it allows changes to be made and studied in one or more of the following:

Inspired oxygen	Breathing capacity
Inspired carbon dioxide	Ventilatory response to arterial PO_2
Cardiac performance	Ventilatory response to arterial PCO_2
Maximum cardiac output	and pH
Whole body metabolic rate	Intrinsic neurogenic ventilatory drive
Respiratory exchange ratio	Inspiratory/expiratory duration ratio
Venous admixture in the lungs	Lung volume
Right to left shunt	Lung elastance
Left to right shunt	Dead space
Tissue ECF volume	End-expiratory pressure
Venous blood volume	Vital capacity
Haemoglobin concentration	Barometric pressure
Packed cell volume	Body temperature
Red cell 2,3-DPG concentration	Threshold for switch to anaerobic
Whole body bicarbonate	metabolism
Brain bicarbonate concentration	

Changes in these parameters* can be specified by the operator, and produce acute changes in the various regulatory mechanisms. Usually a new steady state is reached after a few minutes of simulated time have elapsed. Sometimes a steady state cannot be reached, in which case either sustained oscillations will develop, as in Cheyne–Stokes breathing, or the value of one or more variables may pass outside the range compatible with life. The flexibility of the system is such that expired gases can be collected and analysed, and bag rebreathing experiments performed.

Artificial ventilation of any rate or depth can be used instead of natural ventilation. Simulated normal subjects of any age, size and sex can be created, and clinical disorders can be simulated by the insertion of pulmonary function tests, which change the appropriate internal parameters and allow an unlimited number of different steady states to be obtained. Conditions such as asphyxia, cardiac arrest, ventilatory failure, anaemia, hypothermia, high or

---

* The word 'parameter' is used here in a strict mathematical sense to refer to a quantity which is supplied as a constant, from which the model computes variables such as arterial PO_2 and ventilation.

low barometric pressure, intra-cardiac shunts and muscular exercise can be simulated, and possible therapeutic measures explored with realistic results.

SCHEME OF PRESENTATION

I shall first consider previous work on computer simulation of respiratory processes, then the mathematical treatment of a number of important situations such as the carriage of gases through large blood compartments, tissue metabolism, ventilation control and pulmonary gas exchange. After this I shall try to show how each part is fitted into an integrated working whole. Part II comprises a brief description of some empirical principles of machine/ user interaction, in which I shall attempt to define some general principles of the economical design of interactive dialogue and illustrate some practical applications of the model.

The reader might ask: 'Why a book and not an article in a journal?', but if so he would reveal himself never to have been a journal editor. The programme of a computer model is a precis, virtually in shorthand, of all the facts, relations, and theories which it comprises. Very few computer programmes are published in their entirety, because they are so long and so boring. The full documentation of a programme such as this runs to a length quite beyond the capacity of even a dedicated computer-programme journal. I hope that readers may find this book useful and, for the publisher's sake, that it will justify his time, trouble and expense.

2

Previous Computer Models of Respiration and Main Objectives of MacPuf

In the next chapter I shall restrict my use of the term 'model' to devices incorporating the self-stabilising characteristics of living things. In this chapter I propose to cast my net more widely and to describe the main work which has quantified individual respiratory processes and thus made possible the construction of a large integrative model. Gray (1945, 1950), for example, would hardly have claimed to have built a *model* of ventilatory control, but he came to the conclusion that the stimuli to ventilation from hypercapnia and hypoxaemia were additive and provided the first dynamic analysis of the system. Thus he laid the groundwork for the later more exact mathematical representations which were needed for further progress.

Grodins, Gray, Schroeder, Norins and Jones (1954) in a study correctly described as 'monumental' by Defares (1964) constructed what might be called the original 'chemostat' model of ventilation control. Using an analogue computer they were able to give an accurate description of the ventilatory response to inhaled carbon dioxide. Farhi and Rahn (1955) laid the basis of later models by West (1969), Kelman (1970) and Butler and Mohler (1970) of the effects of different distribution of lung compartments upon the alveolar-arterial gas pressure differences, even though at the time it was not a practical proposition, given the prevailing state of computer art, to turn their theoretical model into a working one. Until very recently, no attempts have been made to put all the main elements of respiration together. Careful measurement of ventilatory responses in man have given greater precision to mathematical representations of ventilatory controls (see Chapter 12).

The mechanical aspects of air flow (excluding gas exchange) have been studied by Gomez (1963), Fry (1968) and Paiva and Demeester (1971) and the distribution and transport of carbon dioxide by Matthews, Laszlo, Campbell and Read (1968). Early attempts to put together the various parts in a single model include the descriptions of Milhorn, Benton, Ross and Guyton (1965) and Grodins, Buell and Bart (1967). The latter model incorporated the novel feature of flow-rate dependent transport delays. Later Milhorn and Brown (1971) incorporated the hypoxic drive to ventilation and non-linear dissociation curves in their model, and also suggested a way of predicting the partition of total ventilation between the tidal volume and respiratory rate. Milhorn, Reynolds and Holloman (1972) by computer modelling and matching ventilatory responses to CO_2 inhalation and to perfusion of the cerebral chemoreceptor with CO_2-rich cerebrospinal fluid suggested that the central chemoreceptor site lay somewhere between deep brain tissue and cerebrospinal fluid.

All these efforts in modelling have intentionally had a restricted scope and have only examined one part of the whole system shown in Figure 1.2. Possibly the simulation of Grodins *et al.* (1967) was the most complete, since it included a cerebral circulation; nonetheless, dead space, respiratory rate, venous admixture and the main tissue compartment circulation were not included. I know of three larger models, but no doubt others are being developed in many places, by independent groups. The model described in this book was demonstrated on an interactive time-sharing computer to the British Physiological Society in March 1972, and has been previously published in abstract form (Dickinson, 1972). Since then it has been further and extensively developed. A similarly comprehensive simulation is well advanced in the basic sciences departments of the University of Michigan at Ann Arbor (Dr. G. Nordby and his associates). The most complete description of a respiratory model yet published in a reasonably extended form is that of Farrell and Siegel (1973). To quote the introduction to their paper: 'There had been a number of important attempts to design computer simulations of the cardio-respiratory system. These past studies have demonstrated that such simulations can reproduce certain interactive physiologic phenomena . . . they were of limited scope . . . and they did not provide any easy way of going from the parameters of the simulation to real patient data so that the assumption and conclusions of the simulation could be checked.'

The advantage of being able to check a complete system by comparing its predictions with physiological and clinical data is an important one, seldom fully appreciated. Since every part of a whole system interacts with every other, it can become very artificial, for example, to consider ventilation controls apart from the exchange and transport of gases. Farrell and Siegel's model has several points of similarity to MacPuf, e.g. in the use of Kelman's equations for interconverting gas contents and pressures and in its description of interactions of tissue metabolism and cardiac output. It is different from MacPuf in that it is a steady state model in which ventilation is described as a continuous process. It uses short iteration intervals (100 ms). This is potentially more accurate, but uses a lot of computer time, and makes it expensive and inconvenient to offer such a model as a teaching tool for wide use. Unlike MacPuf, it incorporates an extensive description of lung mechanics and also uses the relatively sophisticated ten-compartment model for the distribution of ventilation/perfusion ratios described by West (1969). This doubtless increases the accuracy of the final solution, but again at the expense of a great deal more computer time. For most clinical and instructional purposes, I found that I could greatly simplify the description of lung mechanics; and for reasons which I shall explain fully in Chapter 9 I have preferred to use the simplest possible three-compartment model of ventilation/ perfusion matching in the lung (Riley and Cournand; 1949) with some modifications to economise on computer time.

There is one temptation difficult to resist. This is to describe part of the whole model to an accuracy of 99.999% while having to accept the best possible estimate of the performance of some other part, which may be only perhaps 90% or less accurate. I have made a conscious and sustained effort to simplify my description at each stage, aiming for an accuracy in each part of the programme of at least 1–2% where it was obtainable, but avoiding any greater accuracy if it involved extra storage space or execution time unless the errors would be cumulative. Sometimes accuracy which appears excessive costs nothing. For example, room air is given an oxygen content of 20.93 volumes per cent (Haldane and Priestley, 1935) rather than of 21%, because the space allocated in a computer's storage compartment to a floating point number always contains more than four significant figures, and no more storage is needed for 20.93 than for 21. In other respects, however, the reader will find extraordinary liberties being taken with the total description, especially in the use of a basic 10 s interation interval, during which almost all the arterial blood pool is turned over! Once again I have done this to make the model a workable proposition on a small computer, and have extensively used damping techniques, fully described in Chapter 5, to inhibit unphysiological oscillatory behaviour. I do not apologise for this. I hope to convince the reader that the dynamic and steady state performance of MacPuf has not been seriously impaired by cutting a great many corners. This has allowed me in some respects to go much further than Farrell and Siegel and to realise a number of objectives which I shall briefly summarise.

AIMS AND OBJECTIVES OF THE MODEL

1. To describe transient and oscillatory phenomena as well as steady states;
2. To describe every possible variety of disturbance of ventilation control, gas transport and gas exchange, and acid–base regulation which may be seen in disease states;
3. To create a model correct not only for minor deviations within the physiological range, but also for the greater disturbances seen in such conditions as anoxaemia, cardiac arrest, asphyxia, and strenuous muscular exercise;
4. To allow the simplest possible operation by someone without any computer experience;
5. To present the model as a cooperative human subject who will permit any, even lethal, experiments to be performed upon him;
6. To make the model as entertainingly realistic as possible, within the practical limitations of easily available input/output technology;
7. To give it as much clinical relevance as possible, by making provision for the construction of simulated patients by preset routines or by the insertion of respiratory function test results, and for giving different types of artificial ventilation;
8. To allow the simulation of most class experiments and clinical tests involving muscular exercise, bag collection of expired air, rebreathing from a bag, holding the breath, and voluntary hyperventilation;
9. To provide facilities for breaking open feedback loops to allow simplified

types of physiological experiments—just as one may design physiological experiments to hold constant everything except those few things one is studying. This means, of course, that the computer model goes from complex to simple, but this is also just what one does when designing a physiological experiment;

10. To keep the programme itself as simple as possible, written in a standard language (Fortran) available on most mini-computers and immediately transferable to anyone's computer except the very smallest.

SUMMARY

With a few recent exceptions most previous models of respiratory structures and functions have been mathematical descriptions of necessary relationships between blood gas tensions and ventilation, between ventilation/perfusion matching and blood gas composition, or between the mechanical properties of the lungs and the resultant patterns of air flow. In recent years a few more comprehensive models have put these and other components together, thus allowing the behaviour of the whole system to be more readily compared with clinical and physiological observation. The respiratory model described in this book goes much further towards a complete description than any previously described models and is designed to allow simulation of transient as well as steady state responses in a wide range of clinical situations. The key to effective operation of such a model on a small interactive or time-sharing computer is the use of a long (e.g. 10 s) iteration interval.

3
General Principles of Design of a Comprehensive Model of Respiration

I shall try first to justify making a single, large, complete model rather than a number of small models, each covering certain aspects of the field. The use of limited models for instructional purposes is already highly developed. I have seen several imaginative analogue computer simulations of respiratory processes, and Modell, Farhi and Olszowka (1974) have demonstrated the power of a set of limited digital computer models which are already in regular use in the State University of New York at Buffalo, and elsewhere, for doing simulated class experiments in respiratory physiology. These models are written in the BASIC language, and are convenient and economical to run. Since a larger model needs a bigger computer to store the programme, and takes more central processor time to run, I need to explain why a holistic, i.e. comprehensive, approach has more to offer, and why, at the very least, it is complementary to a piecemeal approach. This justification could be extensive; but a simple answer would be that the simulation possible on a holistic model is more realistic and therefore more exciting, and that, as Haldane says, 'A living organism cannot be correctly studied piece by piece separately. . . . A living organism is constantly showing itself to be a co-ordinated self-maintaining whole.'

The advantages of limited models lie in their simplicity. For example, the control of ventilation comprises at least three factors. There is an intrinsic tendency for the respiratory neurones to discharge rhythmically even when separated from all structures above the mid-pons, and even when they are deprived of all sensory input, providing that they are maintained in a suitable chemical environment (see Chapter 12). In addition to this 'central neurogenic drive' which, for reasons still not understood, normally corresponds closely with the body's demands for oxygen (e.g. at different levels of muscular exercise), there is a stimulus to breathing provided by the arterial chemo-receptors, which signal oxygen lack and the prevailing P_aCO_2. Carbon dioxide also stimulates the central respiratory neurones directly. We may envisage a representation of this kind:

Central neurogenic drive ⟶

Hypoxic stimulus ⟶ Resultant ventilation

Hypercapnic stimulus ⟶

Such a scheme could be programmed on a small computer very easily, and equipped with input/output dialogue to make a teaching model. For example, it would be very simple to take one of the many mathematical representations available in the literature, and to construct an interactive 'model' whose output might look like the following (operator's answers in bold type):

SPECIFY PCO_2 IN MM HG   **38**
SPECIFY PO_2 IN MM HG   **71**
SPECIFY OXYGEN CONSUMPTION IN CC/MIN   **500**

****RESULTANT TOTAL VENTILATION = 9.3 LITRES/MIN*****

WHICH DO YOU WANT TO CHANGE......1. PO_2,   2. PCO_2,
3. BOTH?   **2**

OK ... PRESENT VALUE IS 38 – WHAT IS YOUR NEW VALUE?   **50**

****RESULTANT TOTAL VENTILATION = 57.3 LITRES/MIN*****

WHICH DO YOU WANT TO CHANGE ... etc.

Such a teaching exercise could hardly be described as using a model because it amounts to little more than using the computer as a simple calculating machine with predetermined arithmetic, but with the ability to ask text-type questions.

It is also artificial. In practice if one wishes to raise the P_aCO_2 of an animal or man, this can be done by the inhalation of CO_2, by rebreathing from a bag, reducing ventilatory capacity, adding dead space, or chronically administering sodium bicarbonate. Unless one is trying to simulate the physiologically ideal experiment in which a head is perfused from a separate donor, and the resultant ventilation measured in the recipient's trunk, also separately perfused and connected to the head only by the nerve supply, the computer model whose performance is illustrated above will be unexciting and artificial. In practice, the response to CO_2 inhalation is complex, and the prevailing PCO_2 of the arterial blood after a given time may not be at all easy to predict. To take a still more complex example: the addition of a large dead space, e.g. 1000 cc, will immediately reduce alveolar ventilation to zero, and slow oscillatory swings may develop before a steady state is reached.

One might generalise to say that any model which is so simple that it can be described by a few mathematical equations is hardly worth constructing, and perhaps might even do harm by making a student think that the classical experiments of physiology were equally simple. In practice, a great deal of thought has to be devoted to the design of experiments in which all other factors are held constant by some artificial means while the effects of variation in just one of them is measured.

The easy predictability of the results obtained from a simple model makes it difficult to capture a student's interest. He does not feel that he is doing experiments on a simulated human being or animal, but rather simply performing mundane mathematical exercises which have been already designed by his instructors.

Those who are interested enough to read this book will probably be interested enough to set up this programme, or to get it ready-made on magnetic tape or on a card deck from McMaster University (which can supply it in this form at nominal cost*) and can soon discover for themselves that a complete model in which most of the important negative feedback loops are closed allows one to gain useful insight into the ways in which the body reacts in a complex but co-ordinated way to various simple stimuli. Another advantage of a holistic model is that it can be programmed to produce symptoms and signs, which instruct as well as entertain. Tests can be inserted to check for lethal conditions arising, and necropsy reports can be printed if such experiments are accidentally performed.

For these reasons I now believe that the most effective future developments of computer models for *teaching* purposes are likely to be along the lines I have indicated, and that it is well worth the initially greater expense and slight extra running costs to provide lively and reasonably realistic holistic models of biological systems. It is very difficult to make a limited non-circular model at all comprehensive or lifelike. When it comes to research applications, there is no comparison at all. It is easy to scale down or to simplify a complex model, but difficult to get useful insights from an unduly simple model.

If one builds a computer or any other model which relates 30 variables, and specifies that one will be interested in deviations through a ten-step range, e.g. 0, 20, 40, 60, 80, 100, 120, 150, 175 and 200% of the normal value for each variable, a very large number of experiments is possible. Each variable can be independently changed so that 10^{30} possible situations can be examined or simulated experiments performed.

Since in practice it is no more difficult to allow a graded scale for changing each parameter, there is effectively no limit to the number of different experiments or conditions which can be simulated. This situation is both exciting and daunting. It is exciting to the student or researcher because he is in no way constrained in what he chooses to study; but it is daunting to the designer because he cannot be expected to test more than a tiny fraction of all the possible situations which the model can simulate. However, such a model can at the same time be exciting to the designer because it may allow him to make inferences about the size of compartments, constants for rate changes, transfer factors and other quantities which by current techniques are impossible to measure. This in turn allows the possibility of progressively improving the accuracy of the model by supplying it with more accurate functions and parameters, and also allows someone familiar with the model to envisage and test out the practicability of new experiments.

MacPuf has been tested out at each stage, with the help of many friends and colleagues, through a large range of clinical situations. I have also drawn heavily on my clinical experience as a general physician in London, in which respiratory diseases flourish exceedingly. After giving a large number of lectures and demonstrations in many places, I have been able to return to the drawing board, so to speak, and correct inaccuracies of description pointed

* From Computation Services Unit, McMaster University Health Sciences Center, Main Street West, Hamilton, Ontario, Canada L85 4JG.

out by others. To give just one example, I demonstrated the model on one occasion a few years ago to Professor A. C. Dornhorst at St. George's Hospital in London. He pointed out to me that the phase relations of MacPuf's original simulation of Cheyne–Stokes breathing were wrong, and therefore that the assumptions regarding the relative time delays at different points must also be wrong. As a result I was stimulated to read about this subject more extensively, and to write a more accurate description into the programme, after which I found that I had at the same time improved the accuracy of MacPuf's description of the ventilatory changes during rebreathing.

MAIN DESIGN FEATURES OF MACPUF

The main point of originality in the design of this model lies in the use of a long iteration interval of the same order as the respiratory rate. This is quite different, for example, from the simulation of Yamamoto and Hori (1971) who used multiple computing points during each phase of breathing in and out. If respiratory rate is 15 cycles/min, an iteration interval of 4 s allows a single complete respiratory cycle to be described during each execution of the main programme loop, so that the whole tidal volume is moved in and out at each interval. The calculations which are described in greater detail in Chapter 5 indicate that the amount of blood shifted from one main blood pool to another in such a time interval is manageable in terms of the total amounts of oxygen and carbon dioxide transferred. In fact, a rather longer interval still (10 s) proves to be a practicable possibility for resting conditions with a low cardiac output, though in this case damping becomes important to prevent instability of operation. It also proves possible, by careful damping, to represent moderately increased ventilation with a 10 s iteration interval. The techniques discussed in Chapter 8 allow realistic time delays to be created or simulated with minimal complexity or storage capacity.

All this leads to a great saving in computer time, and makes it entirely practical and not unduly extravagant to make the whole model available to a class of medical students on a small dedicated computer or on a larger time-sharing system. It takes a *simulated* time of at least 12 minutes to reach a stable state after changing a number of key parameters, chiefly because of the large size of the body's carbon dioxide stores. If one is using a 0.1 s iteration interval (e.g. Farrell and Siegel, 1973) the time to achieve a steady state would be 100 times longer than it is in MacPuf, using a 10 s interval. I know nothing of what happens inside computers; but in practical terms the user of a time-sharing system such as the Sigma-5 (Cybernet), the CDC 6400 (Intercom and Kronos), the ICL 1900 (Maximop) or the HP 3000 (with all of which I have had long experience) would find that instead of having to wait perhaps a minute to achieve a steady state while such a machine was supporting, say, 30 other users, the time would instead increase to about an hour, which is an intolerable inconvenience and expense except for a well-conceived research project. Effective use of the model would tie up most of the central processor time of a medium-sized computer. Its use on a time-sharing basis would be impossible.

SUMMARY

The relative merits of limited and complete (holistic) models are described, and reasons given for preferring a complete model for most teaching and research purposes, because it is more realistic and entertaining, and because its predictions are much easier to test against physiological or clinical data. The main points of originality of the present model are then described, and the special advantages and economies possible using a long iteration interval (of the order of 2 to 10 s) are enumerated. These are chiefly in the simple representation of the phasic movement of air in and out of the lungs, and in the saving of complexity and computing time. Models need to be accurate, but should also be kept as simple as possible.

4

Units of Measurement—STPD/ BTPS Conversions— Abbreviations, Symbols and Fortran Conventions

Established conventional units of measurement (Comroe, Forster, Dubois, Briscoe and Carlsen, 1962) have been used except where specified. Oxygen consumption and carbon dioxide output, either within the body or measured at the mouth, are expressed in terms of cubic centimetres occupied by the dry gases at 760 mmHg pressure and 0 °C. This unit is referred to by the abbreviation STPD, for Standard Temperature and Pressure, Dry gas. On the other hand the volume of the lungs, the effective 'dead space', the total and alveolar ventilation, and other related quantities are measured and expressed under BTPS conditions, i.e. cubic centimetres or litres measured at Body Temperature and Pressure with the gas Saturated with water vapour. These conventions have been preserved so that the results from the model can more easily be compared with clinical and physiological measurements.

Despite the apparent imminence of a world-wide change to S.I. units, I have retained established units of pressure (i.e. mmHg or torr) for the present, but users will obviously have no difficulty in converting to S.I. units a model which operates through a computer. In the U.K. and in Europe S.I. pressure units (in this case kilo-Pascals, kPa) are already in wide use; but in the U.S.A. and Canada, the mmHg is still preferred. Most working models of MacPuf are in North America at present, so I have not thought it advisable to change the units. I have, however, arranged that kPa as well as mmHg values should be given on the graph scales (e.g. see Figure 25.1). To convert the whole model to kPa would take only a few hours and could be done by any competent programmer equipped with the physiological knowledge which this book provides. In any case subroutine UNITS (which appears at the end of the whole programme—Appendix IV) is called before any output is printed, and allows the model to display output in either S.I. units or mmHg, according to the choice of the user when he first starts to run the programme. (In use, all pressures to be displayed are multiplied by a conversion factor (SIMLT) with a value of 1.0 for mmHg, and of 0.1332 for S.I. units).

To economise computing time any conversion factor which has to be frequently applied is computed only once. The conversion factor used each time a gas volume has to be converted from one unit to another is therefore specified as follows (see subroutine CONST in the full programme listing in Appendix IV):

$$C(11) = BARPR - 1.2703 * TEMP$$
$$C(12) = C(11) * .003592 / (273. + TEMP)$$

In this formulation C(11) is the effective barometric pressure, obtained by subtracting prevailing water vapour pressure, (1.2703 times the temperature in degrees centigrade) from atmospheric pressure (BARPR). TEMP represents the centigrade temperature. In the second expression the constant .003592 is the product of 0.01 and 273 divided by 760. The multiplier '.01' is useful in converting blood gas contents measured in cc/100 ml blood into cc of gas and for converting percentages of inspired gas to simple ratios. I shall use throughout this book the additional (non-standard) convention of referring to gas volumes in cc and volumes of blood in ml, for greater clarity.

Under average conditions in a respiratory laboratory a subject inhales room air which is at a temperature of, say, 18 °C and partly saturated with water vapour. Once in the lungs the air rapidly takes up water vapour to become virtually fully saturated. Measurements of volumes can readily be made at ambient barometric pressure and temperature. Full saturation with water vapour is either arranged, or assumed if the gas has been exhaled. BTPS/STPD conversion allows the volumes to be expressed effectively in terms of the number of molecules of a gas rather than in terms of the volumes the molecules occupy under the special conditions of measurement.

FORTRAN NOTATION

Fortran notation is so similar to that of ordinary arithmetic that it seemed best to write the simple arithmetical expressions in this book in Fortran so that they could easily be identified in the complete programme in Appendix IV. Most of the Fortran conventions used are shown in the expression above for C(12), which in more normal mathematical convention would be written:

$$C(12) = \frac{C(11) \times .003592}{(273 + TEMP)}$$

However, in Fortran the symbol '×' is replaced by '*', which also means 'multiplied by'. The whole expression is written on a single long line, and the slash '/' is used for all division operations. Correct logical sequence of operations is obtained by the extensive use of pairs of brackets, the innermost pair signifying that the expression contained therein shall be executed first. Thus we do not write

$$1 / 760 * (273 + TEMP)$$

because the answer would depend on whether the expression (273+TEMP) was a divisor or a multiplier. Instead, the ambiguity is resolved by writing

$$1 / (760 * (273 + \text{TEMP})).$$

Those interested in Chomsky's celebrated analysis of the general rules describing the syntactical structure of ordinary languages will appreciate that Fortran very exactly conforms to such general rules—which is striking since the development of Fortran and Chomsky's analysis have been proceeding independently. The design of modern compilers has been strongly influenced by Chomsky's theoretical work.

Numbers *without* decimal points represent whole numbers or integers, and when 'floating point' numbers are to be used, as in variable quantities, they are conventionally specified by using a decimal point, even when this is not necessary, e.g. '760.' rather than '760', implying that the number should be regarded as 760.0000, to as many significant figures as the computer is capable of storing. The symbols '+' and '−' have their normal meaning. '**' means 'raised to the power of', and 'SQRT( )' means the square root of whatever is inside the brackets. Finally, although the expression

$$C(12) = C(11) * .003592 / (273. + \text{TEMP})$$

means that C(12) takes up the value to the right of the 'equals' sign, and is a normal arithmetical expression, it would be equally grammatical in Fortran to write an expression such as

$$C(12) = C(12) + C(11)$$

which means 'make the new value for the variable C(12) equal to the previous value of C(12) plus the value of C(11)'.

This description incorporates almost all the Fortran symbolic logic which will be referred to in the text of this book, although naturally other devices such as iterative loops, data statements, subscripted arrays, function statements and other familiar Fortran devices are used in the whole programme, given in full in Appendix IV.

As a simple exercise in Fortran, one may examine the component parts of the full equation specifying the value of the variable, 'C(12)', in a set of expressions such as that which follows, in which the values of local variables C(11) and C(12) successively take up the values of various parts of the expression as they are multiplied, divided or added together. For example, the set of statements below, reading in sequence from top to bottom

$$C(11) = 1.2703 * \text{TEMP}$$
$$C(11) = \text{BARPR} - C(11)$$
$$C(12) = 273. + \text{TEMP}$$
$$C(12) = .003592 / C(12)$$
$$C(12) = C(11) * C(12)$$

correspond exactly in their effect to the original expressions

$$C(11) = \text{BARPR} - 1.2703 * \text{TEMP}$$
$$C(12) = C(11) * .003592 / (273. + \text{TEMP})$$

Symbols for variables used in the programme

In Fortran it is customary to express all variables as strings of one to five (or six) letters or numbers, specifying only that the first character shall be a letter. This allows the variables to be given convenient names to identify them in a complex programme. As far as possible the symbols chosen to represent different components of the system follow standard conventions (e.g. 'V' to signify 'venous', 'A' for 'alveolar') but sometimes a compromise is necessary. Lower case letters are not used in standard Fortran, so that 'a' cannot be used to represent 'arterial.' 'R' has therefore been used to specify immediately available 'arterial' blood. Likewise, Fortran cannot specify a superscript bar to signify 'mean' or 'mixed' (e.g. $\bar{V}$) nor a superscript dot for a time derivative (e.g. $\dot{Q}$). This means that other representations must be used (e.g. 'CO' for 'cardiac output'; 'CBF' for 'cerebral blood flow'). A full list of these non-standard Fortran symbolic names is given in Appendix VI.

Most variables used in the programme contain 5 letters, built up in the following way:

Compartment   Material   Unit of measurement

R	C	2	C	T

The 1st letter refers to the *compartment*, i.e. blood, gas or tissue, according to the following notation:

A = Alveolar; B = Brain; E = Effluent arterial blood going to tissues; P = Pulmonary capillary (idealized); R = Arterial; S = Slow tissue store (for nitrogen); T = Tissue; U = Bubbles in tissues (if present); and V = Venous.

The distinction between E and R will be clarified in Chapter 5, and that between S and T in Chapter 17. The 2nd two letters refer to the *nature* of the material or measurement in the compartment, i.e.

O2 = Oxygen; C2 = Carbon dioxide; C3 = Bicarbonate; N2 = Nitrogen.

The last two letters specify the unit of measurement, i.e.

MT = Amount of something present at cc STPD (for a gas) or in mmol (for bicarbonate)
CT = Content of something measured at STPD/100 ml (for a gas) or in mmol/litre (for bicarbonate or lactate)
PR = Partial pressure in mmHg (torr)
PH= pH (in this case positions 2 and 3 are not used—e.g. 'BPH').

Thus the arterial blood carbon dioxide content is represented as the variable 'RC2CT'; and 'AN2MT' represents the amount of nitrogen in the alveolar compartment. In general, MT = CT × volume of the specified compartment—e.g. VC2MT = VC2CT × VBLVL (where 'VBLVL' is the total venous blood volume). Other abbreviations will be mentioned as they occur and are listed in Appendix VI.

Computation of preset parameters

Not only for the case of the BTPS/STPD correction factor but also in many other cases, certain computations must be executed at every iteration interval of the main programme loop. Inspection of Appendix IV will show that at statement 190 in the main programme subroutine CONST is called, and the array argument 'C', containing 70 elements, brings to the main programme a set of constants for the next set of iterations beginning at the

DO 1590

statement that follows. The values for array C are equivalenced to corresponding named real variables C1, C2, C3, etc. I have shown only partial equivalence of the series. If the computer has a large enough symbol table space to compile the full set of individual addresses for C1, C2, etc., this will run faster; but if not the equivalence statement may be omitted and C(1), C(2), C(3), etc. substituted. The device of LABELLED COMMON might appear better, but I have had trouble with this feature on a few Fortran compilers and therefore recommend the technique shown.

In the remaining text of this book computations of preset parameters will be shown between square brackets.

SUMMARY

Units of measurement and STPD/BTPS gas volume conversion are discussed, and STPD/BTPS conversion is used to exemplify the elementary conventions of the Fortran language in which arithmetical expressions are represented. The choice between S.I. or mmHg pressure units is discussed, and reasons discussed for preferring mmHg at the present time, though the model can be made to display its output in S.I. units if required. Standard symbols are used for variables in the programme. The general way in which parameters are computed outside the main programme is described.

5
Bulk Transport through a Fluid Compartment, exemplified by the Arterial Blood Pool

The mathematical analysis of the rate of change of concentration of a solute in a fluid compartment which is in dynamic equilibrium with other compartments is reasonably simple. The mathematical analysis of fluid flowing into a compartment and out at the other end is rather more complicated, even if the compartment is a uniform tube. The mathematical description of what would happen to blood in the main arterial tree when blood of a different solute composition flowed into it is vastly more complicated. One would need to take account of the branching nature of the vessels, and of different flow rates in different places. A complete description in terms of only ten different branches or compartments would stretch the capacity of the largest computers to solve in a reasonable time. With the added complication of pulsatile flow the problem is in practice insoluble.

Simplification is therefore essential. Acceptance of simplification is a great step forward. One then asks, 'What is the least complex mathematical formulation which will give a reasonably accurate solution?' rather than, 'What have I forgotten in the way of greater complexity which is needed for a complete description?' Problems of scaling and stability in a full description of alveolar gas exchange, blood gas transport and control of ventilation preclude the use of an analogue computer. I have chosen the digital computer rather than a hybrid computer (which might be more suitable) simply because digital computers are widely available, and hybrids are not.

It is fairly obvious that for most applications there is likely to be an optimum time interval between successive digital computations. If the interval is very short, there are no problems with stability or accuracy, but the computational process will be long and expensive. If it is too long, unrealistic oscillations are inevitable. If these are insufficiently damped, no stable state can ever be achieved; and if they are damped excessively changes will be slowed, distorted and out of phase. I propose now to consider flow through the human adult arterial tree, generally reckoned to contain about 1000 ml blood (Green, 1944), and to derive empirically the largest possible computational interval which might be acceptable for a reasonably accurate description of the flow process. The reason for considering the arterial tree first is that it contains a relatively small volume of blood compared with that in the venous side of the circulation, so that problems of numerical stability are likely to be worse.

Two extreme descriptions of flow through the arterial tree

Rather than consider an abstract problem, I shall analyse the situation in which 5.4 litres of blood are flowing into and out of a 1000 ml pool per minute. Thus 900 ml blood flows in and out of the pool each 10 s, and the pool will be almost completely flushed in just over 10 s—certainly by 20 s except in very far distant or slow-flow territories. One may envisage two extreme mathematical descriptions of the first 10 seconds' operation:

Case (1)   1. 900 ml blood flows into the pool, making 1900 ml;
            2. The pool is completely mixed;
            3. 900 ml blood flows out.
Case (2)   1. 900 ml blood flows out, leaving 100 ml behind;
            2. 900 ml blood flows in;
            3. The pool is completely mixed.

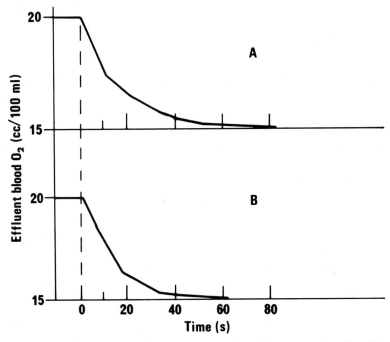

Figure 5.1   Effect of a sudden change in incoming blood O_2 concentration (from 20 to 15 cc/100 ml) on the effluent O_2 content leaving the arterial pool at the time indicated using the Case (1) procedure described in the text. The vertical interrupted line represents the instant at which incoming gas concentration changed. Panel A plotted using a 10 s interval between computations, panel B using a 5 s interval. Plotting was done by the short programme in Appendix I. Cardiac output = 5.4 l/min. Note that effluent blood concentration in A is still not stable even after 40 s of simulated time have elapsed

What is going to happen in each extreme case if the solute concentration of the incoming blood changes abruptly, e.g. from 20 volumes of oxygen per 100 ml blood to 15?

In case (1) above, the oxygen in the whole pool, initially 200 cc, rises to $200 + (15 \times 9)$, i.e. 335 cc. After mixing, its concentration is $(335 \times 100) / 1900$, i.e. 17.6 cc/100 ml. Eventually the volume returns to 1000 ml. In the following 10 s, the volume of oxygen rises to $176 + (15 \times 9)$, i.e. 311 cc, and after mixing its concentration is $(311 \times 100) / 1900$, i.e. 16.4 cc/100 ml—and so on. The whole process is shown graphically in Figure 5.1A, which is plotted by the short programme given in Appendix I.

In case (2) above, at the end of 10 s, the amount of oxygen at first falls to $200 - (20 \times 9)$, i.e. 20 cc, and then rises again, to $20 + (15 \times 9)$, i.e. 155 cc. The new concentration in the pool at this stage is therefore 15.5 cc/100ml. In the next 10 s the volume of oxygen in the pool falls to $155 - (15.5 \times 9)$, i.e. 16 cc, and then rises to $16 + (15 \times 9)$, i.e. 151 cc, with a

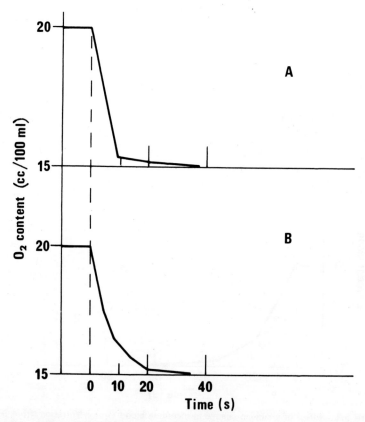

Figure 5.2 Effect of the same acute change as in Figure 5.1, using the same scales and notations, but using the Case (2) procedure described in the text; panel A has a 10 s and panel B a 5 s iteration interval. (Plotted by the short programme in Appendix II. Cardiac output = 5.4 l/min)

Note the improved realism of the output, compared with that of Figure 5.1. (Case (1) procedure)

concentration of 15.1 cc/100 ml, and so on. The process is shown graphically in Figure 5.2A, which is plotted by the short programme in Appendix II.

Figure 5.1B shows the same set of calculations, plotted this time for a 5 s time interval for case (1), and Figure 5.2B shows the effect of a 5 s interval for case (2).

The way that the sequence of events in Case (2) is represented in MacPuf is given in full in Appendix IV (between statements 380 and 410), but in essence consists of considering simultaneously the flow of blood in and out, and not calculating the final oxygen concentration until the computation is complete. Using the Fortran notation already referred to in the last chapter, FT is the fractional time in minutes (0.16667 is 10 s, and 0.08333 is 5 s); CO is the cardiac output in litres/min; PO2CT is the incoming pulmonary capillary blood concentration; EO2CT is the effluent arterial blood concentration; and RO2MT is the total amount of oxygen in the arterial blood pool. At the end of time FT the new amount of oxygen in the pool will be the amount originally present (RO2MT) incremented by the arriving oxygen (FT × CO × PO2CT) and decremented by the departing oxygen (FT × CO × EO2CT). To convert to cc of oxygen, it is necessary to multiply by 10 since CO is in litres/min and EO2CT is in cc/100 ml blood. The content is then derived by dividing by the volume of blood in the pool, in ml. The necessary Fortran statements read as follows:

$$RO2MT = RO2MT + FT * CO * 10. * (PO2CT - EO2CT)$$
$$EO2CT = RO2MT * 100. / 1000.$$

The first statement means 'make the *new* value of oxygen in the pool (RO2MT on the left of the '=' sign) equal to the *old* value (RO2MT on the right) plus the difference in gas contents between incoming and outgoing blood, multiplied by fractional time and cardiac output, adjusting units to cc oxygen'. The second statement means that the content of oxygen (EO2CT) in the blood leaving the pool is then to be made equal to the newly calculated value of total oxygen (RO2MT), divided by 1000 (the volume of the pool in ml) and multiplied by 100 (since contents are measured traditionally in cc/100 ml). In practice, of course, the second instruction would be written

$$EO2CT = RO2MT * .1$$

to save computation time.

The ways in which these calculations are performed over and over again to reach the steady states are illustrated in Figure 5.2. They are illustrated in full in Appendix II and I shall not describe them in detail, since they are written in standard Fortran which would be well known to and easily understood by any programmer.

Although I lack the skill to perform a rigorous mathematical analysis, it is quite obvious, comparing Figure 5.1A with Figure 5.2A, that case (2) (Figure 5.2A) gives a much more realistic representation of the likely change in arterial blood pool oxygen concentration with time than does case (1) (Figure 5.1A). In case (1), for a 10 s iteration interval (Figure 5.1A) it is 50 s before the arterial blood pool is fully flushed, and even with a 5 s interval

(Figure 5.1B) the process takes 40 s. This is absurd, and unrealistically long. By comparison, the representation of blood flow by case (2) (Figure 5.2) is much more satisfactory. By 20 s virtually the whole pool has taken up the new concentration of inflowing blood, and even by 10 s the whole pool has very largely turned over. The reason that case (2) gives a much better result than case (1) is, of course, because the whole arterial blood pool cannot completely mix, even assuming turbulence, within the short time available.

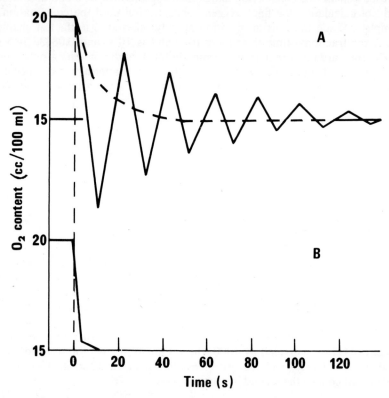

Figure 5.3 Same computations as in Figure 5.2 but using a cardiac output twice as large as in Figure 5.2. Panel A is again plotted with a 10 s iteration interval, panel B with a 5 s interval. (Plotted by the programme in Appendix II. Cardiac output = 10.8 l/min.)

Note the severe oscillation with the longer time interval, which is prevented by using a 5 s iteration interval. The interrupted line in panel A is plotted for the same cardiac output, but using the Case (1) procedure, which though still unsatisfactory is at least free from oscillatory tendency

It is obviously much better to have the incoming blood, as it were, push out the residual blood in the pool. The only advantage of the case (1) representation is that it is inherently stable and free from any tendency to oscillate. The defect of the case (2) representation is that once the volume of blood leaving the pool in the time interval FT becomes greater than that initially in the pool, an unrealistic oscillation is inevitable. This is shown in Figure 5.3A, in which the same computations as in Figure 5.2A are performed, except that the cardiac output is made twice as great, i.e. 10.8 instead of 5.4 l/minute. Using a 10 s computational interval more than 90 s are needed before the oscillation has ceased. The interrupted line superimposed in Figure 5.3A shows the same example, using the case (1) method, which gives a much better and reasonably smooth curve. Alternatively, the computation method of case (2) can still be used, to produce an even better result, as in Figure 5.3B, simply by shortening the iteration interval to 5 s. In this case all the blood pool is cleared by 10 s and indeed more than 95% of it is cleared by 5 s, which seems about right.

However, if the cardiac output was four times normal (i.e. about 20 l/min) the interval between successive computations would have to be no more than 2–3 s, and for 30 l/min no more than 1–2 s. This is wasteful in computing time. Furthermore it makes the handling of alveolar ventilation more difficult, as I shall show in Chapter 10. How can the decisive advantages of the case (2) representation be retained for normal cardiac outputs, but in such a way that large, prolonged, and unphysiological oscillations in gas concentrations are avoided? The answer, obviously, lies either in damping the oscillation by some means, or shortening the interation interval—or (better still) in a judicious combination of both.

Critical damping of blood gas concentration changes

I have determined the ideal degree of damping by trial and error. The essence of damping is to prevent the full change in some variable taking place at once, and allowing it to move only part of the way towards its calculated final value. A simple way of doing this is to determine that the new effective gas content shall be made equal to:

$$\frac{[(\text{Ideal new calculated gas content} \times Z) + \text{old gas content}]}{(Z + 1)}$$

The new gas content, EO2CT, is given by the expression

$$EO2CT = RO2MT * .1$$

as mentioned above (since content is in cc/100 ml, and an arterial blood pool of 1000 ml is assumed). RO2MT is the total amount of O_2 in the pool. The old gas content is the previous value for EO2CT at the end of the preceding iteration interval. Therefore we may write

$$EO2CT = (RO2MT * .1 * Z + EO2CT) / (Z + 1.)$$

The parameter 'Z' could be described as inversely proportional to the amount of damping. If Z is very large there will be virtually no damping, and the new value will be reached at once; if it is very small, a long time and many iterations will be necessary before the new value for EO2CT approaches the value of (RO2MT * .1).

Readers who study the full programme closely (Appendix IV) will observe that since a damping function of this type is used at several places during the

execution of the main programme it is specified as a first FUNCTION statement in the main Fortran programme

$$DAMP\,(X,Y,Z) = (X * Z + Y) / (1. + Z)$$

where X is the new value, Y the old value, and Z the damping factor or
constant. Thus, whenever damping is necessary it is only necessary to write
an expression such as

400              $EO2CT = DAMP\,(RO2MT * .1, EO2CT, W)$

which has the same effect as the previous equation for EO2CT (statement
400 in the main programme). The short programme in Appendix III shows
how such a function is specified and used.

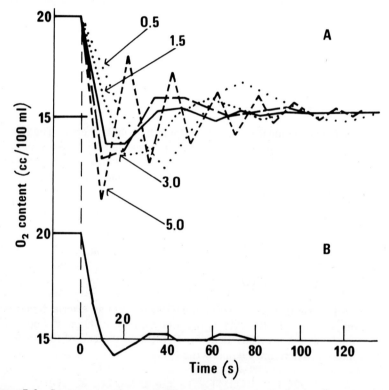

Figure 5.4   Same computations as in Figure 5.3 (Case (2) procedure, with cardiac output
10.8 l/min and, in panel A, a 10 s computational interval, but this time using different values
of damping constant ('Z') between 0.5 and 5.0, as indicated by the arrowed lines. (Plotted by
the programme in Appendix III). The bold line, plotted with a damping constant of 2.5 represents the best compromise, i.e. critical damping, at which there is least overshoot and most
rapid attainment of a steady state. At high values (e.g. 5.0) for 'Z', oscillation is almost as bad
as in Figure 5.3A. At low values (e.g. 0.5) there are slow oscillatory swings taking 2 minutes
to settle. Panel B shows that halving the computational interval to 5 s and using a damping
constant of 2.5 gives a less satisfactory result than that of Figure 5.3, but allows only a slight
and not unmanageable amount of oscillation

Consider again the situation described above (Figure 5.3A) in which there is a step change of incoming arterial oxygen concentration from 20 to 15 volumes %, the cardiac output is doubled (to 10.8 l/min), the iteration interval is kept at 10 s, and case (2) calculations are used. Figure 5.4 shows the effect of different values of damping constant (Z) on the effluent arterial pool oxygen concentration. Given such a large step change in gas concentration, the case (2) computational procedure cannot entirely prevent overshoot at a cardiac output of 10.8 l/min, but it is minimised, and a rapid steady state is attained, if the damping constant Z is made about 2.5. A value less than this (see the curve for 0.5) leads to a slow overshoot, which takes 90 s to settle down. A value of 3 or more leads to an unreasonably large rapid overshoot (see the curve for 5.0). Damping is approximately critical at a value of 2.5. If the computation interval is shortened to 5 s, damping is unnecessary (as was shown in Figure 5.3B) and the inclusion of a damping factor of 2.5 lessens the crisp accuracy slightly (see Figure 5.4B). However, the overshoot and oscillation are both relatively slight. A simple way of arranging that the damping will be no greater than is actually necessary to prevent severe oscillation is to arrange that the damping factor automatically alters as the time interval between successive iterations of the programme is altered. This can be arranged by specifying that the damping factor shall be 0.42/FT. If FT (the fractional time interval in minutes) is 10 s, i.e. .16667, the damping factor Z is then 2.5. If FT is half this, i.e. 5 s, the damping factor is 5.0.

The other dynamic factor which is obviously desirable in a damping function is one related to cardiac output. If cardiac output is low, no damping will be necessary; if it is high, damping will be needed (e.g. cf. Figures 5.2A and 5.3A). This is most easily allowed for by specifying that the damping factor in the equation shall have a value related not only to fractional time, FT, but also to the effective cardiac output (COADJ), normally measured in l/min. If the damping factor is 4.5/(FT * COADJ), it will have a normal value of 5.0 if FT is 0.16667 and COADJ is 5.4 (see the main programme, just before statement 390, in which parameter C22 = 4.5/FT). At a cardiac output of 10.8 l/min (as in the curves of Figure 5.4A) the damping factor will be that empirically found most satisfactory, i.e. 2.5. At a cardiac output of 21.6 it will be 1.25, and at 32.4 (about as high as the cardiac output in man has ever been measured) it would be 0.85. Conversely, at an output of 2.5 the damping factor would be 10.0. The effect of this variable damping on a step change of oxygen concentration from 20 to 15 volumes per cent at different cardiac outputs, and at 10 and 5 s iteration intervals is shown in Figure 5.5A and B.

A desirable consequence of the use of damping is that it creates a similar, though not exactly the same, effect as a time delay, and thus makes some allowance for circulation time. The use of a 10 s computational interval in itself inevitably creates a time delay of 10 s. If the interval is shortened to 5 s or less, the effective time delay is likewise shortened. Rather than introduce extra damping which would be physiologically unrealistic, I have chosen to arrange that on the venous side a time delay network is introduced. This allows consistent results to be obtained with varying time intervals. The techniques will be described fully in Chapter 8.

It is not possible to test directly the accuracy of my description of the

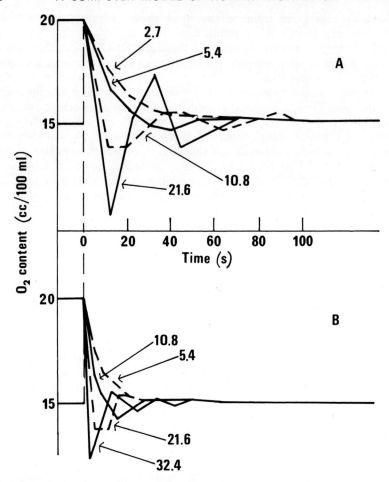

Figure 5.5 Effects of the same step change in inflowing O_2 content as in Figures 5.1 to 5.4 showing the performance of the system using the Case (2) procedure with dynamic damping proportional to fractional time and cardiac output. Panel A—10 s iteration interval; panel B—5 s interval. (All graphs plotted by the programme in Appendix III.) Arrowed lines indicate the curves of effluent O_2 content at the indicated cardiac outputs (given in l/min). Note that the performance at 10 s iteration interval is reasonably good up to 10.8 l/min cardiac output but overshoots rather severely at 21.6 l/min. In B however (5 s intervals) performance is good at 21.6 and only overshoots transiently at 32.4 l/min, which is about the largest cardiac output possible

movement of blood through the arterial blood pool, since there is no single point at which an average and representative sample of blood leaving the pool could be obtained. However, when the description is complete, it becomes possible to check the operation of the whole system. The same expressions as have been described for oxygen are equally applicable to the carriage of carbon dioxide and nitrogen and also to the carriage of bicarbonate, which is the way in which the carriage of blood buffering capacity is described in the programme (see Chapter 14). The necessary computations concerning

CO_2, N_2 and bicarbonate can most conveniently be carried out at the same point in the programme. RC2MT and RN2MT correspond to total amounts of gaseous CO_2 and N_2 in the arterial blood pool. A study of the relevant part of the main programme loop (see Appendix IV between statements 380 and 410) will make the sequence of computational steps clear, since they are carried out in the same way as for oxygen. However, the mixing of shunted with idealised capillary blood is, for economy, incorporated in the expression computing the new value for RO2MT, etc. and a reader puzzled by this statement should read Chapter 9 to appreciate how it is derived.

Despite the inevitable inaccuracy of the expressions which have to be used to obtain stable results with a long time interval, and although the time course of changes also cannot be represented with complete accuracy, the way the whole computation is built up prevents any net gain or loss of solutes from the system. Since oscillations eventually settle, the steady state descriptions must be correct. The interaction of many factors is so complex that the only way in which the whole process can be approximately checked is by a process of trial and error, matching the performance of the model to actual clinical or physiological data obtained during stepwise changes of incoming gas contents. I shall describe some of the applied tests in Chapter 23.

Calculation of gas contents in blood reaching the chemoreceptors

In the next chapter I shall describe the way in which contents of O_2 and CO_2 in blood can be used to compute the respective partial pressures. The preceding section described the means of obtaining a stable and reasonably accurate description of the average contents of gases leaving the arterial blood pool for the tissues. This description is not quite right for the arterial blood reaching the systemic arterial chemoreceptors at the aortic and carotid bodies. These are perfused by a rapid flow of blood, they are close to the heart, and they respond rapidly to changes in blood gas pressures (see Chapters 12 and 13). The size of the arterial blood pool is irrelevant for computation of changes in aortic or carotid blood gas composition, since these are determined simply by the effect of mixing idealised pulmonary capillary and right-to-left shunted blood. A very slight degree of damping and a slight time delay should probably be allowed for, and can be provided by the same damping function described above, using a much larger value for the 'damping factor'. The empirical value chosen was COADJ * FT * 10 (i.e. COADJ * C17). This has a value of approximately 10 at normal cardiac output and 10 s iteration interval; but if cardiac output is very low and the computational interval very short, this value can fall as low as 0.3 (e.g. with cardiac output = 1.0 l/min and FT = 2 s). Once again, the reader will appreciate that this degree of damping is simply a guess, and the appropriate amount of damping could no doubt be better estimated by comparing the performance of the model with the rates of change of arterial blood gas composition resulting from step changes in alveolar gas composition at different levels of cardiac output.

The representation in the main programme (Appendix IV, between statements 400 and 410) is as follows:

$$[C17 = FT * 10.]$$
$$Z = COADJ * C17$$
$$RO2CT = DAMP (PO2CT \ldots, RO2CT, Z)$$
$$RC2CT = DAMP (PC2CT \ldots, RC2CT, Z)$$

The actual computations also include a venous admixture effect, which will be described fully in Chapter 9.

SUMMARY

The passage of blood through the arterial blood pool is discussed. The best simple description involves the simultaneous addition of incoming blood and removal of outflowing blood, followed by a recalculation of the new gas content. Each set of calculations is performed at each iteration interval, usually 5 or 10 s. The necessity of damping arises when large cardiac outputs are being studied; and by trial and error an empirically reasonable damping factor is derived. This depends on both the fractional time interval between successive computations (i.e. the iteration interval) and on the cardiac output. An eventual synthesis of all processes in a Fortran programme is then made. This is precisely accurate for steady state conditions, and sufficiently accurate to form the basis for a complete dynamic representation.

Computation of gas contents in arterial blood reaching the chemoreceptors is necessary for the later determination of partial pressures. This does not depend on the size of the arterial blood pool. Only a very slight degree of damping seems appropriate at this point, and a different description is therefore used.

6
Blood Oxygen and Carbon Dioxide Dissociation Curves

All the calculations about gas transfers through the arterial blood pool which were considered in the last chapter concerned the *contents* of gases in the blood, i.e. the amounts present per unit volume of blood. In the lungs it is likewise possible to consider all the movement of gases in and out in terms of contents, i.e. the volume of each gas present per unit volume of total gas (see Chapter 10). The necessity for computing partial *pressures* arises when the movement of gases between the lungs and the blood-stream is considered. A gas diffuses in bulk from one place to another at a rate proportional to the difference in partial pressure. Bulk movement stops when the partial pressures are equal. In the lungs the partial pressures of each gas are linearly related to the contents of each, and there is no problem. In the blood the presence of haemoglobin is of transcendent importance to the carriage of oxygen, and this and other buffers enormously influence the carriage of carbon dioxide (review by Roughton, 1964). The relations between pressure and content of each gas were determined early this century by driving off the gases from blood in successive steps—hence the term 'dissociation curve', which has puzzled generations of students who might have been happier with 'capacity curve' or some more appropriate description.

The well-known shape of the oxygen dissociation curve (Figure 6.1) can now be explained in terms of the molecular structures of reduced and oxygenated haemoglobin. Unfortunately, the shape of the curve does not lend itself to description by any simple mathematical expression. Furthermore, since in MacPuf's main programme, which is run through at each iteration interval (simulating from 2 to 10 s), it is necessary to convert oxygen partial pressure to content several times, errors involved in representing the curve as a simple mathematical expression might be cumulative. Because at high PO_2 the curve is flat (Figure 6.1) even a small change in O_2 content caused by the normal degree of venous admixture is associated with a relatively large fall in PO_2 between the pulmonary capillaries and the arterial blood. Accurate calculation of the PO_2 shift requires a comparably accurate method of computing the curve. Kelman (1966) published an empirical mathematical description, extending the previous work of Adair (1925) on the curve. This took into account pH, PCO_2, temperature and haemoglobin concentration, and his formulation is now widely accepted as the most accurate and satisfactory

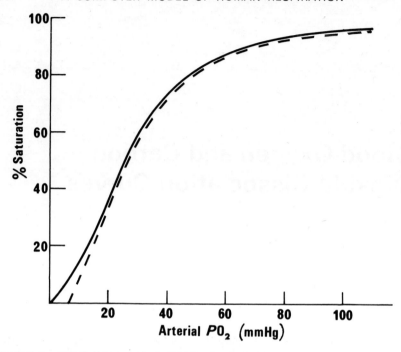

Figure 6.1   Solid line shows the experimentally determined dissociation curve of whole blood at normal arterial PCO_2, pH and temperature. The interrupted line is derived from computations performed by subroutine GASES listed in Appendix IV. (After Kelman, 1966)

available. Roughton (1964) has reviewed other formulations. The closeness of fit can be seen in Figure 6.1 where the interrupted line represents Kelman's formulation. Unfortunately, content is computed from a fourth power expression of PO_2 divided by another fourth power expression. A significant part of the computing time consumed when operating MacPuf results from executing this calculation repeatedly.

Figure 6.2 shows a curve representing the CO_2 dissociation curve of whole blood under average conditions, and the interrupted line in this figure shows the descriptive formulation also published by Kelman (1967), a year later. This curve takes into account haematocrit, pH, temperature and PO_2. Kelman's work is a key which can be turned by a computer to unlock the door which stands between the conception and the completion of a workable holistic digital computer model of respiration and blood gas transport. The present model and the other comprehensive models reviewed in Chapter 2 owe much of their accuracy to Kelman's equations.

The full programme in Appendix IV includes, in subroutine GASES, a short description of the two dissociation curves which is obtained by combining the two formulations published by Kelman. This subroutine computes the gas *contents* expected for the supplied partial pressures, and is called at a number of points in the main programme with 6 'arguments', as follows:

CALL GASES(PO2,PC2,O2CON,C2CON,PH,SAT)

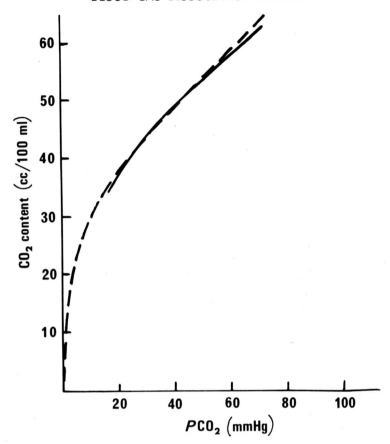

Figure 6.2   Solid line shows the experimentally determined CO_2 dissociation curve for whole blood, oxygenated, changing only PCO_2. The interrupted line shows a typical curve plotted for similar conditions using subroutine GASES, listed in Appendix IV. Most published CO_2 dissociation curves are very slightly more convex than those plotted from Kelman's equations (Kelman, 1967) but in the physiological range they are identical

Before the call or instruction is made, the values of 'PO2', 'PC2' and 'PH' are set to those which are being considered. Thus for brain blood, for example, the call would be:

CALL GASES (BO2PR,BC2PR,BO2CT,BC2CT,BPH,SAT)

The subroutine computes for these values the necessary contents of brain blood oyxgen (BO2CT) and CO_2(BC2CT), which are then available for the next computational step. Saturation (SAT) is also available if needed. The prevailing haemoglobin concentration, haematocrit and temperature are independently supplied by a bank of values COMMON to all parts of the programme.

Conversion of contents into partial pressures

Kelman's equations allow accurate description of the content of O_2 and CO_2 in the blood at different places (tissues, brain and pulmonary capillaries) where the partial pressures have already been determined (by means to be described in Chapters 7 and 13). The arterial chemoreceptors, which are part of the ventilatory control system, are known to be sensitive to gas pressures, rather than contents. In an idealised pulmonary capillary compartment (Chapter 9) the partial pressures of gases are assumed to be the same as those in the alveoli. Some blood behaves as if it had by-passed the lungs and had been added to the pulmonary capillary blood. Normally this slightly changes the resultant contents and very greatly changes them in disease states. It is, of course, easy to compute blood gas contents when two streams of blood with known contents are mixed in known proportion. Computation of partial pressures is more difficult. Unfortunately, no kindly soul has yet provided a simple means of doing for gas content → partial pressure conversion what Kelman has done for partial pressure → content conversion, at least with the degree of accuracy which is needed for representation of conditions of changed haemogloblin concentration, barometric pressure, temperature and pH. To convert contents to pressures it is necessary to proceed as follows— though readers should note that when equally accurate mathematical descriptions have been published for these conversions this part of the programme can be simplified and can also be run more economically.

It is a reasonable assumption that even in acute whole body decompression the pressure of neither oxygen nor carbon dioxide will exceed atmospheric pressure for long, otherwise bubbles would form in the blood. Therefore MacPuf takes atmospheric pressure as a maximum value. Early versions divided the difference between atmospheric pressure and zero pressure by two, made this a first guess at both gas pressures, computed contents, and then adjusted the pressure limits up or down separately for O_2 and CO_2, retesting at each step until the desired degree of accuracy had been obtained. I found it most economical in programme description, and no longer in execution, to combine the computations for the two gases, and to use the same subroutine GASES as was used for the pressure → content conversion (see above).

In the present version of the model a more efficient algorithm has been devised by Dr David Ingram and I am grateful for his permission to include it. This cuts down the repeated iterations of subroutine GASES and greatly speeds up the operation of the model. The algorithm (subroutine GSINV) takes the values of pressures from the preceding iteration as initial guesses. By computing the sign and magnitude of the discrepancy between the old and new contents, a search vector is set up in the 2-dimensional plane of partial pressures of oxygen and carbon dioxide. This is used to search for an improved guess (position on the plane) where the discrepancies are reduced for each gas content. When the discrepancy changes sign between two trial points on the plane a linear interpolation is performed on the corresponding pressure values and a new search initiated for the interpolated solution. The computational process should be clear from inspection of subroutine GSINV (see Appendix IV) since this is appropriately annotated.

Except after major perturbations of the system, only three pressure to content conversions (using subroutine GASES) are needed to achieve an accuracy of about 0.1 mmHg. In typical long runs this results in an overall saving of up to 50% in central processing time over previous versions of the programme.

2,3-Diphosphoglycerate (2,3-DPG) concentration and effects on the oxygen dissociation curve

Since the effects of increases in 2,3-DPG concentration are similar to those of increases in H^+ activity it is easy to arrange that instead of the term 'PH − 7.4' in the composite Kelman equations in subroutine GASES (see Appendix IV) the expression

$$(PH - DPH)$$

is used instead, where 'DPH' represents the influence of 2,3-DPG concentration in mmol/l red cells. DPH is computed before each run by subroutine CONST as follows:

$$DPH = 7.4 + (DPG - 3.8) * .025$$

and a realistic upper limit set for its effect (7.58). The concentration of DPG is allowed to change very slowly from its average value of 3.8 in accordance with the prevailing arterial oxygen content (RO2CT)—see main programme (Appendix IV), between statements 280 and 290. The constant $C10$ in the expression

$$DPG = DPG + (23.4 - RO2CT - DPG) * C10$$

has a value (FT * .005) which gives approximately correct results for the rate of change of DPG concentration in acute anaemic states, although one recent user of the model has suggested that the maximal rate of change of DPG is too fast, and that $C10$ should have a value closer to 0.001 or 0.002 times FT.

SUMMARY

The conversion of blood oxygen and carbon dioxide partial pressures to corresponding contents, allowing for the prevailing pH, temperature, haemoglobin and haematocrit, is described. It makes use of accurate empirical formulae published by Kelman. The corresponding conversion of contents to partial pressures is needed for the arterial blood; and this is accomplished by a method in which about three successive back iterations are performed, starting from previous pressure estimates, computing contents, then retesting and adjusting until an acceptable degree of accuracy is obtained.

Changes in 2,3-diphosphoglycerate concentration are allowed to act by changing effective pH appropriately during computation of oxygen content.

7
Gas Exchanges in the Tissues

Many of the techniques already mentioned in Chapter 5 when considering the arterial blood pool apply equally well to bulk transport of gases through a tissue compartment. Equations can be written in the same general form as before, e.g.

$$TO2MT = TO2MT + FTCO * (EO2CT - TO2CT)$$

in which TO2MT is the total oxygen in the tissues, FTCO is fractional time multiplied by cardiac output, EO2CT the inflowing arterial blood oxygen content, and TO2CT the outgoing tissue blood oxygen content. This equation states that at the end of time FT the new content of oxygen in the tissues will be equal to the old content plus the difference between the amounts going in and coming out. In the case of metabolising tissues other terms are needed to describe the consumption of oxygen and the evolution of carbon dioxide. Oxygen consumption in cc per iteration interval (U) is subtracted at each iteration interval (statement 500). Carbon dioxide production is TRQ * U (TRQ is the tissue respiratory quotient, normally 0.8). This whole term is added to the comparable CO_2 equation, between statements 670 and 690. So much is straightforward. The problem is to compute the concentration of gases contained in the effluent blood from the tissues, knowing the new total amounts of each gas present. It cannot be done simply by dividing the total amount of each gas present by the effective volume of the tissue pool since only part of each gas is held in simple solution in tissues and extra-cellular fluid. Some oxygen is in tissue blood and some is in myoglobin in the muscles; most carbon dioxide is held as bicarbonate. First, some assumptions about the lumped tissue dissociation curves must be made. This will then allow the partial pressures to be computed if the contents are known. Finally the amounts of each gas that will be contained in the blood leaving the tissues at these tissue gas tensions must be calculated.

The calculations offer scope for great inaccuracies, which might appear to be of an order of magnitude rather than a few per cent. Some tissues contain a lot of blood and virtually no myoglobin (e.g. the liver). Others contain only a little blood but a lot of myoglobin (e.g. the skeletal muscles). Any calculation is going to require the conversion of partial pressures to contents, and each such calculation involves the use of the time-consuming GASES subroutine (described in detail in Chapter 5). Thus it is desirable to simplify the programme as far as possible by treating the tissues as a single compartment, though segmentation of compartments might be needed if accurate results are otherwise unobtainable. An intelligent guess about the lumped tissue dissociation curves for oxygen and carbon dioxide is required. The empirical curves which I shall describe began as guesses based on data available in the literature. The curves were later modified to give results for rates of change of arterial oxygen and carbon dioxide tensions in different situations that accord with results obtained from physiological and clinical observations in man.

Lumped tissue dissociation curve for oxygen

Figure 7.1 shows the typical dissociation curves for myoglobin and for haemoglobin plotted on the same axes. The curve for myoglobin is initially steep and levels off at partial pressures above 20 mmHg. I have assumed that there is likely also to be a small linear component comprising oxygen in solution in tissue fluid and in cell fluid, and that the actual curve is likely to be somewhere between that for myoglobin and for blood. The representation in MacPuf is as follows:

$$[C31 = 2.7 / TVOL]$$
$$TO2PR = TO2MT * C31$$
$$IF(TO2MT .GT. 250.) TO2PR = 45. + .09 * (TO2MT - 250.)$$

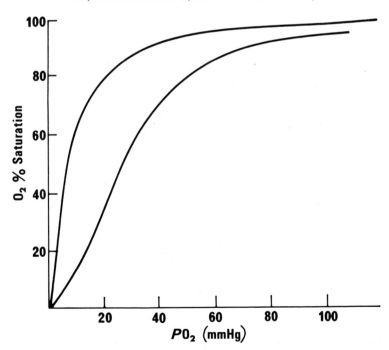

Figure 7.1 Comparison between the dissociation curves for haemoglobin (lower curve) and myoglobin (upper curve) plotted under similar conditions of PCO_2 and pH (after Hill, 1936). Note that very little O_2 is lost by myoglobin until the partial pressure is well below 20 mmHg

TVOL is the approximate extracellular fluid volume, normally about 12 litres. The constants 2.7 and .09 in the expressions above produce a function, relating tissue PO_2(TO2PR) to tissue oxygen mass (TO2MT). This consists of two straight lines (Figure 7.2) and specifies free release of oxygen as tissue

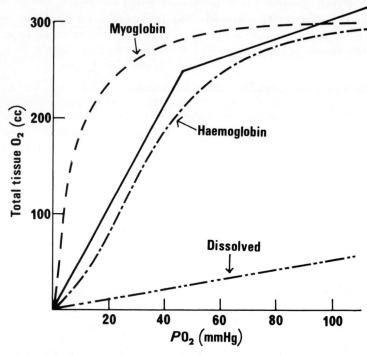

Figure 7.2 Solid line shows the function used to describe the lumped tissue dissociation curve for oxygen in MacPuf. The curves for myoglobin and haemoglobin (at tissue PCO_2) and the line for dissolved O_2 (assuming normal solubility in 35 litres of total body water) are shown in the interrupted lines. Calculation indicates that the dissolved component must be small in relation to haemoglobin and myoglobin stores, and that the total volume of such stores is about the same amount of oxygen as is consumed by the tissues in one minute

PO_2 falls below 45 mmHg, but very little release until this point is reached. When more experimental data are available for the complete curve it can no doubt be made more accurate; but in any case it is generally reckoned that almost all the oxygen of the tissues is likely to be exhausted in about one minute of circulation arrest. Therefore the shape of the curve (Figure 7.2) will not have an enormous influence in any case on the performance of the whole model. In the main programme (Appendix IV, statement 510) there is also a DAMP function (Chapter 5) to prevent oscillatory swings of tissue oxygen when using long iteration intervals.

Lumped tissue dissociation curve for carbon dioxide

Most CO_2 in the tissues, as in the blood, is in the form of bicarbonate, at a concentration of about 24 mmol/l. Estimates of the total readily available

CO_2 in the body are about 12–15 litres (Matthews, Laszlo, Campbell and Read, 1968). This is much less than the total CO_2 in the body (Farhi, 1964), but presumably much of the total is unavailable over short periods, being stored in bone and other inaccessible tissues. In addition, more than half of total bone CO_2 is in the form of carbonate rather than bicarbonate.

Accurate dissociation curves are available for blood (Chapter 6) and are needed for computation of blood gas tensions resulting from venous admixture. A single lumped curve for tissues is likely to have approximately the same form but can be greatly simplified since extreme accuracy is both unattainable and meaningless. Total CO_2 incorporates dissolved CO_2, H_2CO_3, HCO_3^-, and a small carbamino component. If H_2CO_3 and carbamino are neglected then dissolved CO_2 will be given by the difference between total CO_2 and CO_2 present as bicarbonate;

$$\text{Dissolved } CO_2 = \text{TC2CT} * .1 - \text{TC3CT} * 22.4$$

where TC2CT is the content of CO_2 in the tissues (cc STPD per 100 ml blood) and TC3CT the concentration of HCO_3^- present in mmol/l. The constant '.1' converts to litres and '22.4' is Avogadro's constant converting mmol to ml. In its actual form in the programme (Appendix IV between statements 670 and 690) this becomes:

$$[\text{C30} = 520. \, / \, \text{TVOL}]$$
$$[\text{C36} = 7.7 * .9 \, / \, \text{TVOL}]$$
$$\text{TC2PR} = \text{TC2MT} * \text{C30} - \text{TC3MT} * \text{C36} \ldots +$$
$$\text{constant(C33)}$$

The final expression is somewhat more complicated because effective bicarbonate concentration is itself influenced by PCO_2.

The incorporation of distribution volume terms (TVOL) allows subjects of different body size to be represented. The constants '520.' and '7.7' allow the correct pressure to be obtained from measured total amounts of CO_2 and HCO_3^-. The expression '.9 / TVOL' is an assumed effective distribution volume for bicarbonate (see Chapter 14). The constant provides an intercept similar to that shown for blood in Figure 6.2. For an average subject this expression gives a partial pressure of about 45 mmHg for a total CO_2 of about 13 litres and a total bicarbonate of about 400 mmol, with an extracellular fluid space (TVOL) of 12 litres.

It should be noted that for convenience the tissue CO_2 stores of the model are measured in litres, and TC2MT has a normal value of about 13 (litres)—hence the multiplier '.001' in the computation of TC2MT between statements 670 and 690.

I shall return to discuss acid-base regulation more fully in Chapter 14. However, leaving aside metabolic hydrogen ion changes, it is easy to appreciate the truth of Haldane and Priestley's dictum (1935) that 'the chief flywheel of the respiratory centre is the great storage capacity of the tissues for CO_2. There is no such storage capacity in connexion with oxygen'.

Improving estimates of tissue dissociation curves

The expressions for the lumped tissue dissociation curves can only be very approximate since obviously the shape of the curve differs in different regions. Once these guesses have been made, they can be improved later by operating the model and determining, for example, how quickly arterial oxygen content falls after the inspired gas changes to nitrogen, and how quickly the blood PCO_2 or CO_2 content rises with asphyxia or rebreathing of exhaled gases. The dissociation curves of the blood pools are known with great accuracy. The total amounts of oxygen and carbon dioxide in the lungs, and the total oxygen consumption and carbon dioxide production rates are known almost as accurately. The only unknown factors are the tissue stores and tissue dissociation curves. The parameters of MacPuf were chosen to fit clinical and physiological observations as closely as possible (see Chapter 23). Later tests can no doubt improve the estimates and, if it seems worthwhile, subdivisions of tissue compartments can be added.

OTHER ASPECTS OF GAS EXCHANGE IN THE TISSUES

Oxygen cost of breathing and cardiac contraction. A simple refinement which adds little to the computation time and slightly enhances realism is to introduce an extra term for the oxygen consumption and carbon dioxide output of both the heart and respiratory muscles, relating these respectively to cardiac output and total minute ventilation. I have therefore added two terms to the tissue oxygen consumption expression, based on observations by Shephard (1966): the cardiac output (in l/min) specifies the oxygen consumption of the heart, in the same number of cc/min; and a more complex term related to the total ventilation (in 1/min) and to the vital capacity and elastance, has the effect normally of adding to the total oxygen consumption term 0.5 cc/min for each added l/min of total ventilation at low or resting ventilations, and 1.0 cc/min for each l/min at maximal ventilation (e.g. 100 l/min). For those with stiff lungs and severe airways obstruction with reduced vital capacity 15% or less of normal, these figures become about 2 cc/min per 1/min. total ventilation at rest, and 8 cc/min per 1/min at maximal ventilation (15–20 1/min). The method by which this is done will be clear by inspection of the main programme (Appendix IV, statement 490). The term for CO_2 output (TRQ $*$ U between statement numbers 670 and 690) is similar to that for the oxygen consumption calculation (U), multiplied by the tissue respiratory quotient (TRQ), which is normally 0.8.

Whole description of tissue gas exchange. Putting all these calculations together we arrive at the approximate representation of gas exchange in the tissue pool of the body as a whole which is given in Appendix IV between statement numbers 500 and 690. Nitrogen will be discussed in Chapter 17. As can be seen, once the tissue partial pressures have been determined from the amounts and the dissociation curves, the effluent blood is assumed to take up the same tensions as in the tissues. Its contents of O_2 and CO_2 are derived as described in Chapter 6 by the use of subroutine GASES. These newly calculated values for TO2CT and TC2CT are available next time round for the succeeding iteration of the whole programme, so that the difference in contents of arriving and leaving blood can be used again to compute the total quantities of each gas present in the tissue.

Damping of tissue gas changes. As shown in Chapter 5, it is necessary to introduce a damping factor into the arterial blood pool calculations to cope with large cardiac outputs and long iteration intervals. This is unnecessary for CO_2 in the tissues, because of the vast store of CO_2. For oxygen, if we assume a tissue store of about 300 cc, then even in 10 s only one sixth (50 cc) would be used up at an oxygen consumption of 300 cc/min. Problems would only arise at normal cardiac outputs with workloads involving oxygen consumptions of about 2 l/min and upwards, but at these metabolic rates cardiac output would normally increase adequately. The simulation of acute, very intense exercise without matching oxygen delivery (e.g. in the 100 metre dash) would rapidly bring tissue oxygen stores to zero—an example of the insights which a holistic model provides into the importance of rapid circulatory adjustments to exercise. MacPuf incorporates some damping of rate of change of tissue PO_2, and a check to prevent total tissue oxygen falling below zero. If it does so control is passed to statement 940, and subroutine DEATH prints the error message * * * * FACTOR 95 HAS GONE NEGATIVE– TIME INTERVAL PROBABLY TOO LONG. The operator would then have to repeat the run using a shorter iteration interval. Providing TO2MT falls slowly enough, the oxygen-sparing effect of lactic acid generation holds tissue O_2 stores above zero values.

In chapter 15 I shall show how tissue PO_2 is used to determine the rate of production of lactic acid during anaerobic glycolysis.

SUMMARY

The passage of arterial blood through a single lumped compartment representing the systemic vascular bed is described and analysed in terms which can be entered into a digital computer programme. The processes in the tissues whereby oxygen is extracted and carbon dioxide given off are then considered. To determine the gas contents of the effluent blood it is necessary to approximate the lumped oxygen and carbon dioxide dissociation curves of the tissues, and then again compute gas contents from the dissociation curves of whole blood. Once the contents of oxygen and carbon dioxide in effluent blood have been determined, the next stage in the circulation of blood is completed. Damping is not necessary when considering tissue gas stores, because of the large size of such stores.

8
Bulk Transport through the Venous System; Time Delays

Since no gas exchange of any consequence takes place in the venous compartment this can be treated as was the arterial compartment in Chapter 5—but the description has to be a little different. In the arterial compartment sensible results were obtained by the following set of computations, each being performed every 10 s simulated time interval, assuming a cardiac output of 5.4 l/min:

1. 900 ml blood flowed out of the (1000 ml) pool, leaving 100 ml;
2. 900 ml blood flowed in;
3. The pool was completely mixed, and a new value for effluent gas concentration computed.

It is generally reckoned that 60% of the whole blood pool resides in the veins, i.e. about 3000 ml (Green, 1944). A similar treatment, using the Case (2) procedure outlined in Chapter 5, would result in nicely stable operation, since the large pool would prevent sudden unrealistic swings of blood composition. No damping (p. 27) such as that used for the arterial pool calculations would be needed. The whole sequence of operations for a 5.4 l/min cardiac output would be as follows:

1. 900 ml blood flows out of the (3000 ml) pool, leaving 2100 ml;
2. 900 ml blood flows in;
3. The pool is completely mixed, and the new value for effluent gas concentrations computed.

The necessary Fortran representation for oxygen is:

$$[C2 = 100. / VBLVL]$$
$$VO2MT = VO2MT + FT * CO * (TO2CT - VO2CT)$$
$$VO2CT = VO2MT * C2$$

where VO2MT is the total amount of oxygen in the pool; FT and CO, as before, are fractional time and cardiac output; TO2CT is the oxygen content of blood leaving the tissues; VO2CT that of blood leaving the veins; and VBLVL is the venous blood volume in ml. (The factor '100.' is again needed so that contents can be expressed in the traditional units of volumes of gas

44

per 100 ml of blood.) All the computational steps are shown in the Main Programme in Appendix IV, between statements 700 and 710. However, the expressions for VO2MT and VC2MT are complicated by the inclusion of left-to-right shunt terms.

Unrealistic as this description is, it is obviously better than the Case (1) description in Chapter 5, in which the incoming blood is completely mixed with the pool before any blood flows out. It requires no mathematics to perceive what commonsense tells us—that an incoming litre or so of blood cannot possibly mix completely with the two litres or so in the pool. This contrasts with the situation on the arterial side. It seems entirely reasonable to expect that some 10% of the blood there might indeed be mixed, considering the large capacity of the proximal aorta.

TIME DELAYS

At this point I propose to consider the total time delays in the system as it has been analysed so far. The statements or processes simulated are as follows:

$$RO2MT = RO2MT + FT * CO * (PO2CT - EO2CT)$$
$$EO2CT = \text{some function of } RO2MT \text{ (see Chapter 5)}$$
$$TO2MT = TO2MT + FT * CO * (EO2CT - TO2CT) - O_2$$
consumption
$$TO2CT = \text{some function of } TO2MT \text{ (see Chapter 7)}$$
$$VO2MT = VO2MT + FT * CO * (TO2CT - VO2CT)$$
$$VO2CT = \text{some function of } VO2MT \text{ (see above, this chapter)}$$

According to this analysis, a step change in incoming blood oxygen content (PO2CT) will make a change in EO2CT of some 90% of the change in PO2CT after a simulated single 10 s iteration interval has passed (see Figure 5.2A for a graphical example). In the tissues, because there is a relatively large total amount of oxygen the change will be further attenuated, but by the time that the fourth statement above is executed, TO2CT will have taken up some value probably representing some 20% of the initial change in PO2CT which started the sequence. The large venous blood pool, containing another corresponding mass of oxygen, is a further buffer against rapid change. In the end the new content of venous blood entering the right heart and pulmonary circulation might perhaps be immediately changed by a tenth of the total initial change in PO2CT. The only true time *delay* in this whole network resides in the impossibility of changing the value of any variable until one complete iteration of the programme has been performed, and each of the six instructions above acted upon. For reasons fully explained in Chapters 2 and 3, this iteration interval is set at 10 s for normal use, though for large cardiac outputs it may need to be shortened to 5, 4 or 2 s.

In normal use therefore, the circulation time of the model as described so far is short (i.e. 10 s), and at smaller iteration intervals it will be correspondingly shorter still. Ten seconds approaches the fastest arm vein/same arm vein circulation time ever normally seen (12 s). It is nowhere near as large as the normal maximum for resting subjects (28 s) nor the average value of about 25 s (Hess, 1927). The damping which was needed in the arterial blood pool to guard against unrealistic oscillations supplies an impediment to immediate changes around the circulation which is somewhat similar in its effect to a time delay. But it is clearly not the same thing. Unless damping is infinite some rapid change, even if small, can be manifest at once throughout the entire circuit after one iteration of the main programme has taken place.

So far I have not considered passage through the lungs, but in succeeding chapters I shall show that the circulation of blood is completed by statements such as the following, in which 'A' represents the alveolar compartment:

$$AO2MT = AO2MT + FT * CO * (VO2CT - PO2CT)$$
$$AO2PR = \text{some function of AO2MT}$$
$$PO2PR = \text{some function of AO2PR}$$
$$PO2CT = \text{some function of PO2PR}$$

If this short sequence is tacked on to the statements above, the circulation is complete. The final computation gives a new value for PO2CT, which is the starting variable in the first statement—

$$RO2MT = RO2MT + FT * CO * (PO2CT - EO2CT)$$

This means that no further time delays are introduced; and the whole quantity of blood in MacPuf circulates once every 10 s.

If the model was always to be operated at an iteration interval of 10 s, a further time delay of 10 s could easily be inserted by transposing two successive blocks of the programme. For example, if the tissues were considered before the arterial blood pool transit description, the incoming blood to the tissues would not change its composition until two successive iterations had occurred. However, if the model is to operate effectively at shorter time intervals, which is desirable for the most accurate results, such a solution would be unsatisfactory. It is anyway inelegant and illogical.

At first sight the ideal circulation time might appear to be 60 s. After all, 5 litres of blood normally circulate at a rate of 5 litres per minute. However, a much shorter modal circulation time is desirable because there are distant regions in which flow is relatively sluggish and which are contributing little to the whole body oxygen consumption, but in which quite large amounts of the whole blood volume may be pooled. It might eventually prove ideal to have two separate blood pools, one perfused fast and the other perfused slowly. However, this takes us away from the simplest possible description at which I am aiming and would prolong computing time considerably. If allowance is made for the extra and unphysiological damping which has to be inserted into the arterial blood pool for mathematical rather than physiological reasons, it appears sensible to aim for a typical modal value for circulation time of 20 s.

All the foregoing discussion has revolved round the realistic treatment of rapidly changing conditions. Steady states in MacPuf are not affected by damping or time delays. It only becomes possible to check the combined effect of damping and time delays against effective time delays in life by matching the performance of the model to conditions where acute changes have been measured in human subjects. In chapter 23 I shall consider some examples including that of acute reduction of barometric pressure.

Digital computer representation of time delays

The number of operations of the time delay system in MacPuf depends inversely on the fractional time interval and on the cardiac output. Using a 10 s interval, the added time delay is one cycle of 10 s at 5 l/min cardiac output. With a 4 s interval it is 5 cycles of 4, and with a 2 s interval it is 10 of 2— i.e. 20 s in each case. The delay is inserted at only one point in the circuit during venous transit. This saves much time in execution. The insertion of time delays at each point in the whole circuit would be a ludicrous and extravagant refinement unless one was trying to simulate the correct phase relations of rapid changes in one compartment to those in another. The elaborate formulation of Grodins, Buell and Bart (1967) incorporated dyamic time delays dependent on flow rates of blood and gases. In Chapter 23 I shall demonstrate that 'on' and 'off' transients with CO_2 breathing are almost as well represented by MacPuf using a single (venous) time delay as with a more complex time delay system.

Although the digital computer has many advantages over the analogue computer, it is not so convenient for simulating time delays, especially those which need to be variable. Each set of values which is to be used in some later iteration of the whole programme needs extra storage to be set aside for it. Readers who have difficulty in getting the whole of MacPuf into a small computer might take comfort from my observations that the performance of the model without any extra time delays other than those stemming anyway from the long iteration interval and the necessary damping, is not much changed during most simulated experiments. The time delay can be removed by deleting subroutine DELAY, the storage space in the COMMON block assigned to it, and the single call to the subroutine which can be seen in the main programme (Appendix IV) between statements 700 and 710.

Subroutine DELAY (see Appendix IV) provides 10 compartments arranged in a circular fashion. Each compartment has four subdivisions—one each for venous oxygen, carbon dioxide and bicarbonate content and one for venous PCO_2. An integer index (NFT) takes into account the fractional time (FT) and the effective cardiac output (COADJ). This integer index is 10 for a cardiac output of 5.0 l/min and a fractional time of 0.16667 min. It falls to unity for a cardiac output of 1.5 l/min or less or for a fractional time interval of .03333 min, and to some intermediate value for intermediate reductions of cardiac output or time interval. If the value of NFT is 5, the current values of VO2CT, VC2CT, VC3MT and TC2PR are entered into each of the first five compartments. The 'pointer' (INDEX) is then moved on one more compartment, and the values of VO2CT, VC2CT, VC3MT and TC2PR extracted from those previously stored there. Control then returns to the main programme, and the venous blood passes on to the alveolar gas-exchanging compartment. When the subroutine is called again, the originally stored values are released back in similar fashion from compartment 1, creating a time delay of 10 s. If, on the other hand, the value of index NFT is unity, only one box is filled at each call to the subroutine, and the pointer moves on only one space. The effect is then that 10 successive calls to the subroutine have to be made before the originally stored values are released again. If the iteration interval is the smallest permissible (i.e. 2 s) the network contributes a time delay totalling 10×2, i.e. 20 s, making a grand total for the modal circulation time of 22 s. This is virtually the same as the time delay for the longest iteration interval, i.e. 20 (10 s delay and 10 s iteration interval). I shall not describe the subroutine in greater detail, because it is self-explanatory to a Fortran programmer. Interested readers can observe the computational techniques involved by looking at subroutine DELAY in the full programme listing in Appendix IV. Note that the use of a delay circuit such as this, when combined with a STORE or BACKTRACK option (see Chapter 25) means that extra space has to be set aside not only in the COMMON store (the array TDLAY) but also in the dump store (TDUMP). This is necessary if a given set of conditions in the model are to be stored for repeated similar experiments.

Computation of venous blood partial gas pressures

When discussing the interconversion of pressures to contents in Chapter 6 I pointed out that it was necessary to convert content to pressure in at least one part of the circuit, so that the correct PO_2 and PCO_2 of arterial blood could be determined, and have their correct effects on ventilation. Despite much theorising, and much research, there is no general agreement yet that a receptor exists in man or animals which is sensitive to normal physiological changes in mixed venous PO_2 or PCO_2. In early versions of MacPuf I applied the clumsy and time-consuming back iterations of gas contents to determine partial pressures in the venous blood as well as in the arterial. This was wasteful, since the partial pressures were only being computed to make the values available for inspection. Alveolar gas exchanges are computed from blood gas contents and pulmonary blood flow (by techniques which will be described in the next chapter), and the mixed venous partial pressures were not used in any further computational procedures. In later versions of the model, and in the full programme published in this book, therefore, I have placed brackets round the values for mixed venous PO_2 and PCO_2 in the large INSPECT table displaying all computed values (Figure 24.1, p. 146) to remind users that these values are the same as those for blood leaving the tissues, and that no damping is included. Time delay is included for TC2PR only, since this is needed to describe acid-base status of mixed venous blood. It is still possible for a user concerned with exact phase relations to work out the effective time delay operative for his own conditions, then to take as the true mixed venous PO_2 that value obtained for effluent tissue blood PO_2 an appropriate number of iterations earlier. Alternatively, he can take the computed values for oxygen and carbon dioxide *content* in mixed venous blood (which *do* take time delay and damping into account) and separately compute the partial pressures by applying the usual nomograms to the values of contents, pH, temperature and haemoglobin concentration.

SUMMARY

The passage of blood through the venous compartment is considered. The large size of the pool, compared with the arterial pool, means that stability is good and extra damping unnecessary. This leads to consideration of the likely effective time delay, and to the conclusion that making allowance for some inevitable damping, by reason of the long iteration intervals used, a total modal circulation time of 20 seconds is reasonable. With a 10 s iteration interval this necessitates a single further delay of about 10 s. For a 2 s iteration interval, 10 such delays are provided.

The techniques for introducing realistically scaled time delays are considered, taking into account the iteration interval and the cardiac output.

Mixed venous PO_2 and PCO_2 are not separately computed because (1) the values will be similar to those already computed for effluent tissue blood partial pressures, (2) they can be computed individually from the mixed venous blood contents if needed, and (3) the computations are lengthy and slow execution of the programme.

9
The Three-compartment Model; Alveolar Gas Exchange; Completion of the Circulation

Riley and Cournand (1949) showed that it was possible to describe normal and diseased lungs *as if* they contained effectively only three compartments:

1. An 'ideal' gas exchanging compartment in which gas exchange is complete: this contains alveolar gas which in a steady state has a unique composition satisfying the requirement that the respiratory exchange ratio (i.e. volume of CO_2 exhaled divided by volume of oxygen taken up in unit time) is the same as the respiratory quotient of the tissues;
2. A blood compartment which can be visualised as a right-to-left shunt, or 'venous admixture' through which some of the cardiac output passes without making any contact at all with alveolar gas;
3. A gas compartment with no blood flow and therefore no gas exchange. This 'physiological dead space' comprises anatomical (i.e. conducting airways) and alveolar components.

This analysis has been used very extensively in the last two decades to describe clinical disorders. One might say, for example, that in a particular patient the blood gas values are compatible with a 'venous admixture' of 20% and a 'physiological dead space' of 200 cc. This implies:

1. That 80% of the cardiac output perfuses 'ideal' alveoli, the blood leaving which is assumed to take up exactly the same partial pressures of each gas as is present in those alveoli;
2. That this blood behaves *as if* it mixed, in an 80/20 proportion, with blood which has completely bypassed the lungs, thus having unchanged mixed venous composition;
3. That of the total tidal volume of each breath, 200 cc behaves *as if* it is wasted and contributes nothing to alveolar ventilation thus having, on expiration, a composition identical to the inspired gas.

In normal people there is only a small true right-to-left shunt. The physiological dead space may be the same as the anatomical dead space, but it is often considerably more and may even be less at very low tidal volumes.

49

However, the concept of two compartments—'venous admixture' and 'physiological dead space' provides a convenient way of quantifying unevenness in the distribution of ventilation/perfusion ratios in the lungs as a whole. Furthermore, calculations suggest that gaseous pressure equilibrium is normally reached by the time blood has reached the end of a pulmonary capillary (Hill, Power and Longo, 1973) so that the concept of an ideal gas-exchange compartment has some substance in fact.

The major defect of the three-compartment model is the absoluteness of the dead space and shunt compartments, with no gas exchange taking place within them. In reality there is gas exchange in places with both high and low ventilation/perfusion ratios. More complex models (Farhi and Rahn, 1955; King and Briscoe, 1967; West, 1969; Kelman, 1970; Butler and Mohler, 1970), take such compartments into account, and more accurately predict the effects of changes in ventilation, cardiac output and inspired oxygen on the blood gases. For example, patients with severe emphysema may have almost normal arterial oxygen tensions at rest, but on exercise P_aO_2 may fall severely. According to the three-compartment analysis, they have a relatively small 'venous admixture' at rest, and a much greater one during exercise (Jones, McHardy, Naimark and Campbell, 1966).

Most respiratory physiologists would probably now acknowledge that the Farhi and Rahn multi-compartment model describes gas exchange better than the Riley three-compartment model. Why then do I prefer to use the Riley model in MacPuf? The first answer is because of its simplicity. In each gas-exchanging compartment there must be a conversion of gas pressures to gas contents (see p. 33) and each separate compartment adds greater complexity. For example, the 25-compartment model of Kelman (1970) required 10 min on his dedicated computer to calculate the composition of one sample of arterial blood. Maybe this is both acceptable and desirable in a model intended for research as well as for teaching purposes; but there is another reason for avoiding the added complexity of a ten- or more compartment analysis. It is still unduly simplified, and cannot accurately represent every aspect of dynamic behaviour. For example, the pulmonary arterioles constrict actively at low alveolar oxygen tension, thus increasing the ventilation/perfusion ratio of hypoxic parts of the lungs. However subtle and accurate a ten-compartment analysis may be, it cannot deal with these and many other dynamic changes.

The second reason for preferring the three-compartment model is its intelligibility. Most medical students and physicians can understand it, but have difficulty with other models. It is easier for a teacher to put across the *as if* statements describing shunt and dead space than the more complex description of many discretely different ventilation/perfusion compartments.

To mitigate the limitations of the three-compartment model I have specified appropriate changes in 'venous admixture' effect and 'physiological dead space' in accordance with altered alveolar gas tensions, cardiac output, and total ventilation. This is admittedly artificial, but so also would be a multicompartment description if it was to remain correct for a wide range of dynamic changes. I have accepted the limitations of the three-compartment analysis, and have thereby been easily able to arrange that working values of effective venous admixture and dead space can be displayed whenever necessary, and will correspond to values with which physiologists and clinicians have already become familiar.

Equilibration of idealised pulmonary capillary blood with alveolar gas

In the next chapter I shall discuss the derivation of alveolar gas pressures as functions of alveolar ventilation and gas exchange, and in this chapter I shall consider only the computation of pulmonary capillary gas contents, and the mixing with shunted blood. The alveolar pressures of oxygen and carbon dioxide (AO2PR and AC2PR respectively) and the tensions in pulmonary capillary blood are assumed to be the same, according to the definition of an 'ideal' alveolar compartment. Thus to compute the gas contents in idealised pulmonary capillary blood it is only necessary to specify a call to subroutine GASES, as follows:

CALL GASES(AO2PR,AC2PR,PO2CT,PC2CT,PH,SAT)

(see Chapter 6 for further details). This supplies new values for gas contents (PO2CT and PC2CT). The main programme between statements 930 and 960 (see Appendix IV) illustrates the necessary steps, which include a prior estimate of pH from venous blood bicarbonate and alveolar PCO_2 (according to calculations described in detail in Chapter 14).

Specification of the amount of 'venous admixture'

Normal lungs behave *as if* the venous admixture was small, e.g. 3% of the cardiac output. I have chosen to represent venous admixture in two parts. One is a fixed right-to-left shunt, by which, for example, cyanotic congenital heart disease may be simulated. This 'fixed admixture' effect (FADM) is initialised as zero, but can be increased to any desired extent by an operator. The other component of venous admixture (VADM) represents the physiological or dynamic shunt effect. This is initialised to 3 (percent of cardiac output) but is allowed to vary between certain limits. The point here is that changes in apparent venous admixture are needed if a three-compartment model is to behave realistically with changing lung oxygen tensions. A small increase in the PO_2 of a poorly ventilated part of the lung can bring about a marked improvement in the arterial PO_2. Because of this the calculated venous admixture appears to fall. The ventilation/perfusion matching has not improved—merely the PO_2 of areas with low ventilation/perfusion ratios. If the corrections described below were omitted, changes in arterial PO_2 produced by changes in inspired oxygen would not be realistic when the model was simulating patients with lung disease. The designer of a crude make-shift system could take comfort from Haldane and Priestley (1935) who observed: 'It seems probable that by some means at present unknown to us a fair adjustment is maintained normally between air-supply and blood-supply. . . . What seems to matter is the degree of arterialisation not of the blood from individual air-sacs, but of the mixed arterial blood.'

Representation of changes in apparent venous admixture (PW) with changes of alveolar oxygen tension (AO2PR) is made to correspond with the clinical experience of Warrell, Edwards, Godfrey and Jones (1970) (see Appendix IV, main programme, between statements 280 and 370):

$$[C18 = VADM * 80.]$$
$$X = AO2PR$$
$$IF (X .GT. 200.) X = 200.$$
300      $Y = AO2PR$
$$IF (Y .GT. 600.) Y = 600.$$
$$IF (AO2PR .GT. 400.) X = X - (Y - 400.) * .3$$
$$IF (X .LT. 55.) X = 55.$$
360      $PW = C18/X ...$
$$IF (PW .GT. 100.) PW = 100.$$

(Since logical operations are slow in execution, they have been substituted by arithmetic operations in the published programme, but are shown here in logical form for easier intelligibility.) These statements have the effect on a nominal 50% venous admixture* which is shown in Figure 9.1. The fixed

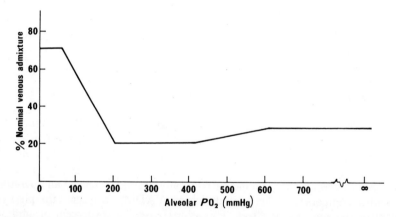

Figure 9.1 Diagrammatic representation of the function used to specify the changes in effective venous admixture resulting from variation of alveolar PO_2 between zero and infinity. At a normal PO_2 of 110 the operative venous admixture is the same as the 'nominal' venous admixture (in this case 50%), but as the PO_2 goes down so the operative venous admixture rises to a maximum. Up to 200 mmHg venous admixture falls, but tends to rise slightly with high PO_2 values (see text)

shunt, FADM, is added to the total effective shunt PW right at the end (see Appendix IV, statement 360), so that its contribution is unaffected by alveolar PO_2. An upper limit of 100% shunt is applied to prevent arithmetic errors through ridiculous values being entered by an operator. The full programme has another term C19 (incorporating two other parameters, PD and RVADM) added to the final expression for PW

$$(PD - 90.) * RVADM * .05$$

* 'Nominal' here means 'that operative at normal alveolar PO_2'

The parameter PD represents metabolic rate, and can be increased by the operator to simulate muscular exercise. RVADM has the normal value of zero, so that apparent venous admixture does not normally change with exercise; but if the values supplied by respiratory function tests (see Chapter 22) specify changes which indicate a gas-exchange disturbance (e.g. in emphysema) RVADM takes a positive value, increasing effective venous admixture in proportion to the exercise.

The other modification to effective venous admixture is brought about by the use of positive end-expiratory pressure (PEEP) and the artificial ventilation option (see Chapter 19). PEEP is allowed to have some value, in cm water, between zero and 15, and slightly and proportionately lessens effective venous admixture as pressure is increased, to simulate the opening of previously unventilated alveoli. Finally, before PW is used in computation, it is augmented by any value which may have been specified for fixed right-to-left shunt (FADM).

Statement 360 in the main programme (Appendix IV) incorporates all the terms described above.

Mixing of shunted and idealised pulmonary capillary blood

The gas contents of mixed venous blood have already been computed as described in Chapter 8, and it only remains to mix the two streams of blood— that from the 'idealised' pulmonary capillary bed, and that from the 'venous admixture' which has bypassed the lungs. The venous admixture will contain gases with contents VO2CT and VC2CT; the idealised pulmonary capillary blood will have contents PO2CT and PC2CT. Mixing is accomplished by the main programme between statements 380 and 390 (see Appendix IV). The values of two constants are first calculated, X being the venous admixture and PC the non-shunted blood, each incorporating a division by 100 to get standard units for content measurement

$$X = PW * .01$$
$$PC = 1. - X$$
$$V = X * VO2CT + PC * PO2CT$$
$$RO2MT = RO2MT + FT * CO * (V - EO2CT)$$

A similar system of mixing determines the P_aO_2 and P_aCO_2 of arterial blood reaching the chemoreceptors (see p. 31).

COMPLETION OF THE CIRCULATION

Chapters 5, 7, 8 and 9 together complete the description of the bulk circulation of gases starting with blood entering the systemic arterial pool from the lungs, and finishing, as described in this chapter, by the specification of some new composition for arterial blood gas content in terms of dynamic venous admixture. Figure 9.2 shows in diagrammatic form the steps making up the whole circulation. Inspection of the complete programme in Appendix IV will

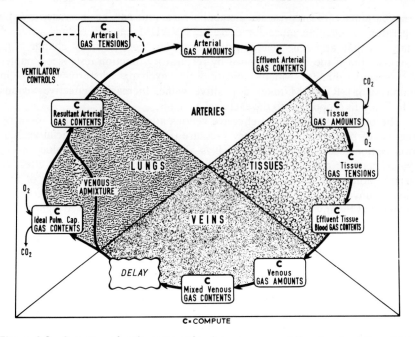

Figure 9.2 Summary of main computational processes completing the circulation. (Note that the computation in each compartment involves a new estimate of gas amounts and finally of gas concentrations which are passed on to the next compartment in sequence)

show that all the steps are contained in the main programme loop, between statements 190 and 1590 controlled by the index MORAN which is executed a number of times corresponding to the length of simulated time requested by the operator. Each repetition simulates the passage of FT minutes of time, which may vary between 0.16667 (i.e. 10 s) or 0.03333 (i.e. 2 s). Since the circulation is closed it makes no essential difference which part of the whole description is placed first, but there proves to be a slight advantage for the representation of chemoreceptor function in having the arterial blood composition determined before the ventilatory response is computed (see Chapter 12), thus allowing accurate phase relationships to be simulated during Cheyne–Stokes respiration.

Some users of previous versions of MacPuf have chosen to make the iteration interval (FT) dynamic, and inversely dependent on the rate at which some sensitive computed variable is changing. This is easily arranged, but makes more complications in time delays and graph scales than, to me, seems justified. However, such a scheme is easy to introduce, because FT is COMMON to all parts of the programme.

SUMMARY

The completion of the circulation demands consideration of passage of blood through the lungs. In the last 20 years the Riley three-compartment model has been a popular method of analysing functional disturbances of ventilation/

perfusion matching. Several improved multi-compartmental analyses have been published, but they prove to be both complex and less intelligible, and slow down execution speed. Although strictly speaking it is less physiological, the three-compartment model is preferred for its conceptual value, simplicity and comprehensibility. The concepts of an 'ideal' alveolar compartment and an effective 'venous admixture' are defined, and the ways in which the Riley analysis is applied to analysis of pulmonary gas exchange are described. Mixing of the two (hypothetical) streams is described, and the circulation is completed by the computation of a new value for blood entering the systemic arterial tree. The physiological processes described in Chapters 5–9 are summarised in diagrammatic form.

10
The Determination of Alveolar Gas Tensions by Alveolar Ventilation and Gas Exchange

In the last chapter I defended the use of a three-compartment model, the essence of which was an 'ideal' compartment in which all gas exchange takes place. In this chapter I shall assume that the amount of true alveolar ventilation is already known, and consider the way in which this, together with alveolar gas exchange, determines the characteristic alveolar gas tensions.

The complete analysis which follows is given in considerable technical detail to make clear every step in the computations carried out in the main programme (Appendix IV, between statements 720 and 900). General readers are therefore advised to skip over the rest of the technical description in this chapter, and simply appreciate that the sequential steps in the computations are as follows:

1. Start from resting lung volume (i.e. functional residual capacity, FRC), with known volumes of O_2, CO_2 and N_2;
2. Allow alveolar ventilation to fill the lungs with appropriate amounts of each gas present in the inspired air;
3. Determine the gas tensions present at the end of mixing;
4. Allow gas exchange to occur, with amounts of each gas being added or taken away from the ideal gas exchanging compartment in accordance with pulmonary blood flow and with the difference in contents between incoming mixed venous blood and outflowing pulmonary capillary blood;
5. Allow lung volume to return to resting level (FRC);
6. Recompute the new gas tensions now present;
7. Take as the representative gas tensions in ideal alveolar air a damped average of the two values for tensions at end-inspiration and at end-expiration;
8. Assume that these gas tensions are equal to those in idealised pulmonary capillary blood, and use them to determine new outflowing contents of each gas (as already described in the last chapter).

In a comprehensive model which is to represent the bulk carriage of gases and their delivery to the tissues, the time scale is such that individual breaths count for very little. Construction of a model in which each breath is separately considered leads to unnecessary complexity. It is simpler for most purposes, and almost equally effective, to represent all processes in the model as if there was a known amount of alveolar ventilation per unit time interval. I have already explained in Chapter 3 that an important feature of MacPuf is the use of an iteration interval of the same order of magnitude as the interval between breaths. This allows a far simpler and almost equally realistic representation of the flow of gases into and out of the alveoli at each breath than does a more complex analysis in which a shorter iteration interval is used (e.g. Yamamoto and Hori, 1971).

In the complete programme (Appendix IV, statements 1360 and 1400) alveolar ventilation in cc (BTPS) per iteration interval is represented as a variable, AVENT. Alveolar ventilation in l/min (FVENT) is given by the expressions:

$$[C56 = .001 / FT]$$
$$1400 \qquad FVENT = AVENT * C56$$

where FT is the fractional time interval in minutes (usually 0.16667, i.e. 10 s). The simplest situation is an iteration interval corresponding exactly to the average interval between breaths. For example, if the respiratory rate is 12 breaths/min the fractional time interval should ideally be 0.083333 minutes (i.e. one twelfth of a minute). I shall consider first ventilation *in*, then gas exchanges, and finally ventilation *out*, taking account of changes in total amounts of oxygen, carbon dioxide and nitrogen in the alveoli at each stage, and their respective partial pressures.

Ventilation in

Let us assume that incoming air has three parts: oxygen, making up FIO2 per cent (normally 20.93); carbon dioxide, comprising FIC2 per cent (normally 0.03); and nitrogen, comprising (100 − FIO2 − FIC2) per cent (normally 79.04). For the purposes of the model 'nitrogen' is taken to include other relatively inert gases, which are not specified separately. But the type of analysis used lends itself equally well to the handling of any volatile material which can be inhaled as a gas and dissolved in the blood; and MacPuf could easily be adapted to simulate the handling of anaesthetic or other gases by incorporation of a few extra statements at each appropriate point in the main programme.

If AO2MT is the total amount of oxygen present in the alveoli at the beginning of ventilation *in*, this will be augmented by AVENT * FIO2 / 100. cc of oxygen after inspiration is complete; i.e.

$$X = AVENT * C12$$
$$U = X * FIO2$$
$$AO2MT = AO2MT + U$$

Similar equations can be written for CO2 and N2. The parameter C12 is a conversion which needs to be applied to cope with atmospheric pressure and temperature changes, because all gas volumes are considered at STPD (see Chapter 4). Total and alveolar ventilation are conventionally considered at BTPS. In Chapter 4 I derived the conversion factor C12 which takes account of both barometric pressure and temperature differences and also incorporates the constant divisor '100'. In the full programme, given in Appendix IV (between statements 740 and 750), the value AVENT * FIO2 * C12 is computed first and stored as another variable 'U' (the oxygen intake)— because this value will later be needed to work out the respiratory exchange ratio. A similar computation is written for CO_2 uptake (V). For nitrogen, the comparable expressions are:

$$Z = 100. - FIO2 - FIC2$$
$$AN2MT = AN2MT + AVENT * C12 * Z$$

The total amount of gas in the lungs, at STPD, is then stored as another variable

$$W = AO2MT + AC2MT + AN2MT$$

This is the same volume as VLUNG (the resting alveolar volume in cc) plus AVENT (the total alveolar ventilation in time FT), if BTPS/STPD correction is made.

For reasons which will be made clear later, but are in any case easy to appreciate, the average alveolar gas tensions must lie somewhere between those prevailing at the end of inspiration and those at the end of expiration. It is therefore necessary at this point to store all these values as further local variables for use later. Given an effective barometric pressure of C11 mmHg (making due allowance for water vapour pressure—see Chapter 4), the partial pressure of each gas is proportional to the amount of each gas divided by the total amount of all gases present (W) as follows:

$$X = C11 / W$$
$$PO2 = AO2MT * X$$
$$PC2 = AC2MT * X$$

(To avoid needless repetition of calculations, the expression 'C11 / W' is computed first, stored as a local variable 'X' and then used in each expression). PN_2 at this point could be obtained similarly, or by subtracting (PO2 + PC2) from C11. The steps in the computations so far appear in the main programme (Appendix IV) following statement 740.)

Gas exchange

Alveolar gas exchange is continuous, but it is convenient to sandwich it between inspiration and expiration. Since it is governed by average alveolar gas pressures it makes little difference at which point in the whole computation it is placed. However, if the amount of a particular gas present at end-expiration is very small, gas exchange during a long iteration interval may give impossible negative values, which are less likely to occur if the lungs are full *before* exchanges take place. This phenomenon is an artefact of a long iteration interval, and can in any case be prevented by using a shorter one.

In Chapter 9, when the exchange of gases between the 'idealised' pulmonary capillary blood and alveoli was considered, the amount of oxygen delivered into the arterial tree after passing through the lungs was given by the expression

$$FT * CO * (100. - PW) * PO2CT$$

where FT is fractional time, CO cardiac output, PO2CT the idealised pulmonary capillary oxygen content and PW the effective per cent venous admixture. The delivery of oxygen to the lungs in time FT is $FT * CO * (100. - PW) * VO2CT$, where VO2CT is the mixed venous blood oxygen content (see Chapter 8). Therefore, the net uptake of oxygen from the lungs is given by the first expression minus the second. To avoid needless repetitive calculations, the expression for fractional time multiplied by pulmonary blood flow is computed first as a local variable, as follows:

$$[C14 = SHUNT + 1.]$$
740 $$PC = FT * CO * C14 * PC$$

(Statement 740 in the main programme also incorporates the parameter C14 describing a left-to-right shunt, and parameter PC (previously computed between statements 380 and 390) describes venous admixture or right-to-left shunt).

The total amount of oxygen in the alveoli (AO2MT) after gas exchange has taken place is then given by:

$$AO2MT = AO2MT + PC * (VO2CT - PO2CT)$$

Comparable expressions describe similar exchanges for other gases. Inspection of the whole programme in Appendix IV (between statements 740 and 750) should make clear the processes so far described.

Once each gas volume in the alveoli has been appropriately augmented or diminished according to its diffusion gradient, a new total volume of the alveolar compartment (PC) is then computed as before by adding together the total amounts of each gas present:

$$PC = AO2MT + AC2MT + AN2MT$$

Ventilation out

Normally expiration proceeds until resting alveolar volume (VLUNG) is reached again, so that the total amount of gas ventilated out in FT time (XVENT) is the difference between PC and VLUNG. Since VLUNG and also the expired volume in time FT are measured at BTPS a correction (C35) is needed:

800                    $XVENT = PC * C35 - VLUNG$

The new value for total lung oxygen can then be computed:

$$AO2MT = AO2MT - AO2MT * XVENT * C25 / PC$$

This states that the amount of oxygen in the alveoli is diminished by the oxygen breathed out, which is given by the ratio of oxygen to total volume of gas, multiplied by XVENT.

As this expression is applied also to CO_2 and N_2, the expression simplifies to

$[C25 = C12 * 100.]$
810                $DVENT = XVENT * C25 / PC$
                   $Y = DVENT * AO2MT$
                   $Z = DVENT * AC2MT$
840                $AO2MT = AO2MT - Y$
                   $AC2MT = AC2MT - Z$
                   etc.

Once again, inspection of the whole programme should make the steps clear, if the intervening statements are, for the moment, ignored.

At this stage, the new partial pressures could be obtained, as before, by determining the ratio of each gas volume to total gas volume, and multiplying this by the effective barometric pressure, e.g.:

$$PN2 = AN2MT * C11 / PC$$

This is not entirely accurate, for reasons which will now be explained. (The description from now on becomes more technical, and could be skipped by those readers willing to accept that the final effective average alveolar gas tensions are going to lie somewhere between the two computed tensions, and that some 'damping' (see Chapter 5) to prevent unacceptable oscillations of alveolar gas pressures may be needed).

Calculation of effective alveolar partial pressures

If the iteration interval (FT) is approximately the same as that between each breath (e.g. 5 s), the alveolar ventilation in time FT will be on a breath-by-breath basis. There are two different gas tensions to take into account, one at resting lung volume (see above), and one at full inspiration. Alveolar and arterial gas tensions do, in fact, fluctuate during the course of the respiratory cycle. The phase as well as the amplitude of oscillatory change may influence the rate of discharge of arterial chemoreceptors, though this possibility is not at present allowed for in MacPuf. The simple formulation as it stands is far from perfect since gas exchange is not confined to that portion of the cycle in which the lungs are fully inflated, but continues throughout the respiratory cycle. Rather than have to take into account two partial pressures for each gas, I have assumed that the blood in its passage through the lungs makes contact with an alveolar compartment having a unique gas composition. The average partial pressure for each gas in this compartment must lie somewhere between the pressures at end-expiration and end-inspiration. Assuming that during

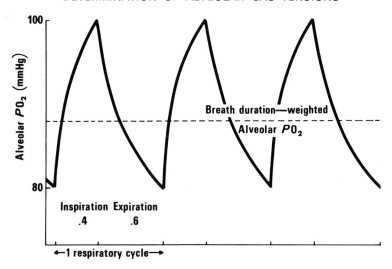

Figure 10.1 Diagrammatic representation of fluctuations of mean alveolar PO_2 during 3 breaths. If all changes are linear, and expiration occupied twice as long as inspiration, the average alveolar PO_2 over a long period of time would be closer to the end-expiratory rather than to the end-inspiratory value (see text). In the schematic diagram inspiration occupies 40% of the whole cycle time, and the mean alveolar PO_2 is taken to be end-expiratory PO_2 plus 40% of the difference between end-expiratory and end-inspiratory PO_2

normal breathing there is slightly longer between breaths than there is during the breath itself, the prevailing gas tensions ought to lie closer to those at residual lung volume than to those present at end-inspiration (Figure 10.1). Taking an estimate of average conditions, with 60% of the cycle time spent in expiration and 40% in inspiration, the average oxygen tensions, for example, would be approximately given by the expression

$$PO2(EI) * .4 + PO2(EE) * .6$$

where PO2(EI) is end-inspiratory PO_2 and PO2(EE) is end-expiratory PO_2. Another way of writing this expression would be:

$$PO2(EE) + (PO2(EI) - PO2(EE)) * .4$$

which is exactly the same in effect, and has the advantage of expressing the ratio of inspiration to cycle duration as a single parameter, in this case 0.4.

Earlier in this chapter the values for PAO_2 and $PACO_2$ at end-inspiration were computed and the values stored as local variables 'PO2' and 'PC2'. At the end of the last section, I showed that the end-expiratory tensions were given by expressions of the form

$$PZ2 = AZ2MT * C11 / PC$$

where 'Z' stands for O, C or N. Therefore, a complete expression which gives the breath-duration-weighted average tension for oxygen, for example, would be

$$AO2PR = AO2MT * C11 / PC + (PO2 - AO2MT * C11 / PC) * .4$$

Since exactly similar expressions are used to compute AC2PR (and also AN2PR if needed), intermediate values are computed, e.g.

850        $U = C11 / (AO2MT + AN2MT + AC2MT)$
           $Y = AO2MT * U$
           $AO2PR = Y + (PO2 - Y) * .4$

The inspiration/cycle duration ratio (0.4) is a parameter specifiable by the operator, and included in the COMMON storage space of the model, in which its value can be changed as desired. The COMMON variable 'SPACE' in the main programme (Appendix IV) is this inspiratory/cycle duration ratio. It is normally set at 0.4.

Time weighting of the effective inspiratory/expiratory duration ratio

The description of breath by breath changes in gas volumes and partial pressures which has been given in this chapter has so far assumed that the interval between successive computations is the same as the interval between successive breaths. For reasons fully explained in earlier chapters I have allowed the iteration interval to be lengthened to a maximum of 10 s, to save computation time in normal use, and to be shortened to a minimum of 2 s, to allow accurate handling of extremely large cardiac outputs. Clearly this will foul up any carefully chosen unique value for the factor representing the simulated subject's inspiratory/cycle duration ratio. If, for example, the subject is breathing 12 times per minute, and computations are performed only 6 times per minute, as they would be with a 10 s interval, the swings between resting conditions and end-inspiration would be excessive. In effect the lungs would be treated as if they distended by twice the real volume of alveolar ventilation *in* at each breath. The opposite situation would occur at a shortened time interval.

This potential source of inaccuracy can be reduced by incorporating some function of fractional time (FT) in the expression for the effective duration ratio. It is necessary also to include some function of respiratory rate, for the same reason, and inspection of the main programme in Appendix IV (between statements 850 and 890) will show that the value for the weighted duration ratio V is given by the following expressions:

$$(C37 = SPACE / FT)$$
$$V = C37 / RRATE$$

SPACE has a normal value of 0.4 and $RRATE * FT$ has a value of unity if iteration interval and breath interval are equal. This expression should make some allowance for different respiratory rates and different iteration intervals, though artefacts in solution could arise. It remains true that the most accurate representation of alveolar gas tension changes in MacPuf will be given when the iteration interval is the same as the interval between breaths. The full programme includes tests to limit the maximum value of V to 4.0 and to make it zero when alveolar ventilation (AVENT) is very small, so that extreme conditions cannot produce absurd results.

Damping of rates of change of alveolar partial pressures

Despite the care taken in the computational descriptions given above, excessively large swings in computed partial pressures are almost bound to occur if the iteration interval is long, unless at the same time alveolar volume (VLUNG) is considerably larger than normal. Commonsense indicates that in normal lungs there will be small delays while gases mix by bulk movement, as for example, during lung movement communicated by the beating heart. In life it is improbable that average alveolar gas tensions can change quite as rapidly as the description so far has allowed them to do. In Chapter 5 I described a simple description of damping which was applied to the transit of gases through the arterial blood pool. This allowed reasonable results to be obtained with long iteration intervals, even at relatively large cardiac outputs. I have used a similar technique to damp slightly the speed of change allowed to alveolar gas tensions. A damping factor 'X' is first computed, taking into account the fractional time interval, the tidal volume and the lung volume. This factor is entirely empirical. A value was first chosen on the basis of what I hoped was intelligent guesswork. It was then refined by applying a number of dynamic tests (some of which are mentioned in Chapter 23). No doubt the accuracy of this, as of most other factors in the model, can be improved by later more stringent dynamic testing and adjustment.

The final computation for AO2PR (between statements 890 and 900) reads as follows:

$$[C38 = 20. / VLUNG]$$
890          $$X = (TIDVL + 100.) * C38$$
$$AO2PR = DAMP((Y + (PO2 - Y) * V), AO2PR, X)$$

There is a similar expression for AC2PR, and one for AN2PR can be included if it is needed, or it can be computed by difference. As mentioned in the previous section, V is the weighted duration ratio.

Diffusion respiration (aventilatory mass flow)

Sometimes in clinical practice alveolar ventilation is so slight that net gas uptake by diffusion exceeds it and expired volume (XVENT) becomes negative in sign; i.e. the processes of ventilation in and gas exchange result in a fall in the volume of gas in the lungs below resting lung volume (FRC). Another situation where this would occur is after an acute increase of barometric pressure. In either case, it would clearly be necessary that air should enter the lungs to make up the deficit and restore resting lung volume.

The simplest way to arrange this is to apply a test to XVENT so that if it is found to be negative, control is passed to a further set of statements which determine that the deficit shall be made up of inspired air with the same concentrations of oxygen and carbon dioxide as was previously inspired.

$$Z = 100. - F1O2 - FIC2$$
$$IF (XVENT .LT. O.) GO TO 720$$
720          $$FD = XVENT * C12$$
$$AO2MT = AO2MT - FD * FIO2$$
$$AC2MT = AC2MT - FD * FIC2$$
$$AN2MT = AN2MT - FD * Z$$

The test is made between statements 800 and 810 (main programme, Appendix IV).

Calculation of the expired respiratory quotient

'U' was earlier defined (p. 57) as the oxygen uptake and 'V' as the CO_2 uptake during ventilation *in*. The amount of CO_2 output (Z) is given by the expression

$$DVENT * AC2MT$$

and the amount of oxygen breathed out (Y) by

$$DVENT * AO2MT$$

DVENT was previously defined as

810          $$DVENT = XVENT * C25 / PC$$

Total net uptake of oxygen (QA), net output of carbon dioxide (QB) and expired respiratory quotient (PC) are then computed (between statements 810 and 920):

$$QA = U - Y$$
$$QB = Z - V$$
IF (QA .EQ. O.) GO TO 930
920   PC = QB / QA
930   . . . .

(The test of QA being zero is of course necessary to prevent the computer trying to divide by zero!)

The whole of this highly concentrated and somewhat lengthy chapter describes only some 50 statements (between statement numbers 720 and 920 in the main programme, Appendix IV); but the representation of physiological mechanisms is so highly compressed and so complex that I hope the general reader will forgive the full documentation here, since it would be needed by anyone wishing to introduce modifications, e.g. for adding in a realistic treatment of the handling of other gases or anaesthetic agents. It would also be needed to disentangle any inaccuracies which may later be revealed by checking MacPuf's performance against experimental or clinical results.

SUMMARY

The processes by which alveolar ventilation and pulmonary gas exchange cause changes in the gas composition of an ideal alveolar compartment are reduced to their simplest possible terms. There is first ventilation *in* of gases in proportion to their respective concentrations in inspired air, then gas exchange with an idealised pulmonary capillary circulation, and finally ventilation *out*, in which the altered gas is exhaled and the lung volume returned to its original value. The problem arises as to which alveolar gas pressure to take as the average, and this problem is resolved in a way which takes account of the iteration interval and also of the respiratory rate. Some damping of the rate of allowable alveolar partial pressure changes is desirable, and is empirically determined, taking into account tidal volume and lung volume.

The possibility of diffusion respiration (aventilatory mass flow), when gas exchange reduces total volume of alveolar gas below residual volume, is allowed for in a short extra section of the whole programme, brought into operation only when such conditions apply.

11
Determination of Alveolar from Total Ventilation—the Concept of 'Dead Space'

In the last chapter I showed how alveolar gas tensions could be computed if alveolar ventilation was already known. In this chapter I shall move a step back and consider how alveolar ventilation itself can be computed if total ventilation is already known. The main problem is to determine the effective 'dead space'—the third compartment of the Riley three-compartment model. Strictly, dead space can be defined as comprising those parts of the gas-filled lungs and upper airways which have ventilation/perfusion ratios greater than that of the ideal alveolar compartment (defined in Chapter 9). The simplification of the three-compartment model requires that dead space be treated *as if* it behaved as a single compartment with infinite ventilation/perfusion ratio— i.e. no blood perfusion at all.

In the complete programme (Appendix IV) tidal volume is a variable (TIDVL), dead space another (DSPAC), and respiratory rate another (RRATE). It follows not by logic or mathematics, but simply by the definition of dead space that alveolar ventilation (AVENT) in cc per fractional time interval (FT) is given by the expression:

1360 $$AVENT = (TIDVL - DSPAC) * RRATE * FT$$

'FVENT' is another variable, giving alveolar ventilation in litres/min. FVENT and AVENT are related by the expressions:

$$[C56 = .001 / FT]$$
$$FVENT = AVENT * C56$$

The variable FVENT is not used in any subsequent computation but is simply provided to give a value for alveolar ventilation in the same units in which it is commonly measured and recorded.

In the next chapter I shall describe how the various stimuli to ventilation summate and interact. It appears from available evidence that the respiratory neurones function *as if* they set out to determine total ventilation in the first instance and that respiratory rate is to some degree independently determined by other factors. I have followed the same logical sequence in MacPuf and have made known ventilatory stimuli first determine total ventilation. Lung elastance and arterial oxygen saturation are subsequently allowed to determine respiratory rate. The computation of tidal volume is then simply a matter of taking total ventilation (DVENT) and dividing by respiratory rate (adjusting units since DVENT is in l/min and tidal volume in cc):

1350   TIDVL = DVENT $*$ 1000. / RRATE

There is one more factor to consider—the limitation of tidal volume by mechanical factors. The relative importance of each (e.g. lung compliance, chest wall compliance and respiratory muscle power) varies in different clinical circumstances, but their summated effect is taken into account by using the vital capacity and making use of the observation that tidal volume does not normally exceed two thirds of the vital capacity.

I shall describe later (Chapter 22) the way in which MacPuf can be made to take account of data from respiratory function tests. These allow the specification of vital capacity, in litres, as a variable (VC). The normal value for this is set at 5.0. Once tidal volume has been determined from total ventilation and respiratory rate, it is tested against maximal tidal volume. If the maximum has been reached, tidal volume is thereafter fixed however great the total ventilation may be, and respiratory rate is adjusted accordingly. This type of behaviour has been described by many authors. In British respiratory physiological jargon it is often known as the 'Hey plot' (Hey, Lloyd, Cunningham, Jukes and Bolton, 1966). Although this behaviour is not what occurs—tidal volume rising asymptotically, rather than linearly, to a maximum value of about two thirds the vital capacity—the approximation does not lead to serious errors. The following sequence of statements (Appendix IV, main programme) represents the determination and limitation of tidal volume in the model:

```
            [C20 = 650. * VC]
1350        TIDVL = DVENT * 1000. / RRATE
1360        AVENT = (TIDVL − DSPAC) * RRATE * FT
            X = TIDVL − C20
            IF (X .LE. .0) GO TO 1380
1370        TIDVL = C20
            RRATE = DVENT * 1000. / TIDVL.
            GO TO 1360
1380        CONTINUE ... etc.
```

No correction is at any stage necessary from BTPS to STPD, since conventionally total ventilation, alveolar ventilation, tidal volume and dead space are all expressed at BTPS.

DETERMINATION OF TOTAL EFFECTIVE DEAD SPACE

At first sight it might appear that the total effective dead space should be the total volume of the upper airways, trachea and all lung branches down to alveolar level, because it is this volume which has to be flushed before any fresh air can enter the alveoli. This volume has been measured in.cadavers by making casts of the airways. The measurements of Weibel (1963, 1964) suggest average volumes of large conducting airways of at least 170 cc, and a volume for the 'respiratory zone' in which gas exchange takes place of about 3000–3500 cc. At rest dead space is effectively less than 170 cc in healthy supine subjects; in exercise it is appreciably more than studies of gross anatomy would predict.

To allow a simple model to give realistic results it is necessary to take account of those factors which alter the apparent or physiological dead space.

A. Factors tending to diminish physiological dead space

1. Distribution of total ventilation during quiet breathing only to certain parts of the lungs (e.g. preferential ventilation of the lower well-perfused zones in an upright subject).

2. Axial streaming of air at low flow rates, in the absence of turbulence— thus allowing a lining film of air to remain relatively stationary. Presumably this influence would be greater in the smaller airways.

3. Narrowing of the calibre of small, and to some extent large airways during expiration. The taking of casts to estimate airway volume requires the application of pressure. This must distend the bronchi, so that cadaver measurements may overestimate the resting volume of larger airways.

B. Factors tending to increase dead space

1. Dilation of airways during deep breathing, e.g. during exercise, simply through distension of the whole lung.

2. Turbulence of airflow during hyperventilation.

3. Mismatching of perfusion to alveolar ventilation, with relatively inadequate perfusion. This will be more likely to occur during hyperventilation when in some cases air may be moved out of alveoli before there has been enough time for gas transfers to have reached equilibrium.

As Haldane and Priestley (1935) remark: 'The "effective or virtual dead space" is neither a definite anatomical dead space nor a fixed dead space in any sense, but a value dependent on several variable factors.'

From the definition of physiologically effective dead space, i.e. that portion of each tidal volume which behaves *as if* it made no contribution to alveolar ventilation, it is possible to work out dead space under a variety of conditions providing that tidal volume, respiratory rate and net gas exchanges are known. Empirically, the values for average normal-sized healthy subjects range from 100 to 150 cc at rest (approximately 2 cc/kg body weight), rising with exercise to values of 500 cc or more. It has been noted that dead space tends to increase when lung perfusion is inadequate. Although quite big changes in cardiac output of themselves have little effect on pulmonary gas exchange, empirically it is observed that when cardiac output is low, there tends to be a loss of uniform distribution of blood flow in the lungs, particularly failure to perfuse the upper zones, leading to increase in effective dead space. Again empiricially it has been observed that the apparent dead space tends to rise as alveolar PO_2 is increased.

Table I   List of components added up to compute total effective dead space (BTPS)

	Normal average value (cc)
1. A component describing upper airway volume, related to lung volume (VLUNG * .025 − 20.), and incorporating a manually variable component (BULLA) allowing the operator to specify increases (e.g. in airways obstruction) or decreases (e.g. tracheostomy)—normally BULLA has a value of zero.	69
2. A component related to tidal volume computed from DVENT * 100. / RRATE ** 1.12.	35
3. A component related to total ventilation and cardiac output, computed by 20. * DVENT / (5. + COADJ).	14
4. A component dependent on alveolar oxygen tension (U), computed as described in the text.	18
5. A component which is added in, and becomes positive only in the event that more gas goes out than in (FY)—normally having a slightly negative value (see text).	−5
6. An added component, taking account of the amount by which specified FEV1 falls short of predicted FEV1 (XDSPA)—normally has a value of zero unless results of respiratory function tests have been entered and are compatible with emphysema (see Chapter 22).	0
Total value for normal average physiologically effective dead space, (BTPS).	—— 131

I have therefore tried to make due allowance for all these factors and to design an empirical equation (perhaps, in this context, more truthfully described as a 'multiple fudge factor') to determine changes in apparent dead space in a number of different conditions, taking due account of all the empirical relationships already discussed. The term describing total effective dead space comprises a number of terms, which are added together as shown in Table I. The formulation in Fortran notation is as follows:

$$[C52 = VLUNG * .03 − 20. + BULLA]$$
$$[C54 = XDSPA * .001]$$

1340 $$DSPAC = C52 + DVENT * 100. / RRATE ** 1.12 + 20. * DVENT / (COADJ + 5.) + U + FY + C54 * (TIDVL + 500.)$$

The six consecutively added terms correspond to the list in Table I. All the terms have been derived empirically to fit available data and experience as accurately as possible. The second term, a function of total ventilation (DVENT) and respiratory rate (RRATE) is related to tidal volume, and the divisor exponent (1.12) has the effect that the dead space rises increasingly rapidly as tidal volume increases. The third term (20. * DVENT / (5. + COADJ)) comprises a ratio of total ventilation to cardiac output. If cardiac output is disproportionately low in relation to total ventilation, this component of dead space rises. The fourth component (U) is derived as follows:

1320   U = AO2PR * .15
             IF (U .GT. 70.) U = 70.

This component has the effect of increasing effective dead space as alveolar oxygen tension rises, to an arbitrary and empirically-derived maximum.

Many readers will have objections to what appears to be an arbitrary assignment of components of dead space to factors 1–4 in Table I and they might be happier with some more familiar formulation such as

ANDSP (anatomical dead space) = 2. * WT (body weight)
DSPAC = ANDSP + (ANDSP * .5) * (TIDVL − 450.) * .001

(which is essentially a Fortran representation of the observations of Jones, McHardy, Naimark and Campbell, 1966). Empirically I found it easier to segment descriptions of the other appropriate factors so as to allow very simple arithmetical representation of changes in exercise and various disease states. It should not be assumed that factors 1–4 represent anatomically or functionally discrete components, but only that, added together, their summated effect corresponds closely to physiological and clinical observations.

The fifth component (FY) is more complex and needs slightly more explanation, especially since its very existence is physiologically deduced and since it would be difficult to measure. During the computations of alveolar gas exchange described in the last chapter an end-inspiration value for total lung volume was computed (W). Then gas exchange with the bloodstream was allowed to occur, following which a new value for total lung volume was computed (PC). Under normal steady state conditions W would be slightly less than PC because more oxygen is taken up than carbon dioxide evolved. However, in unsteady states and certain special conditions the volume of gas might actually increase. This would move part of the alveolar gas, already equilibrated with the ideal alveolar compartment, out of the alveolar compartment and up into the bronchioles and bronchi. The movement of fresh inspired air to the alveoli in the next breath would be impeded by the coincident evolution of this stale alveolar gas. It appears that this must increase effective dead space slightly during the period that these conditions obtain. Once again the representation is empirical and based on what I hope is reasonable guesswork. I have designated a term FY as follows (see main programme, statement 760):

             [C34 = .004 / (FT * C12)]
760   FY = (PC − W) * C34 / RRATE

To give an example with realistic values: suppose that RRATE is 12 and FT is 0.083333 (i.e. one twelfth of a minute). The product RRATE * FT is unity. C12 converts the gas volume at STPD to BTPS (see Chapter 4), and contains a multiplier (0.01). Thus the expression .004 / (FT * RRATE * C12) has a value of about 0.5, which has the effect that the dead space is increased by half the total extra gas in the lungs, assuming that inspiration takes about half the cycle time. This proportion is nothing more than a reasonable guess about the size of this 'pushing back' of gas out of the lungs. The effect of the term is normally likely to be small. In strenuous muscular exercise, for example, when the expired respiratory quotient might be, say 1.15 and total oxygen consumption 2000 cc/min the amount of CO_2 exhaled per minute over and above the amount of oxygen taken up would be 2000×0.15, i.e. 300 cc. Assuming that half this amount went to increase dead space, the residual 150 cc would be split up between perhaps 20 breaths, and would contribute therefore 7.5 cc per breath. An extra dead space term of this magnitude (i.e. 7.5 cc) is negligible, and would contribute almost nothing to the total increase in effective dead space during exercise. However, conditions might be quite different in a situation where large amounts of carbon dioxide were being evolved, with only slight uptake of oxygen—e.g. after the institution of artificial ventilation in chronic ventilatory failure. The increase of effective dead space might be of some importance in cutting down effective alveolar ventilation for a time. Note, incidentally, that FY can be negative as well as positive. If there is a net uptake of gas during gas exchange, (as there normally is), this will diminish the effective dead space.

The sixth component of dead space (XDSPA * .001 * (TIDVL + 500.)) is used simply when the results of respiratory function tests are being specified, as described in Chapter 22, and specifies an extra component of dead space in airways obstruction, related to tidal volume. The manually changeable component (BULLA), incorporated in parameter C52, allows an operator to study the effects of any amount of added dead space, to simulate physiological experiments of different kinds and the attachment of a mouthpiece and gas tubing to a subject or patient. The name 'BULLA' is just a Fortran symbol and does not signify a bulla in the clinical sense. Specification of a value for BULLA of −70 (cc) would allow simulation of tracheostomy since it is generally reckoned that tracheostomy diminishes the effective dead space by this amount.

By trial and error I found that if the value for dead space is allowed to vary widely and rapidly from one iteration interval to the next, unrealistic oscillations may arise simply as a computational artefact of the long interval. Empirically this can be prevented by the application of a small amount of damping (see Chapter 5) to the permissible rate of change of effective dead space. This seems not too unreasonable. The concept of 'effective dead space' is an artificial one, even though it is useful. Limiting its rate of change seems no more unrealistic. The DAMP function is therefore again used, as elsewhere in the programme, the damping constant being related to fractional time (see the main programme in Appendix IV, statement 1340).

SUMMARY

Alveolar ventilation can be derived from total ventilation providing that the effective dead space, and either tidal volume or respiratory rate are known. The various known and theoretically deduced influences on effective dead space are combined in the model to provide a multi-factorial expression taking account of lung volume, adequacy of lung perfusion, rate of airflow, alveolar oxygen tension, net change of lung gas volume during gas exchange, and results of respiratory function testing. The expression also provides for alterations in total dead space by specification of changes by an operator. No pretence of physiological realism is made for what is essentially an empirically determined and artificial quantity; the computational procedures are justified by correct matching of model behaviour to physiological observations.

12
Factors determining Total
Ventilation and Respiratory Rate

In this chapter I shall consider how total ventilation is determined, then the way this is partitioned between tidal volume and respiratory rate. Perhaps the central respiratory apparatus does not work like this—but the advantage of this approach is that total ventilation has been used by most workers to quantify the ventilatory responses to stimuli such as CO_2 inhalation, rebreathing from a bag, muscular exercise and hypoxia.

The control of breathing in general and the relation of chemical and non-chemical factors is too vast a subject to review, and has been done by others (e.g. Defares, 1964). I have based the simulation technique in MacPuf on the following observations:

1. Experimentally, hypercapnia, acidaemia and hypoxia stimulate breathing. The magnitude of their effects can be expressed in terms of the change in total ventilation with changes in P_aCO_2, P_aO_2, or arterial hydrogen ion activity—i.e. as the slopes of the respective response curves. These slopes vary a lot between individuals, but remain reasonably constant in given individuals over long periods of time, given the same initial chemical environment.

2. There is more to the control of ventilation than blood or even brain chemistry. Thus a high $P_{\bar{a}}O_2$ and a low P_aCO_2 do not usually abolish breathing; during exercise there is increased ventilation despite normal arterial PO_2, PCO_2 and pH; possibly in normal circumstances, and certainly in abnormal ones, breathing may be driven by stimuli from many sites—the lungs in particular—and also from higher brain centres.

3. A single expression of the ventilatory response to any stimulus is of uncertain physiological significance. Any interference with neuromuscular transmission, mechanical coupling, or chest or lung mechanics will lessen the response.

4. Chemical stimuli act on different parts of the nervous system in different ways and at different rates. Hypoxia acts almost exclusively on the peripheral arterial chemoreceptors, in which a small mass of tissue is bathed by a rapid flow of blood. The neural signal passed to the brain is

thus extremely rapid. Current opinion about the effects of hypercapnia may be summarised by saying that although the peripheral arterial chemoreceptors are sensitive to changing P_aCO_2 under certain conditions, the central brain chemoreceptors eventually dominate long term changes, and the total ventilatory response of animals to a rising PCO_2 is only slightly impaired by total chemoreceptor denervation. It is also agreed that all respiratory neurones are not equally sensitive to changing PCO_2, but that the response is largely, perhaps exclusively, mediated by central chemosensitive receptors in the area postrema on each side, at a site which may be as close to cerebrospinal fluid as to arterial blood (and hence as sensitive to changes in CSF chemistry as to changes in blood chemistry). It seems likely that an important stimulus from changing arterial PCO_2 is exerted by a change of hydrogen ion activity at this central site. Brain receptor pH must depend importantly on the bicarbonate concentration as well as on prevailing PCO_2 of the cerebrospinal fluid.

5. The rate of change of arterial PCO_2 influences the ventilatory response, and a rapidly rising P_aCO_2 increases ventilation more than a slowly rising value.

Empirically the relationships between arterial pH, PCO_2, PO_2 and ventilation have been put together by a large number of authors who have obtained data from normal subjects during rebreathing and other procedures. Since the subject is so controversial I shall list most of the important papers, so that those who object to the formulation used in MacPuf can easily substitute another one. Recent authors include Katsaros, Loeschcke, Lerche, Shoenthal and Hahn, 1960; Lerche, Katsaros, Lerche and Loeschcke, 1960; Grodins and James, 1963; Grodins, 1963; Lloyd and Cunningham, 1963; Clegg, Goodman and Fleming, 1964; Kellog, 1964; Milhorn, Benton, Ross and Guyton, 1965; Horgan and Lange, 1965; Severinghaus, 1966; Grodins, Buell and Bart, 1967; Yamamoto and Hori, 1971; Swanson and Bellville, 1974. Kellog (1964) for example, produced a formulation in which ventilation was a linear function of arterial PCO_2 with an intercept dependent on arterial pH. This type of formulation was also used by Farrell and Siegel (1973) in their model. To fulfil the purposes I had in mind such a formulation is inadequate even after the response to hypoxia is added in. It accurately describes steady state conditions in normal subjects over a relatively small range of acute alterations in P_aCO_2 and arterial bicarbonate concentration, but it falls down seriously in other respects. For example, it fails to simulate chronic states of hypo- and hyperventilation. It fails to simulate properly chronic metabolic acidaemia, in which, for example, a resting total ventilation of 35 l/min would be predicted by a P_aCO_2 of 20 mmHg, HCO_3^- of 6 mmol/l and pH of 7.1. Such a resting ventilation is clinically unrealistic and in any case logically impossible unless dead space or metabolic production of CO_2 is much increased (otherwise P_aCO_2 would be less than 20). However, it would be very reasonable for a state of acute metabolic acidaemia with increased CO_2 production.

Against a background of generally agreed knowledge and disputed mathematical formulations I have adopted the simulation which follows. No particular merit is claimed for it except that so far it has answered the requirements of an effective simulation: i.e. the speed and magnitude of responses to various physiological manoeuvres performed on MacPuf correspond to those observed in the laboratory, and the ventilatory patterns and responses in various pathological states can be accurately reproduced. Some of the dynamic tests applied to the whole model are discussed in Chapter 23. As I pointed out in Chapter 3, MacPuf is flexible enough to allow at least 10^{30} discretely different experiments to be performed upon it so that I have not been able to test this, or indeed any other part of the model, as fully as I would wish. Therefore the description of ventilatory responses which follows should be regarded as a working hypothesis which is a first approximation, and is capable of being progressively improved as new data become available. In accordance with my previously stated general philosophy of model-building I have aimed at the simplest possible mathematical representation which fits the facts. Readers who wish to review other mathematical descriptions of ventilatory responses should consult some of the authors listed above.

Representation of the ventilatory response to carbon dioxide

Let us suppose that the total stimulus to ventilation in a normal subject (measured in l/min total ventilation and assuming normal lungs) is represented as TVENT, and arterial PCO_2 as RC2PR (see Chapters 4 and 5). We could write a description as follows:

$$\text{TVENT} = 7. + 2. * (\text{RC2PR} - 40.)$$
$$\text{IF (TVENT .LT. 0.) TVENT} = 0.$$

This says that total ventilation is normally 7 l/min, and that for every mmHg that arterial PCO_2 rises above 40 mmHg a further 2 l/min is added to total ventilation. This ventilatory response corresponds to an average figure for normal adults given CO_2 to breathe. This expression also operates in reverse. At an arterial PCO_2 of 37 the total ventilation would be only one l/min, and at any lower P_aCO_2 it would be zero (Fig 12.1).

There are some problems about this simple formulation. The inhalation of CO_2 is an unnatural stimulus, and such a relationship does not hold under all physiological conditions. In exercise, particularly, ventilation rises enormously with little if any rise in average arterial PCO_2 and with no significant arterial oxygen desaturation. A possible explanation is that the fluctuations of P_aCO_2 in arterial blood during the respiratory cycle may be accentuated because of increased cardiac output and CO_2 production. Perhaps the changing phasic relationship might increase total ventilation in a subtle centrally integrated fashion, as some investigators have suggested. There is disagreement whether breathing ever stops if P_aCO_2 falls low enough. It certainly does in anaesthetised animals, and in some human subjects, though in the latter the effects of suggestion are difficult to eliminate. When experts disagree, it seems reasonable to arrange the working of the model in such a way that breathing ceases only under extreme circumstances of diminished CO_2 stimulus.

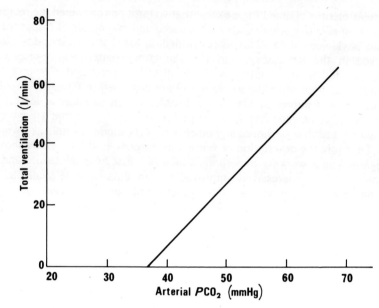

Figure 12.1   Ventilatory response to changes in arterial PCO_2 using the simplest possible representation with linear response discussed in the text. Note that at a PCO_2 below 36 mmHg ventilation would stop altogether

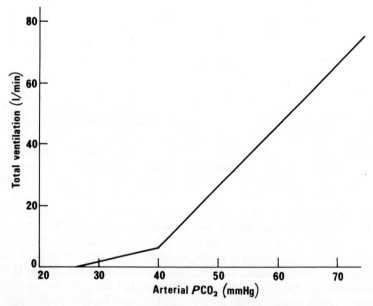

Figure 12.2   Basic CO_2/ventilation response curve used in MacPuf (though the final common path is a function of arterial and brain pH). Note that the slope of the function curve above 40 mmHg $PaCO_2$ is steep and linear, and that below 40 the slope flattens off so that below a $PaCO_2$ of approximately 25 mmHg ventilation ceases (unless driven by hypoxia or some other stimulus)

This requirement makes inadequate a single slope to describe the CO_2 response curve. At the very least two curves are needed: a steep one to describe ventilatory responses to rising PCO_2 and a shallower one, only reaching the baseline at very low values for P_aCO_2, to describe ventilatory responses to falling PCO_2.

The first formulation with the single slope described above produces the response curve shown in Figure 12.1. An improved formulation might be:

$$IF\ (RC2PR\ .GE.\ 40.)\ TVENT = 7. + 2. * (RC2PR - 40.)$$
$$IF\ (RC2PR\ .LT.\ 40.)\ TVENT = 7. + .5 * (RC2PR - 40.)$$
$$IF\ (TVENT\ .LT.\ 0.)\ TVENT = 0.$$

This gives the response curve illustrated in Figure 12.2.

However, the description of the CO_2 response curve is not yet adequate. There is the interesting and not completely solved problem of acclimatisation to high altitudes. It has been repeatedly found that people who chronically hyperventilate at high altitudes (because of hypoxaemia, which will be discussed later in this chapter) continue to do so for a time after returning to sea level, even though the stimulus from hypoxaemia has been removed. It has also been observed that people breathing carbon dioxide for days or weeks tend to hypoventilate for a time after returning to normal air breathing. In a more extreme form failure to respond to normal stimuli may be seen in people with 'primary' alveolar hypoventilation who do not hyperventilate despite a high P_aCO_2.

The kidneys adapt to the prevailing PCO_2 of the blood perfusing them in such a way that blood pH tends to be preserved. The arterial pH is not much if at all reduced in chronic ventilatory failure, because of renal bicarbonate generation or retention. The cerebrospinal fluid (CSF) also adapts to high blood PCO_2, and its own pH tends to be partly stabilised. Much recent experimental work suggests that the central PCO_2 or H^+ ion receptor is influenced not only by the chemical properties of arterial blood but also by the prevailing chemical environment of the brain tissue, as reflected by the composition of the CSF. Perfusion of CSF of different compositions through the ventricular system of animals shows that changes in pH can importantly influence ventilation. Cerebrospinal fluid is a secretion and it appears that its bicarbonate content, for example, can change with chronic changes in the prevailing PCO_2 in such a way that bicarbonate is retained in chronic ventilatory failure, thus reducing the central response to elevation of arterial PCO_2 as well as stabilising CSF pH.

All these considerations make it desirable to include a simplified brain circulation in a holistic model which is to describe ventilatory changes in a large variety of clinical states. This not only makes possible a more realistic and dynamic description of local chemical changes due to the interaction of cerebral metabolism and incoming gas contents, but also allows the continuous assessment of cerebral oxygenation, which must be adequate if any natural ventilation is to take place at all. The account of the simulation which follows leans heavily on the work of other authors who have incorporated a cerebral circulation in their models of ventilatory control (e.g. Defares, Derksen and Duyff, 1960; Horgan and Lange, 1965; Grodins, Buell and Bart, 1967).

Control of ventilation by a central brain H⁺ ion receptor

As a first approximation to a more exact description I have assumed that the central receptor site is situated part-way between arterial blood and brain tissue, so that its pH (BPH) is given by the expression

$$BPH = PHFNC(2. * BC3CT + RC3CT, 2. * BC2PR + RC2PR)$$

(This pH function is defined as a Fortran function at the start of the main programme—it will be further described below and in Chapter 14.)

BC3CT and RC3CT are the brain tissue and arterial blood bicarbonate concentrations and BC2PR and RC2PR are the brain and arterial blood partial pressures of CO_2. Twice as much weight is given to brain as to arterial blood values. Before this computation is made, the prevailing values of BC3CT and RC3CT are worked out from the bicarbonate concentration, measured at a standard PCO_2 of 40 mmHg, by adjusting these concentrations in accordance with the titration curve, e.g.

$$W = BC2PR - 40.$$
$$Y = BC3CT + BC3AJ + .2 * W$$

where Y is the effective bicarbonate content of brain tissue or CSF. (See main programme, Appendix IV, between statements 1060 and 1080). The multiplier '.2' is a guess, which is half-way between the characteristic constant for whole blood (0.3) and that for tissues generally (0.1). The computation of the effective value for arterial blood bicarbonate concentration (RC3CT) and the adjusting constant BC3AJ will be discussed further in Chapter 14.)

In practice, since the pH function above is used at a number of points in the programme, it can be economically specified by a generic function PHFNC (bicarbonate, PCO_2). Empirically I have found a small amount of damping (p. 27) to be desirable, and this can be specified by the DAMP function discussed previously. The total description then reads as follows:

```
        [C17 = FT * 10.]
        W = BC2PR - 40.
        Y = BC3CT + BC3AJ + .2 * W
        . . . . . .
        X = PHFNC(2. * Y + RC3CT, 2. * BC2PR + RC2PR)
        Z = ((ABS(X - BPH) + .00001) * 100.) ** 2 + .04
        IF (Z .GT. C17) Z = C17
1080    BPH = DAMP(X,BPH,Z)
```

The complex damping factor Z is proportional to the rate of change of BPH and is designed to represent the fast contribution of the arterial chemoreceptors as well as the steady state central responses to increased H⁺ or PCO_2. Empirically it allows reasonably accurate simulation of both acute CO_2 inhalation and Cheyne-Stokes breathing.

Having thus derived a value for brain receptor pH which takes into account both brain blood flow and metabolism, and arterial blood composition, the way is now open to describe the ventilatory responses to H⁺ ion and PCO_2 changes according to the following formulation, which gives a composite curve of the general shape previously illustrated in Figure 12.2. This comprises a steep slope corresponding to acute ventilatory responses to rising

PCO_2 and a shallower slope corresponding to falling PCO_2. The formulation is as follows:

```
          [C65 = 7.324 − CZ * .00005]
          [C66 = C65 − .002]
1100      Y = (118. − PJ) * .05
          Z = Y * .002
          X = (C65 + Z − BPH) * 1000. * Y
          IF (X .LT. 0.) X = 0.
1120      W = (C66 + Z − BPH) * 150. * Y
          IF (W .LT. 0. .AND. CZ .GT. 30.) W = 0.
1150      Z = (BC2PR − 120.) * .25
          IF (Z .LT. 0.) Z = 0.
...       Total ventilatory stimulus = function of (X + W) − function
          of (Z)
```

The first six statements specify a variable slope and intercept. The seventh statement (1150) determines the potential suppressant effect of increased brain PCO_2 on breathing.

PJ is arterial oxygen saturation. If this is low, the sensitivity to brain pH is increased by the multiplier 'Y' which also alters the intercept. The next two statements redefining 'Z' supply a progressively more powerful depressant effect on ventilation once brain PCO_2 has risen above 120 mmHg. I shall describe the complex function involving breathing capacity later (p. 79) after hypoxia and other stimuli to ventilation have been described.

Representation of the ventilatory response to hypoxia

The peripheral arterial chemoreceptors, as already mentioned, are sensitive to P_aO_2 and virtually not at all to oxygen content, since they have such a high rate of blood flow. However, the stimulus from changing PO_2 is non-linear and as Rebuck and his colleagues have shown (e.g. Rebuck and Campbell, 1973) a straight line relationship between total ventilation and hypoxia is obtained if arterial saturation rather than P_aO_2 is used. This is a great mathematical convenience. The alternative is a complex quartic equation giving ventilation in terms of P_aO_2 (Grodins, Buell and Bart, 1967). Since it appears to hold in a wide range of conditions, and simplifies the total description I have used it in MacPuf, as follows:

```
1170      Y = (98. − PJ) * (RC2PR − 25.) * .12
          IF (Y .LT. 0.) Y = 0.
...       Total ventilatory stimuli = ... + function of (Y)
```

In this formulation PJ is the percentage arterial oxygen saturation. (Readers of Chapter 6 will have noted that although a value SAT is returned every time the subroutine GASES is called, the value of SAT will change each time the subroutine is used for a different compartment, e.g. arterial blood, tissues, brain and venous pool. Therefore, another variable, PJ, is made equal to SAT for arterial blood earlier in the programme—see between statements 470 and 480). Rebuck's description not only specifies a response linearly dependent on the degree of desaturation but also specifies that the slope of the response curve will depend on the prevailing arterial PCO_2. This accords with recent physiological information about the way in which the peripheral arterial chemoreceptors signal a complex integrated signal from arterial oxygen desaturation and PCO_2. The values given are approximately normal average ones, such that half-saturation of the arterial blood at normal PCO_2 and normal effect or response would produce about 20 l/min extra total ventilation.

I have not inserted any central brain stimulus by hypoxia since this is known in animals not to be a natural stimulus to ventilation once the chemoreceptors are denervated; but I have retained an index of brain oxygenation to ensure that once the brain has run out of oxygen breathing will cease. This damped index of 'brain oxygen adequacy' is computed from the partial pressure of oxygen in the brain, as follows:

$$[C7 = O_2 \text{ consumption term}]$$
$$[C63 = FT * C7 * .12]$$
1190 $$U = BO2PR - 11.$$
$$IF (U .GT. 0.) U = 1.$$
$$IF (U .LE. 0.) U = 0.$$
1220 $$BO2AD = DAMP (U,BO2AD,C63)$$
$$SVENT = BO2AD * \text{Damped total stimulus (U)}$$

In these equations, BO2AD is the arbitrary index of brain oxygenation, and the constants are derived empirically in such a way that breathing stops from cerebral anoxia within about 30 s of complete circulatory arrest.

'Central neurogenic' drive to ventilation

Much animal evidence, dating from the last century (e.g. Geppert and Zuntz, 1888) suggests that muscular exercise supplies a stimulus to breathing independent of changes in arterial PCO_2, PO_2 and pH. This is strongly supported by many physiological studies in man. Most such studies concur that arterial PCO_2 and PO_2 are little changed even by strenuous exercise, and that even the slight fall in bicarbonate concentration and pH resulting from accumulation of lactic acid is quite inadequate to bring about the large increases in ventilation observed.

Once again we can take refuge in an *as if* description. I have assumed that if the system is working perfectly, ventilation would be proportional to the metabolic needs of the body, as expressed by the total oxygen consumption. This is implied by normal arterial gas tensions despite hyperventilation. As Barcroft (1934) elegantly put it '... it seems impossible to escape from the conception that the adaption to exercise is an integration of a large number of factors, no one of which could alter sufficiently to be completely effective'.

In the full programme (Appendix IV), subroutine CONST computes an index of O_2 consumption (C7) taking into account resting O_2 consumption (CONSO), specified metabolic rate (PD—as percentage normal resting value) and temperature (TEMP); then this index (C7) is used to compute a central neurogenic drive (C46). This is allowed to affect the total ventilatory stimulus in a slightly damped manner. 'CZ' is an overriding manual control. The damping of XRESP prevents an operator bringing about unrealistically rapid changes of central neurogenic drive.

$$[C7 = CONSO * PD * .00081 * (TEMP - 26.) ** 1.05]$$
$$[C68 = FT * 3000. / (PD + 200.)]$$
$$[C46 = CZ * .78 * ((C7 * .00051) ** .97 + .01)]$$
$$XRESP = DAMP(C46, XRESP, C68)$$
$$\text{Total ventilatory stimulus} = \ldots + XRESP \ldots$$

(see main programme between statements 1220 and 1230, and subroutine CONST). The nominal oxygen consumption CONSO (in cc/min) is specified in MacPuf for resting conditions. This is changeable by an operator either directly, or indirectly by specifying a subject of a particular height, weight, age and sex (see Chapter 21). The total metabolic rate is specified as another parameter (PD), also manually changeable, which expresses total metabolic rate and oxygen consumption as a percentage of normal. When an increase in metabolic rate is called for by increasing PD or TEMP, C7 increases proportionately. The expression given subsequently for U (total ventilatory stimulus) incorporates C46, which specifies that the central neurogenic drive to ventilation is almost linearly proportional to oxygen consumption, though not quite exactly so, because the exponent '.97' in the expression for C46 above is slightly less than unity. Empirically all these constants have been chosen to give normal average results for exercising subjects. For moderate exercise the performance of MacPuf corresponds to the measurements of Cotes (1966) who observed an increased ventilation of 2.1 l/min for each 100 cc increase in oxygen consumption. Departures from strict equivalence of metabolic rate and total ventilation will naturally occur if coupling of ventilatory stimuli to the movement of air is impaired.

It should be noted that Grodins, Buell and Bart (1967) criticise the inclusion in a model of any central neurogenic drive to breathing (because its nature is obscure)—but without such a 'black box' representation, correct behaviour of a holistic model is impossible. My personal guess is that the preservation of normal gas tensions in exercise is predominantly a learned rather than a chemically-mediated response. If so, a 'black box' description is not only inevitable but, in our present state of knowledge, correct.

Coupling of the total ventilatory stimuli to the ventilatory response

In the preceding sections I have shown how an estimate may be made of the total stimuli to ventilation, summed together to give the index (U) which corresponds to l/min total ventilation. We have to envisage the possibility that these stimuli may fail to exert their full effects on actual movement of air because of mechanical factors, chiefly airways obstruction. This factor can be very simply allowed for by multiplying the whole expression by a function of the 'breathing capacity' (PR—see below). I have also introduced into the relationship another variable depending on body temperature, which makes ventilation increase according to the amount by which body temperature (TEMP) exceeds 29 °C. In addition, a term (X) is incorporated to take account of the increased viscosity of gases under pressure. Since the two main gases considered (O_2 and N_2) have similar viscosities (Radford, 1964) this expression would only need modification for helium breathing. The index has been chosen to give average correct values for arterial PCO_2 in divers, but the choice of a mathematical representation is somewhat arbitrary since some of the increased P_aCO_2 of habitual divers can be attributed to diminished central ventilatory response to CO_2 (Lanphier, 1958).

The total formulation of ventilatory stimuli is now as follows (all stimuli are added together):

1120 $\left.\begin{array}{l} W) \\ X) \end{array}\right.$ previously defined stimuli from brain pH.

1150   Z = previously defined depressant effect of high brain PCO_2

1170   Y = previously defined stimulant effect of hypoxia

XRESP = previously defined 'central neurogenic drive'

[C11 = effective barometric pressure]

[X = .5 + 356. / C11]

[IF (X .GT. 1.) X = 1.]

[C47 = PR * .000214 * (TEMP − 29.) ** 1.5 * X]

U = (C44 * (X + W) + C45 * Y + XRESP − Z) * C47

[C6 = FEV * 25. + 29.]

IF (U .GT. C6) U = C6

1240   . . .

(As before all statements in square brackets are pre-computed as parameters before any run, by subroutine CONST.) An arbitrary but empirically realistic limitation to total ventilation is afforded by parameter C6, related to FEV.

Over-riding manual controls of ventilatory responses and limitation of maximal breathing capacity

To enable an operator to dissect the responses of the model, and to create his own subjects with different types of ventilatory response, each component of the system described in this chapter (i.e. the stimuli from PCO_2 and pH, from PO_2, and from 'central neurogenic' drive) has been made independently variable. Three factors, AZ, BZ and CZ, which each have a normal value of 100 (per cent) are used as multipliers of each individual ventilatory stimulus. By means of instructions supplied by the operator while running the model any or all of these factors may be changed to any degree. (The techniques used for factor changing are described in Chapter 24.) This allows, for instance, simulation of normal subjects with high, average or low ventilatory responses to CO_2 inhalation. As well as allowing simulation of specific ventilatory defects in disease, it is also possible to simulate changed CO_2 sensitivity (e.g. the reduced CO_2 sensitivity of some individuals, mentioned above). AZ, BZ and CZ are incorporated in the pre-computed multipliers C44, C45 and C46 (see between statements 1220 and 1230).

The coupling of the summated ventilatory stimuli to resultant total ventilation is also independently variable, by a further parameter described as 'breathing capacity' (PR) which also has a normal value of 100. (This is incorporated in parameter C47.) The units may be thought of as 'percentage of the normal total response', but might also be considered as reflecting approximately the maximum steady state breathing capacity in l/min.

Total description of ventilatory responses to known stimuli; damping of speed of response

The whole sequence of steps appears in the main programme between statements 1240 and 1280 (see the main programme, Appendix IV). The main steps are given by the following expressions:

$$[C48 = .04 * (TEMP - 26.) * VC]$$
$$[C62 = FT * 240000. / (CZ + 300.)]$$
U = total potential ventilatory stimulus (see above)

1240
$$X = (COADJ + 5.) * C62 / (TIDVL + 400.)$$
$$SVENT = BO2AD * DAMP(U,SVENT,X)$$

1300
$$DVENT = SVENT$$

1250
IF (SVENT .LT. C48 .AND. natural ventilation in use and trachea not obstructed) DVENT = 0.

It will be noted that a DAMP function is again used, with a damping coefficient chosen empirically to give stable and lively responses to changing stimuli which correspond to realistic behaviour as closely as possible (see Chapter 23). The damping coefficient (X) takes into account fractional time (FT), effective cardiac output (COADJ) and tidal volume (TIDVL). Without this damp function the breathing pattern of MacPuf oscillates unduly unless the iteration interval is made inconveniently small. The DAMP function has been adjusted to give a good description of the correct phase relationships observed in Cheyne–Stokes respiration and at the same time allows a not unduly rapid ventilatory response to CO_2 inhalation. As previously mentioned, the influence of rate of rise of the brain pH stimulus was allowed for by making the damping coefficient itself a DAMP function (p. 27).

Another requirement for satisfactory simulation of Cheyne–Stokes breathing is that if the ventilatory drive is less than a certain low value, breathing will cease altogether. This is accomplished by statement 1250.

Factors influencing respiratory rate

Milhorn and Brown (1971) reviewed previous descriptions of the relationship between respiratory rate and total ventilation, and arrived at the formulation:

$$TIDVL = .134 * DVENT ** .7$$

from which respiratory rate could be determined simply by dividing total ventilation (DVENT) by tidal volume (TIDVL). In MacPuf I have adopted a slightly more complicated approach, to allow greater flexibility in operation of the model to simulate disease states, and have incorporated a term describing the stiffness of the lungs, or elastance (ELAST)—usually measured in cm H_2O/l. This term can be manually varied, as described in Chapter 24, to simulate abnormal stiffness of the lungs, and can also be used artificially to drive breathing faster than it might otherwise be driven, e.g. by nervous reflexes from the lungs. A term related to arterial oxygen saturation is also included because it is known since the work of Haldane, recently verified and quantified by Rebuck and his colleagues (personal communication), that a hypoxic ventilatory response is typically accompanied by a faster respiratory rate than the same total ventilatory response to other stimuli.

The whole description is as follows (see between statements 1300 and 1310 in the main programme):

$$[C49 = 9 + SQRT(ELAST * 1.25)]$$
$$[C50 = (150. + PR) * .0275 * (TEMP - 17.)]$$
$$RRATE = (C49 + DVENT ** .7 * .37) * C50 / (PJ + 40.)$$

As before, PR represents breathing capacity and PJ oxygen saturation. Normal subjects vary a lot in their characteristic respiratory rate both at rest and on exercise. The manual overriding control provided by the parameter ELAST provides an easy way of changing the pattern of breathing from the normal average pattern which this whole expression provides. ELAST has a normal value of 5.0 but it is obvious that it can be used to change respiratory rate to any desired extent. Once the respiratory rate has been computed, tidal volume is worked out, and the test previously described on p. 80 applied to check that tidal volume has not exceeded its maximum, in which case respiratory rate is forced to increase, whatever original value had been computed for it.

Programme symbols for ventilatory responses and total ventilation

The reader may have become confused by the multiplicity of Fortran symbolic names (U, SVENT and DVENT) used to represent different aspects of total ventilation control in the model. The justification for what might appear to be unnecessary complexity lies in the desirability of preserving an index of the ventilatory stimuli even during artificial or forced ventilation (Chapter 19), or tracheal obstruction (Chapter 20) so that if artificial ventilation is turned off and the trachea no longer obstructed, the stimuli present at that moment can immediately determine an appropriate level of resultant ventilation. This value is kept as variable (SVENT) derived as a damped function of U. The final value used in later computations of alveolar ventilation (Chapter 11) is yet another variable, DVENT. This is also measured in l/min, and represents the final common path, i.e. movement of air in and out of the lungs. The use of an artificial ventilation option acts directly upon DVENT, and disconnects the influence of SVENT (as described in Chapter 19), even though SVENT is still computed at each iteration interval.

SUMMARY

The normal stimuli to ventilation, operating directly upon the respiratory centres in the brain stem, are considered in turn. The hypercapnic stimulus is assumed to be exerted principally in the brain, at a receptor site between the arterial blood and the brain tissue, and to be dependent ultimately upon intracellular hydrogen ion activity. This formulation also takes into account a small and rapidly-acting contribution from direct arterial chemoreceptor stimulation from increased PCO_2. In addition to the central CO_2 stimulus, another additive stimulus is considered—that from hypoxaemia. This is arranged to depend on arterial blood O_2 saturation, and to be influenced by the prevailing arterial blood PCO_2, in a complex but empirically defensible formulation. In addition to the hypercapnic and hypoxaemic stimuli, there is deemed to exist a 'central neurogenic' drive to ventilation which depends upon a stimulus from unknown mechanisms and which behaves *as if* it is closely matched to the prevailing whole body metabolic rate. An empirical formulation is derived from known data in the literature to represent this relationship. An index is computed for the adequacy of oxygenation of the brain, which reduces and eventually stops all ventilation when the brain has run out of oxygen. The whole description incorporates a factor dependent on body temperature and also incorporates a small amount of damping to inhibit unrealistic oscillation when operating the model at a long iteration interval.

The stimuli are finally coupled to the actual movement of air through a controllable variable described as 'breathing capacity' which relates the effective coupling of ventilatory stimuli to total ventilation and also supplies an upper limit for maximum breathing capacity. Respiratory rate is made dependent on lung elastance, total ventilation, breathing capacity and oxygen saturation in another empirical formulation.

13
Brain Blood Flow and Gas Tensions at the Central Chemoreceptor Site

The reasons for including a simulation of the cerebral circulation are:

1. To be able to describe changes in hydrogen ion activity at the central chemosensitive site in the medulla, taking into account the bicarbonate and CO_2 content of arterial blood, cerebral blood flow, and cerebral metabolic rate;
2. To maintain an index of cerebral oxygenation so that when the oxygen available to the brain falls below some critical value ventilation becomes depressed and eventually ceases.

Unless these two possibilities are allowed for any model will behave unrealistically in extreme conditions.

When cardiac output and blood pressure are low, cerebral blood flow falls; but at perfusion pressures above about 70 mmHg cerebral blood flow remains constant despite further elevations in arterial pressure or increases in systemic blood flow to other territories. Cerebral gas tensions, especially cerebral PCO_2, are one link in a negative feedback chain. As cerebral blood flow begins to fall, cerebral PCO_2 and H^+ concentration rise. These supply a strong vasodilator stimulus by which reduction of flow is partly corrected. When tensions of oxygen in arterial blood or cerebral tissue fall, cerebral blood flow increases, though to a lesser extent (see reviews by Lassen, 1959 and Patterson, 1965).

Factors determining cerebral blood flow

The systemic arterial blood pressure is not represented in MacPuf since it is irrelevant to the main problems, i.e. gas exchange in the lungs and bulk transport of gases round the circulation. However, there is likely to be some relationship of the following type between cardiac output and cerebral blood flow:

$$Z = SQRT(COADJ) * .5$$
$$IF (Z .GT. 1.) Z = 1.$$

1010 $$CBF = CBF * Z$$

This states that cerebral blood flow remains at its normal value (in practice about 55 ml/100 g brain/min) until effective cardiac output (COADJ) falls below about 2.5 l/min. When cardiac output falls to one l/min, cerebral blood flow would fall to about 27 ml/100 g/min, and thereafter more rapidly still. This formulation takes some account of the body's adaptation to shock, i.e. a life-threatening fall of cardiac output, in which blood tends to be diverted from other territories to maintain the cerebral and coronary circulations.

Although the cerebral circulation is known to be exquisitely sensitive to changes in arterial PCO_2 in acute experiments, it appears from the available literature that in state of chronic CO_2 retention the cerebral blood flow is less increased, and the cerebral vascular resistance behaves as if it depended more on local extravascular hydrogen ion activity. I have allowed for this by providing a damped adjustment of cerebral blood flow in accordance with brain receptor pH (BPH—defined in Chapter 12) as follows:

$$[C55 = .1 / FT]$$
970
$$Y = (7.4 - BPH) * (BC2PR * .0184 . . .)$$
$$IF (Y .GT. 0.) Y = 300. * Y ** 2$$
$$IF (Y .GT. 4.4) Y = 4.4$$
1010
$$BF = DAMP ((Y - .12) * 42.5 * Z, CBF * Z, C55)$$

Note that the final statement of this series includes the factor 'Z' (related to cardiac output—see above) and a function of brain pH. The response to brain hypoxia is mediated by switching on anaerobic metabolism (see below).

This representation is less mathematically sophisticated than that of Grodius, Buell and Bart (1967) who used a quartic equation with constants fitted to data from the literature; but it allows for adjustments of extracellular fluid pH of brain and thus for greater accuracy in states of chronic CO_2 retention. Its accuracy is tolerable in most other situations, and it is economical in execution.

Slow brain bicarbonate adjustments

Normally the brain (or at least cerebrospinal fluid) has a slightly lower bicarbonate concentration than that of blood or other tissues. This changes slowly with chronic change of brain PCO_2, and is one of the adaptive changes at high altitudes, and in chronic ventilatory failure. In the first case CO_2 sensitivity is increased, in the latter decreased. This possibility is allowed for by an adjustment index, BC3AJ, in mmol of HCO_3 per litre, which is added to brain bicarbonate concentration before gas tensions and effluent gas contents are computed. BC3AJ slowly changes, as follows:

$$[C1 = 1000. / VBLVL]$$
$$[C42 = .003 * FT * .0039 * WT ** .425 * HT ** .725]$$
$$BC3AJ = BC3AJ + ((RC3CT - 24.) * .3 - BC3AJ) * C42$$
$$BC3CT = BC3CT . . . + BC3AJ$$

(see main programme between statements 1060 and 1070).

BC3AJ normally has a value of zero, but it slowly rises if arterial bicarbonate (or PCO_2) rises, and falls slowly if it falls. C42 is a parameter related to body surface area and the iteration interval.

Determination of cerebral gas tensions and effluent blood gas contents

Providing that there is a value available for cerebral blood flow, cerebral contents of oxygen and carbon dioxide can be calculated from the cerebral metabolic rate and the difference between gas content between arterial and cerebral venous blood. An average sized brain consumes about 50 cc O_2/min. In MacPuf the constant C41 represents an estimate of the effects of temperature on cerebral O_2 consumption. This is multiplied by the index of brain O_2 adequacy (BO2AD—see Chapter 12). If brain oxygenation is normal $Z = X$, and the final expression '2. * Z * (BO2AD + .1)' corresponds to 50 cc/min O_2 consumption (main programme, statement 1040):

$$[C39 = FT * .127]$$
$$[C41 = FT * (TEMP - 24.5) * 1.82]$$
$$Y = CBF * C39$$
$$X = C41 * (BO2AD + .25)$$
$$Z = X$$
$$IF \ (BO2PR \ .GT. \ 18.) \ GO \ TO \ 1040$$
$$Z = X * (BO2PR * .11 - 1.)$$
$$X = X * (19. - BO2PR)$$
$$IF \ (Z \ .LT. \ 0.) \ Z = 0.$$

1040
$$BO2MT = BO2MT + Y * (RO2CT - BO2CT) - 2. * Z * (BO2AD + .1)$$
$$BC2MT = BC2MT + Y * (RC2CT - BC2CT) + 2.15 * X$$

For CO_2, '2.15 * X' amounts to about 98% as much CO_2 produced as O_2 consumed (the cerebral RQ being about 0.98). However, if brain PO_2 falls below 18 mmHg, cerebral O_2 consumption slows, though CO_2 is still generated. In fact the rate of generation of CO_2 is much increased since by this time cerebral metabolism is anaerobic. The factor 'X' is a guess about the rate of generation of CO_2 (from lactic acid) during cerebral anoxia. *In vitro*, lactic acid production in the brain is switched on at higher PO_2 (20–25 mmHg)—but I have assumed in MacPuf complete cessation of oxygen consumption below a certain threshold, which I have set arbitrarily somewhat lower at 9 mmHg. This description could obviously be improved by exact data if such became available.

The remaining problem is to determine the effluent brain gas contents. For this the partial pressure needs to be determined from the amounts of each gas present in the brain, according to the dissociation curves of brain. Making the assumptions that there is little blood in the brain itself, that over ranges of clinical and physiological interest the dissociation curves are likely to be straight, and that the brain runs out of oxygen in a short time, I have used the following approximations:

$$BO2PR = BO2MT * 1.6$$
$$BC2PR = BC2MT * .078$$

These allow for the much greater solubility of carbon dioxide in brain tissue and give reasonably correct results in dynamic tests involving cardiac arrest, asphyxia and nitrogen breathing. Even so, the amount of O_2 present in the brain (18–20 cc) may be overestimated.

Once the partial pressure has been determined, it is a not unreasonable assumption that the effluent cerebral venous blood contents will have the same partial pressures as those of the tissue itself, and that the contents can be determined by the 'GASES' subroutine (p. 34). However, before this can be done and 'brain pH' determined, brain bicarbonate must be computed. The statements between 1060 and 1090 (Appendix IV) complete the description of the cerebral circulation. The value for 'Y' (brain bicarbonate) is derived as described in the next chapter (p. 93). The pH function (PHFNC) calculates pH in blood from the prevailing bicarbonate concentration and PCO_2, and is also described fully in the next chapter.

SUMMARY

The determination of cerebral blood flow in terms of cardiac output, cerebral tissue pH and arterial oxygen content is described. Outflowing contents of gases in the cerebral venous blood are computed from the brain partial pressures, which are themselves computed from cerebral blood flow, metabolic rate and extraction or addition of gases to the blood.

14
Whole Body Hydrogen Ion Regulation and Bicarbonate Space

The reasons for including a description of whole body hydrogen ion regulation in a comprehensive model should have become clear from the preceding chapters. Oxygen carriage by haemoglobin is importantly dependent on pH, and ventilation is probably dependent on the pH of a central chemosensitive site (Chapter 11).

Considering the reaction:

$$H_2CO_3 \rightleftharpoons H^+ + HCO_3^-$$

The Law of Mass Action states:

$$[H_2CO_3] \propto [H^+] \cdot [HCO_3^-]$$

(Square brackets represent concentrations.) Since the amount of undissociated carbonic acid is proportional to the partial pressure of carbon dioxide, the equation above can be rewritten

$$PCO_2 \propto [H^+] \cdot [HCO_3^-]$$

Rearranging these terms, changing the signs, supplying a constant, and taking logarithms gives one of the familiar forms of the Henderson–Hasselbalch equation:

$$pH = 6.1 + \log_{10}\left[\frac{[HCO_3^-]}{0.03\, PCO_2}\right]$$

(The constant '6.1' is itself slightly influenced by pH, and also by temperature.)

Since this function is used repeatedly in the model, it is specified at the start of the main programme as a generic function (PHFNC) defined as follows:

$$PHFNC(X,Y) = 6.1 + ALOG(X / (.03 * Y)) * .434294482$$

In this function 'X' represents HCO_3^- concentration in mmol/l, 'Y' is PCO_2 in mmHg and '.434294482' is a constant converting natural logarithms into base 10 logarithms (or ALOG10 could be used instead). The value returned by this function is in standard pH units. When the pH, of say, arterial blood is needed, it can be obtained as follows:

$$RPH = PHFNC(RC3CT, RC2PR)$$

The changes in pK with pH and temperature are not allowed for by this function, but in practice the inaccuracy is only slight, and tolerable. Corrections would be advisable if the model was to be used for research study of blood gas transport in hypothermia, for example. In that event instead of a pK of 6.1 being specified, one would need to compute (after Kelman, 1967)

$$pK = 6.086 + 0.042(7.4 - pH) + (38 - temp) \cdot (0.0047 + 0.0014(7.4 - pH)).$$

Arterial H^+ ion activity in nanomolal units is displayed at the end of each run (e.g. Fig. 25, 1, p. 155) and calculated as follows:

$$PPH = 10. * 2. ** ((8. - RPH) * 3.33)$$

(see sub-routine DEADY, Appendix IV, between statements 370 and 390). The values for CO_2 tension have already been computed at each point in the circulation, as described in preceding chapters. It remains only to describe the computation of bicarbonate concentrations for each compartment whose pH has to be determined. It is also necessary to arrange for the transport of bicarbonate from one compartment to another to allow bicarbonate to be added or taken away in the tissues in accordance with variations in lactic acid concentration, and also to allow bicarbonate or strong acid to be added to the venous blood pool to simulate the effect of acid or alkali infusions.

Transport of carbon dioxide in all forms

I have already described in Chapters 5–9 the means by which gas transport through the body pools in a closed circuit is represented. The necessary equations for carbon dioxide transport cover the tranport of carbon dioxide in all forms, i.e. dissolved CO_2, carbonic acid, carbamino and bicarbonate. The carbonic acid is too small an amount to be significant and most CO_2 is present as bicarbonate. In general the transport of CO_2 through a pool might be exemplified by the venous compartment, e.g.

$$VC2MT = VC2MT + FT * CO * (TC2CT - VC2CT)$$
$$VC2CT = VC2MT * 100. / VBLVL$$

These equations are similar to these already described in chapter 8 for the carriage of oxygen. It remains necessary to choose some other index either of hydrogen ion activity, bicarbonate, or dissolved CO_2 itself to enable the appropriate acid-base state of the blood or extra-cellular fluid at each point to be determined. For reasons of convenience, particularly because of the reciprocal relation between the amount of bicarbonate and the amount of lactic acid present in the tissues, and because I wished to make it possible for bicarbonate to be added to simulate bicarbonate therapy, I chose to describe the transport of 'standard bicarbonate', i.e. the mass of bicarbonate which would be present if the PCO_2 was 40 mmHg. Mass transport equations are all given in terms of standard bicarbonate, but at each point in the circulation the effective bicarbonate concentration also depends on the prevailing PCO_2 as discussed below.

Transport of bicarbonate

Starting in the tissues, we can write an equation comparable to that already discussed for CO_2 as follows:

$$TC3MT = TC3MT + FT * CO * (VC3MT / VBLVL - TC3MT / (1.1 * TVOL)) . + . . .$$

(see main programme between statements 670 and 690). To avoid repetitive computations and divisions 1./VBLVL, with adjustment of units, is performed in subroutine CONST so that the first term within the brackets reads VC3MT * C1. The second expression is similarly simplified. The equation above states that the total mass of bicarbonate in the tissues (measured in mmol) after time FT is equal to the previous amount plus the amount of standard bicarbonate delivered by the incoming blood, less the amount going out in the blood leaving the tissues. Since only standard bicarbonate is concerned, the change in PCO_2 during passage through the lungs is immaterial and the concentration in the blood in the pool will be, at least after a short time delay, given by the expression VC3MT / VBLVL where VC3MT is the total mass of bicarbonate in the venous blood pool, and VBLVL is the volume of that pool. A constant can be inserted so that the concentration of standard bicarbonate is given in the usual clinical (and SI units), mmol/l. The concentration of standard bicarbonate in blood leaving the tissues is given by the expression TC3MT * .9 / TVOL, the latter being computed as C13. In this expression TVOL refers to the approximate extracellular fluid volume of the tissues, and the distribution of bicarbonate is taken to be approximately equivalent to the volume of extracellular fluid. The actual volume of distribution is, of course, greater than this since there is some bicarbonate in cells, but allowance needs to be made for the lower concentration inside cells. The distribution volume chosen has been arrived at empirically in such a way that a correct figure is obtained for the whole amount of immediately available bicarbonate in the body. The normal concentration of standard bicarbonate is approximately 24 mmol/l.

In addition, another term is necessary to describe the molar equivalent reduction of tissue bicarbonate mass by the generation of an equivalent amount of lactic acid, and by the regeneration of bicarbonate if the mass of lactic acid in the tissues falls. This factor is taken account of by the subtracted variable 'V * .4' whose derivation will be described in detail in the next chapter.

In the venous blood pool a similar description is used. When the total mass of standard bicarbonate in the pool has been estimated its concentration is then determined by dividing the mass by the volume of the pool. There is again an extra term in the expression (ADDC3) which represents the number of mmol of bicarbonate which may be added to the venous blood pool according to instuctions specified by an operator. The addition of strong acid can likewise be simulated by assigning to ADDC3 an appropriate negative value. To allow the bicarbonate to be added gradually, the amount to be added during the course of a specified run is assumed to be infused into the venous compartment in small equal amounts at each iteration interval (computed in subroutine CONST), so that by the end of NREPT repetitions the whole amount specified has been added. The expression for the new value of bicarbonate in the venous blood pool should thus be clear.

No exchange of standard bicarbonate takes place in the arterial pool or during passage through the lungs. All that happens is that the PCO_2 changes. I have therefore not included an analogous computation for the arterial compartment but simply assumed that the concentration of standard bicarbonate in the arterial pool is the same as that coming in from the venous side, and later leaving the arteries for the tissues, i.e. VC3MT / VBLVL.

Computation of effective total bicarbonate concentration

If whole blood is studied *in vitro* and the PCO_2 is acutely changed, the titration curve of whole blood with a normal haemoglobin content shows that the effective bicarbonate concentration rises or falls in parallel with changing PCO_2 so that a 1.0 mmHg change in PCO_2 brings about a change in bicarbonate concentration of 0.3 mmol/l. Since this constant is related to haemoglobin, we may write for the arterial blood passing to the chemoreceptors and to the brain the following expression:

$$RC3CT = VC3MT / VBLVL + .0203 * HB * (RC2PR - 40.)$$

The parameters .0203 $*$ HB compress to 'C3' (see main programme, Appendix IV between statements 400 and 410). This equation specifies that the arterial bicarbonate concentration (RC3CT) is the same as the concentration of standard bicarbonate in the mixed venous blood, plus an adjustment up or down according to the haemoglobin concentration and the amount by which the arterial PCO_2 exceeds or falls short of 40 mmHg. The effective venous bicarbonate concentration (VC3CT) is likewise given by the standard bicarbonate concentration in the venous pool (VC3MT $*$ C1) plus a comparable expression based on tissue (i.e. mixed venous) CO_2 tension.

In the tissues the situation is slightly different since, for the body as a whole, the bicarbonate titration constant is approximately one third of that in whole blood, i.e. the tissues behave as though they were a fluid with a haemoglobin concentration one third that in blood. I have allowed for this by determining the amount of change in tissue PCO_2 by the local variable FY (see between statements 670 and 690, main programme, Appendix IV). If P_aCO_2 goes up 1 mmHg, RC3CT goes up, in blood *in vitro*, by 0.3 mmol/l; but the effective tissue buffering is less than in blood, so the tissue bicarbonate pool (TC3MT) is reduced by an appropriate function of FY, incorporating haemoglobin concentration (HB) and tissue volume (TVOL):

[C3 = .0203 * HB]
[C13 = .9 / TVOL]
[C64 = .01488 * HB * (TVOL + VBLBL * .001)]
TC3MT = TC3MT − FY * C64 (see between statements 700 and 710)
Y = (TC2PR − 40.) * C3

690   TC3CT = TC3MT * C13 + Y

For the local extracellular tissue of the brain I have assumed a comparable relation with a titration constant of 0.2, midway between blood *in vitro* and the pooled titration constant of the tissues as a whole (see local variable 'Y' between statements 1060 and 1070). This estimate is obviously something of a guess at present but could be readily modified if sufficient data became available. A more detailed description of brain pH computation has already been given in the preceding chapter.

Calculation of pH in each compartment

The means by which PCO_2 at each point can be computed has already been discussed in the preceding chapters. If PCO_2 is known and effective bicarbonate is known, then pH can be readily computed by the pH function described earlier in the chapter. For example, in the arterial blood pool it is only necessary to write:

410   RPH = PHFNC(RC3CT,RC2PR)

RC2PR here is the already computed arterial PCO_2 and RC3CT the effective bicarbonate concentration derived from PCO_2 and bicarbonate according to the formula already mentioned (statement 410 in the main programme).

It will be obvious to the reader that a certain amount of inaccuracy in rapidly changing conditions is bound to result from alternately computing pH from PCO_2 and CO_2 content, and then computing PCO_2 from content and pH. However, artefacts caused by this artificial sequence are minimised and can indeed be eliminated by a small enough iteration interval. In practice, except in rapidly changing conditions, it is usually possible to employ a 10 second interval without obvious oscillation occurring from this cause. Since the CO_2 dissociation curve is somewhat complex mathematically, an exact solution would be difficult, and an iterative solution at each fractional time interval would consume a great deal of time, though it could be done if extremely accurate computation was necessary.

Distinction between effective bicarbonate in tissue and brain blood pools and in blood leaving tissues or brain

In the tissues, although the titration constant is 0.1 for blood leaving the tissues it is necessary to apply the already described titration constant related to haemoglobin (normally 0.3) to compute the effective bicarbonate concentration, and thus the pH of blood leaving the tissues for the venous system. This is done by the sequence of statements (see main programme, Appendix IV, between statements 670 and 700).

	TC2PR = function of TC2MT and TC3MT (see chapter 7)
690	TC3CT = see above
700	TPH = PHFNC(TC3CT,TC2PR)

In the brain the effluent blood likewise must be treated in the same way as blood anywhere else is treated, to bring the effective bicarbonate concentration of blood leaving the brain to the correct value. (See Appendix IV, between statements 1080 and 1090.)

1080	BPH = DAMP(X,BPH,Z)
	Z = PHFNC (VC3MT $*$ C1 + (BC2PR − 40.) $*$ C3, BC2PR)
	CALL GASES(BO2PR,BC2PR,BO2CT,BC2CT,Z,SAT)

SUMMARY

The use of a pH function to determine local pH from bicarbonate and PCO_2 is described. Previous chapters have discussed the transport of CO_2 in all forms and the determination of PCO_2 in each main systemic pool. This chapter considers the distribution and transport of 'standard bicarbonate', i.e. that bicarbonate which would be present at a PCO_2 of 40 mmHg. Before this value can be used to compute effective bicarbonate concentration, it must be corrected for deviations of PCO_2 above and below 40 mmHg, and this is done separately for arterial, venous, tissue, and brain blood.

The transport of standard bicarbonate round the circulation is considered independent of changes in CO_2 tension, and provision is made for the addition or subtraction of bicarbonate as such from the venous pool to simulate the intravenous infusion of acid or alkali.

Care has to be taken that the titration constants appropriate for blood, tissues and brain are applied at each point so that the effective bicarbonate concentration is changed to an appropriate extent by changes in the local PCO_2. For the body as a whole a separate adjustment to the bicarbonate pool is required. The dilemma that arises in computation because pH affects the operative bicarbonate concentration, and bicarbonate concentration in turn affects pH, is resolved by the consideration that, if the time interval is sufficiently short, iteration will lead to a reasonably exact solution providing that the changes in bicarbonate concentration are not occurring too rapidly.

15
Tissue Oxygen Debt and Lactic Acidosis

A full mathematical description of the generation of lactic acid by anaerobic metabolism and muscular exercise in different tissues at different metabolic rates would consume considerable space in a complete programme. However, an accurate description of hypoxic conditions such as cardiac arrest and strenuous muscular exercise is impossible without some description of lactic acid metabolism. In the last chapter I described the way in which chronic sustained metabolic acidaemia as in diabetic ketosis and chronic renal failure can be simulated (by reduction in the pool of standard bicarbonate). Such changes take place with no reference to the tissue stores of oxygen, though they have effects on those stores because the carriage of oxygen by haemoglobin depends on the hydrogen ion activity of the blood. Evidence from the literature (Pernow, Wahren and Zetterquist, 1965; Meyer, Ryu, Toyoda, Shinohara, Wiederholt and Guiraud, 1969) suggests that when the mixed venous body or brain PO_2 falls below 25–27 mmHg there is a rapid switch from aerobic to anaerobic metabolism. This conserves oxygen but leads to the much less efficient production of ATP. Lactic acid accumulates rapidly and, being a relatively strong acid, displaces bicarbonate which is evolved as CO_2. Much literature suggests that the mixed venous oxygen tension only rarely falls below 20 mmHg except during very strenuous exercise or in terminal states.

Lactic acid is normally being produced during metabolism and turned over at a relatively rapid rate. It is, therefore, not enough simply to specify the generation of lactic acid under extreme conditions of tissue hypoxia, but it is also necessary to take account of its normal turnover. Studies of the rate of disappearance of radioactively labelled lactate from the bloodstream (Hubbard, 1973) suggest that there is first a dilution into a fluid pool approximately half the body weight, in litres, followed by a slower metabolism with a half life of ten minutes. The rate of metabolism is much increased with exercise (Hermansen and Stensvold, 1972). It seems reasonable to suppose that the normal relatively small turnover of lactate represents spillage from the normal tissue pool of lactate. This is in dynamic equilibrium with the pyruvate pool which lies on the pathway between glucose and its complete metabolism to carbon dioxide and water. At rest the liver removes most of the lactate, and to a reasonable approximation the rate of lactate removal corresponds to first order kinetics, i.e. the rate of removal by the liver and probably also by other adequately oxygenated tissues such as the kidneys is directly proportional to the plasma concentration (Eldridge, 1975).

From the observations already summarised, it is apparent that under conditions of mild hypoxia or increased lactic acid production for any reason an equilibrium would normally be established comparable to that in chronic renal failure, in which the concentration of urea in the blood is related to the amount of protein ingested, in steady state conditions. Other factors can be taken into account, e.g. the spillover of lactate into the urine at very high plasma concentrations, but such effects are probably of little quantitative significance and much more important are the constraints upon lactic acid catabolism imposed by high hydrogen ion activity (i.e. low pH).

The description which follows and its quantitative translation into a workable Fortran notation owes a great deal to the help of Dr. Gerald Partridge. I am most grateful to him for permission to use his formulation of lactic acid metabolism in the complete programme. As a result of his work I have been able to substitute for my previous 'black box' description of lactic acid metabolism a much more accurate total picture which gives results which correspond well with clinical observation and exercise testing.

Lactic acid synthesis

The concentration of lactate in its 35 l pool is usually about 1.0 mmol/l or slightly less. It can be calculated that the normal rate of production in a well oxygenated subject at rest is approximately 1.0 mmol/min, corresponding reasonably closely to a half-life of 10 min. The major contributors to lactic acid production are skin, red blood cells, brain and muscle (Kreisberg, 1972).

The basal production or spillage of lactate is augmented by an additional factor depending on the fourth power of the difference between an average tissue oxygen PO_2 threshold (25–30 mmHg) and the actual mean tissue oxygen pressure. The reason for the choice of a fourth power term for this function rather than a linear or quadratic function was that when the total description of lactic acid metabolism was inserted into the whole model, the best simulations of strenuous muscular exercise were obtained on the assumption that the switchover from aerobic to anaerobic metabolism took place rather suddenly below a critical partial pressure of oxygen. To make this correspond to available data in the literature, it was necessary to arrange that there was virtually a trigger effect.

The whole description in Fortran can be reduced to the following terms (see main programme—Appendix IV—between statements 530 and 640). Note that some parameters, as before, are pre-calculated as members of array C in subroutine CONST:

$$[C29 = FT * .0039 * WT ** .425 * HT ** .725]$$
$$[C40 = C29 * (PD - 25.) * 1.3]$$
$$[C42 = .003 * C29]$$
$$W = C29 \text{ (in effect)}$$
$$V = FITNS - TO2PR$$

```
        IF (V .LE. 0.) GOTO 570
560     W = W + C42 * (V. + 1.) ** 4
570     ......
        IF (W .GT. C40) W = C40
        TLAMT = TLAMT + W
```

W is the basal spillage rate of lactate, related to body surface area. TO2PR is mean tissue PO_2, which is compared with parameter 'FITNS'. This represents the average tissue PO_2 at which anaerobic metabolism begins. It has a normal value of 33 (mmHg). Raising it simulates unfitness, lowering it simulates increased fitness, relative to average normal. If V is greater than zero, a fourth power function of V is added to W. W is then limited to a maximum rate (C40) dependent on body size (C29) and on specified metabolic rate (PD). Finally, W is added to the previous quantity of lactate (TLAMT). Production is increased when PCO_2 is low by using the variable CBF, which changes in an appropriate way (statements 530–540).

This formulation ignores the fact that lactic acid production is small in anoxic resting muscle. Most of the metabolic acidosis of cardiac arrest derives from the liver. In strenuous exercise with tissue anoxia, however, the maximum rate of production is much higher because the active muscles dominate. Prof. R. H. T. Edwards (personal communication) calculates that maximum lactic acid generation at maximal exercise probably exceeds 1000 mmol/min.

It must be admitted that the formulation of lactic acid production as a basal value augmented linearly by increasing metabolic rate during muscular exercise, and increasing very rapidly as by a trigger effect when PO_2 of tissues falls below 25–30 mmHg is a guess or, more correctly, a hypothesis. It is, however, not only compatible with presently available data from the literature but also gives quantitatively reasonable and consistent results when placed in the context of a whole descriptive programme.

Lactic acid catabolism

At rest the liver is quantitatively the most important organ in catabolism of lactic acid but the kidneys also play some part. Apart from the ability of the kidneys to excrete lactate in the urine at high plasma concentrations (above a tubular reabsorptive maximum), we can assume that at the normal plasma concentration of 1.0 mmol/l the rate of lactate removal by liver and kidney corresponds to the production rate, i.e. about 1.0 mmol/min. According to data previously summarised the rate of catabolism of lactic acid by liver is linearly related to its concentration in body fluids and hence to its concentration in the blood perfusing the liver. The total description is as shown in statements 530 to 640 (main programme, Appendix IV).

```
        [C24 = CONOM * .3]
530     Y = RLACT * C29
        X = TPH * 10. − 69.
550     Z = Y * (X * .8612 + .0232 * 2. ** ((8. − TPH) * 3.33) +
        COADJ * .01)
```

610
$$IF\ (TO2PR\ .LT.\ FITNS)\ Z = Z * TO2PR * .04$$
$$X = C24 - COADJ$$
$$IF\ (X\ .GT.\ 0.)\ Z = Z * COADJ / C24$$
......
$$TLAMT = TLAMT + W - Z$$

RLACT represents tissue (or blood) lactate concentration in mmol/l, and as before C29 makes catabolism proportional to body size. 'Y' is a local variable and 'Z' the rate of lactate catabolism in mmol per iteration interval. The expression in brackets in statement 550 represents liver catabolism (.8612), reduced by low tissue pH (TPH); plus a renal metabolic contribution (.0232), *increased* by low tissue pH; plus a small contribution related to cardiac output and representing the contribution of non-hypoxic muscles and other tissues. Normally, the whole expression in brackets has a value of approximately unity. Liver catabolism is reduced by hyperventilation and in those conditions, in general, in which cerebral blood flow tends to be low (see extra statements between 530 and 550).

Two constraints are applied to the removal of lactate by the liver and other tissues in proportion to its plasma concentration. The work of Cohen, Lloyd, Iles, Simpson, Strumm and Layton (1973) and Cohen and Yudkin (1975) suggests that at pH below about 7.0 in liver extracellular fluid (H^+ activity greater than 100 nmol) the rate of catabolism of lactate falls off rapidly, even if the concentration of lactate is high. At pH about 6.9 in the liver catabolism ceases altogether. Cohen and his associates suggest that at this point lactate catabolism gives way to lactate production—but it seems perhaps simpler to assume that lactate production continues unimpaired whereas lactate catabolism ceases. In the kidney the rate of catabolism is increased in linear proportion to the rise in H^+ ion activity. (The complex $(8 - TPH)$ term converts pH to nanomolal units). The two effects are compounded in proportion to the approximate contributions of liver, kidneys and other tissues by the formulation in statement 550.

As previously mentioned there is increased turnover of lactate with exercise, normally with little rise in plasma lactate concentration. This is represented by the third term, proportional to the increased oxygen consumption of exercise and representing the increased catabolising power of muscles through the increase in capillary endothelium surface made available by the increased circulation. The value for this term is at present a very approximate estimate. At about the same level of exercise that lactate concentration increases sharply, the rate of lactate removal begins to decrease. On the assumption that this is due to tissue hypoxia, 'Z' (the catabolic rate) is multiplied by a factor which decreases linearly from 1.0 to zero as tissue oxygen partial pressure falls from 25 mmHg to zero (Tashkin, Goldstein and Simmons, 1972). These authors found a decrease in lactate uptake in the liver when hepatic venous PO_2 was less than 24 mmHg. The effective cardiac output (COADJ) is also taken into account to make lactate catabolism fall off rapidly as cardiac output becomes less than half the nominal resting value (CONOM). The steps in the main programme (Appendix IV, between statements 530 and 640) should be self-explanatory.

Lactate excretion

Although the kidney catabolises lactate to some degree, as already mentioned, it has a tubular maximum corresponding to 10 mmol/l. At plasma concentrations above this level, lactic acid is excreted in the urine at an increasingly rapid rate. Quantitative data are difficult to come by but the observations of Cohen and Yudkin (1975) suggest that about one quarter of the lactate in glomerular filtrate is excreted at a resting glomerular filtration rate of 120 ml/min at lactate concentrations greater than 10 mmol/l. The contribution of urinary excretion seems too small to be worth inclusion, since kidney metabolism is normally more important, especially in acidaemia.

Summated effect of lactic acid production, metabolism and excretion

The amount of lactic acid remaining in the metabolic pool of the body (35 l) at the end of a specified iteration interval FT is given by the expression

630         $V = W - Z$
$$TLAMT = TLAMT + V$$

where the local variables have already been defined (see above).

One important possibility arising from the way the description is formulated is that the local variable V represents the value of the change up or down which may have occurred in the total pool of lactic acid. In the last chapter I have described the way in which bicarbonate is handled in the form of standard bicarbonate. Since lactic acid is a much stronger acid than carbonic acid, it could be assumed in the absence of other buffer systems that for each mmol of lactic acid generated one mmol of standard bicarbonate is removed from the pool. Since the total amounts of carbon dioxide are unchanged, this means that much more CO_2 is present as carbonic acid and as dissolved CO_2 (with a consequent elevation in partial pressure) and less is present as bicarbonate.

In the complete programme description, I have assumed that each mmol of lactic acid displaces 0.4 mmol of bicarbonate. This makes a reasonably realistic assessment of the influence of other buffers (see Chapter 14). Accordingly, if V increases (i.e. if the lactic acid pool is increased) the tissue pool of standard bicarbonate (TC3MT) is decreased, as follows:

$$TC3MT = TC3MT + FTCO \ldots - V * .4$$

(see main programme, Appendix IV, between statements 670 and 690). The speed of this process will obviously depend on the rate of change of the lactic acid pool. Naturally, if lactate concentration falls (by liver catabolism) the bicarbonate pool is approximately increased.

Plasma lactic acid concentration

The lactic acid concentration of the pool can be simply calculated by dividing the total amount of lactate by the volume of the pool (approximately 35 l). However, it is not possible to measure whole body tissue lactate concentration, but rather that in mixed venous or arterial blood. The use of a DAMP function (Chapter 5) related to cardiac output allows this:

$$[C15 = 2. / WT]$$
$$[C55 = .1 / FT]$$
$$RLACT = DAMP(TLAMT * C15,RLACT,COADJ * C55)$$

(see main programme between statements 630 and 640). WT is body weight, giving a distribution volume of 35 l in a normal subject. If cardiac output is zero, RLACT cannot change; and it will reflect the prevailing mass of lactic acid in the body only if the blood is circulating, and even then only after some time delay.

Oxygen sparing effect of lactic acid production

As a first approximation, I have assumed that the evolution of carbon dioxide continues unabated during lactic acid production. However, the switch to anaerobic metabolism has the effect of, and indeed probably has the main function of saving oxygen consumption. Therefore, during the computation of changes in lactic acid production and destruction a term XLACT is computed and stored as a COMMON variable whose value from one iteration interval to the next corresponds to the extent to which oxygen is spared. Empirically I found that some damping was necessary in this function, otherwise the production of lactic acid oscillated grossly from one computation to the next, unless the iteration interval was made inconveniently small. I have therefore used a DAMP function of the type described in chapter 5 to prevent unrealistic oscillations developing.

```
         [C29 = FT * .0039 * WT ** .425 * HT ** .725]
         [C32 = C29 + .0000001]
         [C53 = .8 / FT]
570      X = 2.04 * (W − C32)
         IF (X .GT. U) X = U
590      XLACT = DAMP(X,XLACT,C53)
         .
         .
500      TO2MT = TO2MT + ... − U + XLACT
```

The rate of production of lactate (W) is compared with the basal rate (C29) and the difference multiplied by 2.04, which is 22.4 (mmol to cc conversion) divided by 11 (less efficient ATP generation in anaerobic metabolism). X is not allowed to exceed actual (aerobic) oxygen consumption (U) and finally a DAMP function is used as described. In the tissue oxygen pool, where total O_2 consumption (U) is subtracted, XLACT is added. If anaerobic metabolism alone is going on then U and XLACT have the same value.

During operation of the whole model in conditions of high oxygen consumption or poor oxygen delivery, the effect of this constraint is that lactic acid metabolism is switched on rapidly below a tissue oxygen tension of about 25 mmHg and the oxygen sparing is such that the mixed venous PO_2 almost never falls below 20 mmHg. This appears to conform closely with numerous observations in the literature of strenuous exercise.

Examples will be given in chapter 23 of total model simulations using this description but so far it appears that the whole body descriptions of lactic acid production in conditions such as cardiac arrest and muscular exercise are accurately simulated. (Muscular exercise is simulated by increasing metabolic rate (PD) and, when exercise is strenuous, raising respiratory quotient (TRQ) to unity. PD as a percentage corresponds roughly to kpm/min work load.)

It is easy to appreciate the necessity for giving sodium bicarbonate after cardiac arrest. Beyond a certain level of tissue acidosis it has a life-saving effect by preventing the vicious circle which occurs when catabolism of lactate becomes seriously impaired.

SUMMARY

The bulk production, metabolism and excretion of lactic acid is described and is a function principally of tissue oxygenation, but also of tissue extracellular pH and blood flow. The distribution of lactate throughout a body pool is described and the changes in the total mass of lactic acid are assumed to displace an appropriate amount of bicarbonate and to spare a molar equivalent amount of oxygen, leaving CO_2 production unabated.

The total programme description in the whole model allows accurate representation both of cardiac arrest and different levels of strenuous muscular exercise, as well as allowing reasonable predictions of the generation of lactic acid in hypoxaemic states.

16
Regulation of Cardiac Output and Representation of Intra-cardiac Shunts

The final description of cardiac output in MacPuf is a compromise between a number of previous representations, each of which had both advantages and drawbacks. In earlier versions of the model cardiac output was specified simply as a number of l/min and initialised at 5.0 for an average subject. The operator could alter this value at will, but it did not undergo spontaneous changes. As the rest of the descriptions in the whole model became more realistic and results began to resemble real-life situations more closely, the constancy of cardiac output, which was an advantage for a student using MacPuf to study basic respiratory and circulatory physiology, became an annoyance. While changes in ventilation were dynamically determined by known stimuli, without an operator having to specify them for each run, the behaviour of the heart began to seem absurd.

In some later versions I added a measure of dynamic behaviour to cardiac output, in such a way that output increased appropriately in conditions of moderate hypoxia. At this time I retained the option of removing the hypoxic influence, so that cardiac output could be fixed at will. This might be said to bring cardiac output in line with ventilation. I have already described the way in which known ventilatory stimuli are summed to produce a resultant total ventilation (Chapter 12). In Chapter 19 I shall describe an artificial ventilation option which allows an operator to control ventilation at will, at any rate or depth. For physiological reasons it might seem desirable to retain the possibility of similarly fixing cardiac output; but in my observation of extensive use of MacPuf by students and staff over some three years, at University College and St. Bartholomew's Hospital, and at McMaster University, no-one to my knowledge has ever used or wanted to use the option formerly provided of disconnecting natural cardiac output variation and fixing cardiac output for the purposes of doing simulated physiological experiments.

The reason is not far to seek. The artificial control of ventilation is an everyday event in the operating theatre and in the intensive care unit. Its effects are well known. On the other hand, there is no simple way for a machine to take over the circulation of blood and allow comparable changes to be made in cardiac output. One might generalise and say that most people are not interested in artificial experiments, but only in examining or simulating those which could be performed in man, with presently available techniques. The natural experiments of disease do not involve fixed changes of output. The cardiac output of a damaged heart is never exactly fixed at 3 l/min, for example; a damaged heart still has a Starling function curve relating output to filling pressure. It still has a sympathetic and vagal innervation.

When considering 'venous admixture' (Chapter 9) I pointed out that the term is an abstract concept, useful in quantifying certain aspects of the mismatching of perfusion to ventilation. Nevertheless, in some congenital heart diseases there is a true shunt of blood from right to left side of the heart, completely bypassing the lungs. A fixed right-to-left shunt is easily added to the 'venous admixture' expression, and it is not much more difficult to represent the more common situation of a left-to-right shunt, which I shall also describe in this chapter.

Normal variations in cardiac output related to metabolic rate and oxygen consumption

The changes in cardiac output of normal subjects at different levels of exercise are well known. To allow changes to apply not only to standard normal subjects, but also those of different age, sex and size (see Chapter 21) I have made the dynamic changes in cardiac output with exercise relate not directly to percentage changes in metabolic rate, but rather to the amount by which oxygen consumption during exercise exceeds resting oxygen consumption. Once an operator has specified a particular metabolic rate and body temperature, the total oxygen consumption, in cc/min (STPD) is computed by the following expression

$$C(7) = CONSO * PD * .00081 * (TEMP - 26.) ** 1.05$$

in which C(7) represents that resting oxygen consumption for the subject at a body temperature of 37 °C (see Appendix IV, subroutine CONST). Temperature influences will be discussed in Chapter 18. PD specifies a percentage change in metabolic rate, from a normal value of 100 (%) and TEMP is the body temperature in degrees centigrade. Another changeable parameter (C9) represents the difference between exercise and resting oxygen consumption multiplied by a conversion factor:

$$C(9) = (C(7) - CONSO) * .01$$

Subsequently (at statement 240 in the main programme, Appendix IV) the effective cardiac output is computed as follows:

[C8 = (30. − PEEP * 5. / ELAST) * .0016 * CONOM *
(TEMP − 12.2)]
[C16 = CO * .01]
240   COADJ = Function of C8, C9 and C16

The need for inclusion of positive end-expiratory pressure (PEEP) in relation to lung elastance (ELAST) is justified in Chapter 19. 'CONOM' is the characteristic average value of cardiac output, in l/min, at rest. 'TEMP' is body temperature. COADJ returns a value of l/min, which may be above or below resting value. For example, the effect of the relationships itemised above is that if oxygen consumption is increased by, say, one l/min over the resting value, the cardiac output rises by 6 l/min. Over a wide range of exercise in normal subjects such values match recorded observations, and also correspond with average expectations in fever and hypothermia.

The changes in cardiac output with hypoxia have been less well studied, but I have taken the combined clinical experience of my colleagues at McMaster to derive the following representation in terms of arterial oxygen content and saturation:

$$[C61 = .22 / FT]$$
$$Y = RO2CT * .056$$

220   IF (Y .LT. .35) Y = .35

240   COADJ = DAMP((C8 / Y + C9 / (Y ** 2) * C16,COADJ,C61)

The effect of these statements (see Appendix IV, main programme, between statements 210 and 240) is that when arterial oxygen content (RO2CT) falls, cardiac output is increased, up to a certain realistic limit. At high oxygen contents, it is appropriately decreased. The other terms C8, C9 and C16 have been described above. A damp function prevents unrealistically rapid swings of cardiac output.

Manual control over cardiac output is provided by another parameter (CO), incorporated in C16, which can be taken to represent 'percentage normal cardiac function'. This factor is initialised as 100(%). If it is made zero, cardiac output is likewise zero. If it is made 200, cardiac output under any given conditions is twice the normal average value for those conditions. If it is made zero, the damp function is bypassed and COADJ made equal to E(.00000001), effectively to stop movement of blood but at the same time to prevent arithmetical errors in the computer. Finally, COADJ is limited by 'COMAX' (the maximum cardiac output) which is initialised at 35 l/min—perhaps somewhat optimistically! If nominal cardiac output is lower than normal (e.g. if a small subject is specified by options described in Chapter 21) COMAX is appropriately reduced.

The statements are self-explanatory and appear in the main programme (Appendix IV) between statements 240 and 270. Then a local variable, FTCO, is computed, to comprise cardiac output in unit time, and adjustment of units to speed later computations. An index of fitness (FITNS—see Chapter 15) determines some degree of inadequate tissue perfusion. Effective tissue perfusion is given by FTCOC (see main programme after statement 280).

Representation of right-to-left intracardiac or intrapulmonary shunts

The representation of effective 'venous admixture' was discussed in Chapter 9, p. 51. A fixed right-to-left shunt, FADM, is initialised as zero for normal subjects, but can be changed to insert an extra term at the end of the equations representing effective right-to-left shunt. This is subject to no limitation other than that the total amount of shunt cannot exceed 100%! I will not reiterate the statements, which appear in Appendix IV in the main programme, between statements 280 and 370.

Representation of left-to-right shunts

The presence of a shunt from left to right has no effect on arterial gas tensions providing that:

1. The distribution of ventilation/perfusion ratios throughout the lungs remains the same;
2. The cardiac output measured in the aorta remains the same;
3. The gas contents of blood coming back from the tissues remain the same.

Changes due to a large left-to-right shunt may be visible in an X-ray, e.g. as engorged lung fields, but can be reflected in MacPuf only in the composition of mixed venous blood. The whole representation requires the specification of a single parameter, 'SHUNT', which has a normal value of zero, i.e. 0:1. If SHUNT is made 2, for example, a 2:1 left-to-right shunt is specified. This conforms with the normal way such shunts are described clinically and quantified. For convenience this parameter is made to specify another one (C14) as follows:

$$C(14) = SHUNT + 1.$$

This computation is performed in subroutine CONST. The equations shown below only apply to oxygen, but exactly similar equations apply to carbon dioxide, and can be seen by referring to the complete programme (between statements 700 and 710).

$$[C2 = 100. / VBLVL]$$
$$VO2MT = VO2MT + FTCOC * TO2CT - FTCO *$$
$$(VO2CT * C(14 - RO2CT * SHUNT) + X * EO2CT$$
$$VO2CT = VO2MT * C2$$

The first statement increments the total amount of oxygen in the venous pool by the blood coming in from the tissues, diminishes it by the blood flowing through the lungs (incorporating the shunted blood), and increments it again by the arterial blood flowing through the shunt. The final multiplier 'X' takes account of wasted tissue perfusion, related to fitness (see above). The second line computes the effective mixed venous oxygen content. A modification is also needed to describe alveolar gas exchange, to allow for the increased pulmonary blood flow:

740   PC = FTCO * C14 * PC

The rest of this statement was originally described in Chapter 10, and its context can be seen by inspecting statement 740 in the main programme. PC is a local variable describing the proportion of total blood flow which passes through an idealised alveolar mixing compartment.

During operation of the model this left-to-right shunt will give correct results only for the mixed venous *contents* of oxygen and carbon dioxide. For reasons which were spelt out in detail in Chapter 8, the programme economises on execution time by taking the mixed venous tensions to be the same as tissue tensions. This approximation is usually correct, except in the case of a left-to-right shunt. To remind the operator about this limitation when the full INSPECT table (see Chapter 25, p. 157) is printed, the values for partial pressures of mixed venous blood appear in brackets.

Because a left-to-right shunt increases the amount of blood available for gas exchange, the iteration interval has to be reduced from 10 s to 2 s for shunts exceeding 0.5:1. This is done automatically by subroutine DEADY when a change in SHUNT is requested.

SUMMARY

Reasons are given for representing cardiac output as a dynamically variable function rather than giving it a value fixed during operation of the model. A function is described which takes into account the increment of cardiac output with increased tissue oxygen consumption and with diminished oxygen content or increased PCO_2 of arterial blood (up to a certain limit). This function is damped to allow stable operation, is subject to overriding manual controls by an operator, and is also subject to a preset limit of maximum cardiac output.

The representation of a fixed right-to-left anatomical shunt is described. Left-to-right shunts involve modifications to the computation of mixed venous gas contents and of pulmonary blood flow.

17
Representation of Changes in Atmospheric Pressure; Body Nitrogen Stores

The amounts of each gas present inside the body are considered exclusively in terms of the volumes they occupy at STPD (see Chapter 4). The effective barometric pressure (C11) remains constant during any particular run, i.e. during a set of iterative computations; but it is changeable between each individual run by techniques to be discussed in Chapter 24. Before the iterative computations begin in the main programme, the value of the conversion factor (C12—see p. 18) is computed in subroutine CONST. This allows gas volumes measured at BTPS to be converted to equivalent volumes at STPD. Since C12 is used at every point in the programme at which conversion is necessary, and since its value incorporates barometric pressure changes, few other adjustments are necessary.

Inside the body I have made the assumption that the partial pressures of nitrogen cannot (except very briefly) exceed atmospheric pressure. In blood or tissues, if this gas is present in an amount greater than the compartment can hold at the prevailing atmospheric pressure, the excess is removed and stored in the form of bubbles. There has been a recent interesting suggestion that supersaturation of blood and tissues with gases may last longer after decompression than is generally believed, and that ionising radiation may be needed to initiate bubble formation. Though this may be true for small decompressions, the consistent formation of bubbles (and symptoms) with sudden large decompressions (exceeding $1\frac{1}{2}$ atmospheres) is well known.

The descriptions of alveolar gas exchanges, discussed at length in Chapter 10, take into account the effective number of molecules of a gas inhaled or exhaled. Ventilation volumes, measured at BTPS, are converted to STPD by the correction factor before being used. An effective alveolar ventilation of 4.2 l/min, at normal barometric pressure, for example, would bring into the alveolar compartment 21/100 of 4.2 l of oxygen, BTPS, equivalent to about 17/100 of 4.2 l STPD (i.e. about 700 cc of oxygen). If the barometric pressure was doubled, to 1520 mmHg, the amount of oxygen brought in for the same alveolar ventilation would be 35/100 of 4.2 l STPD of oxygen (i.e. about 1400 cc). Similarly, the amounts of each gas present in the lungs at resting volume would automatically be corrected to standard units by the set of equations in the main programme (between statements 720 and 900).

Though I cannot pretend to have tested MacPuf through more than a small range of the possible situations of altered barometric pressure, some of the dynamic tests carried out will be discussed in Chapter 23. So far these have not disclosed any serious errors of description, and rapid changes of alveolar gas tensions after decompression are accurately simulated.

EFFECTS OF ACUTE ATMOSPHERIC DECOMPRESSION; REPRESENTATION OF TISSUE NITROGEN STORES

The need for representing the volume of nitrogen in the lungs at different stages of alveolar ventilation and gas exchange was made clear in Chapter 10. Only one variable, specifying the alveolar volume of nitrogen, was mentioned (AN2MT). This referred to the STPD volume in cc. The addition of a few further lines of Fortran and the addition of a few more variables to the COMMON store of the programme allows MacPuf to give a tolerably accurate account of the carriage of nitrogen to and from the tissues, and its storage there. The description is not needed for operation of the rest of the model, and could be left out of the main programme with no effects other than failure to simulate the ill effects of acute decompression. I have thought it worth while to include this small section, however, because of the intrinsic physiological interest of atmospheric pressure changes, their importance in clinical medicine and research and their potential application to practical problems.

I have assumed that nitrogen in the blood has a solubility corresponding to 0.71 cc/100 ml blood at its normal partial pressure (570 mmHg) (Farhi, 1964) and that it is possible to describe its carriage through the arterial compartment as follows (between statements 380 and 410):

$$RN2MT = RN2MT + FTCO * (\text{incoming aortic } N_2$$
$$\text{content} - EN2CT)$$
$$EN2CT = DAMP(RN2MT * .1, EN2CT, W)$$

The effluent arterial nitrogen content (EN2CT) in cc/100 ml blood (STPD) is given by a damped expression exactly comparable to that described for oxygen and carbon dioxide in Chapter 5, p. 27. The mixing of ideal and shunted blood is performed as described in Chapter 9. EN2CT in the DAMP function on the right side is the previously computed value for this variable. 'W' is the damping constant (see Chapter 5). Note (main programme, after statement 380) that alveolar partial pressure of nitrogen is obtained by difference (C11 − AO2PR − AC2PR) and that the partial pressure of nitrogen in the idealised alveolar compartment is, by definition, the same as that in the idealised pulmonary capillary blood issuing from that compartment. The full statement in the main programme (Appendix IV) is as follows:

$$RN2MT = RN2MT + FTCO * ((X * TN2PR + PC *$$
$$(C11 - AO2PR - AC2PR)) * .00127 - EN2CT)$$

'X' here represents the shunted blood, coming from the tissues with partial pressure TN2PR; 'PC' is the non-shunted blood perfusing the ideal alveolar compartment with PN_2 of $(C11 - AO2PR - AC2PR)$. The multiplier '.00127' converts mmHg to content of N_2 in cc/100 ml.

The tissues are assumed to contain two normal compartments: a small one in intimate contact with the bloodstream containing TN2MT cc of nitrogen (about 75 cc), and a much larger one very slowly equilibrating with the first and containing SN2MT cc of nitrogen (about 950 cc). These values correspond with data on whole body nitrogen content (Haldane and Priestley, 1935; Farhi, 1964). These compartments hold nitrogen at partial pressures of TN2PR and SN2PR mmHg, respectively. In addition, a third (abnormal) compartment, containing UN2MT (also representing cc of nitrogen) represents the volume of free nitrogen held either in supersaturation or as bubbles in the bloodstream, brain and other tissues. This volume is monitored, as described in Chapter 26, and used to determine symptoms and lethal conditions.

The interaction is described in the following set of equations, which appear in the main programme between statements 640 and 680:

$$[C23 = 20. * SIMLT / BARPR]$$
$$[C26 = 7. / TVOL]$$
$$[C27 = FT * .1]$$
$$[C28 = 30000. / (VBLVL + 1000.)]$$
$$[C60 = FT * .008]$$

640	$X = (TN2PR - SN2PR) * C60$
	$TN2MT = TN2MT + FTCOC * (EN2CT - TN2PR * .00127) - X$
	$SN2MT = SN2MT + X$
	$Y = (SN2MT * C26 - C11) * C27$
	IF (Y .GT. 0.) GO TO 660
650	$Y = Y * .3$
	IF (UN2MT .LE. 0.) GO TO 670
660	$SN2MT = SN2MT - Y$
	$BUBBL = UN2MT ** 1.2 * C23$
	$UN2MT = UN2MT + Y$
670	$SN2PR = SN2MT * C26$
	$TN2PR = TN2MT * C28$

The first local variable (X) describes the amount of nitrogen transferred between the fast compartment (T) and the slow (S) in time FT. The rate is proportional to the previous differences in partial pressure. The second statement is analogous to those considered for O_2 and CO_2 in the tissues (p. 38), except that the effluent nitrogen content is computed directly from tissue N_2 pressure (TN2PR) and a solubility factor. The second local variable (Y) is normally negative—i.e. the sum of the partial pressures of nitrogen in the tissues plus local PO_2 and PCO_2 is less than atmospheric pressure. If Y becomes positive it is added to the bubble store (UN2MT) and taken away from the slow tissue store (SN2MT). If Y becomes negative at a time when bubbles are still present, they redissolve (though at $\frac{1}{3}$ the speed—see statement 650) and get carried away, first into the fast compartment (TN2MT) and eventually into the bloodstream. The partial pressures in each compartment are finally computed assuming that the slow space is related to tissue volume (TVOL) in litres, and the fast space to the venous blood volume (VBLVL), in cc.

The constants have been empirically adjusted so as to bring into line real data from compressed air work (the Dungeness B Harbour experience, kindly provided by Professor D. N. Walder). However, an intermediate compartment is also needed to allow assessment of the risks involved with short dives at 5–10 atmospheres pressure.

I am actively engaged at present on the further improvement and refining of an index for decompression symptoms (BUBBL) which will, I hope, eventually allow MacPuf to provide a flexible, quick and accurate way of analysing virtually any dive and decompression schedule, using any mixture of gases. For the time being, however, the performance of MacPuf should be regarded as a rough guide only.

The reader of the preceding chapters will appreciate that the description of nitrogen transport is greatly simplified, when it is compared with the expressions derived in previous chapters for the carriage and exchange of oxygen and carbon dioxide. This is not only the consequence of nitrogen being an inert gas, with linear dissociation curves in all compartments, but is also a deliberate oversimplification to allow MacPuf to describe economically the physiological events associated with diving and resurfacing.

SUMMARY

The BTPS / STPD conversions already specified throughout the gas-exchanging compartments of the model means that it can without further special instructions describe accurately the exchanges and transport of oxygen and carbon dioxide. A simple three-compartment model to describe nitrogen storage in the tissues (comprising a fast and slow compartment, with a third potential compartment to describe bubble formation) is added to enable the model economically but realistically to simulate the physiological changes associated with compression and acute decompression.

18
Representation of Changes in Body Temperature

The main effects of changed temperature on respiratory components of the body are:

1. Alteration of water vapour pressure;
2. Changes in the solubility of gases in body fluids;
3. Changes in the oxygen and carbon dioxide dissociation curves of blood;
4. Alteration in metabolic rate;
5. Change in cardiac output;
6. Change in total ventilation in response to known stimuli;
7. Changes in acid-base equilibrium and hydrogen ion activity.

The effects of (1) above are small, but easily allowed for when computing effective barometric pressure C11 by subtracting water vapour pressure (see subroutine CONST):

$$C(11) = BARPR - 1.2703 * TEMP$$

Subsequently, the effective barometric pressure is used to compute C12, the universal correction factor for BTPS / STPD conversion (Chapter 4).

The effects of (2) and (3) are likewise fairly small, and were empirically incorporated by Kelman in his equations describing the O_2 and CO_2 dissociation curves of blood. These were fully described in Chapter 6, and the temperature corrections will be clear on inspecting subroutine GASES in Appendix IV; temperature (TEMP in the main programme) appears in this subroutine also as the COMMON variable TEMP.

The effects of altered body temperature on metabolic rate are well known. A change of body temperature of 1 °C within the clinically encountered range brings about an approximate 12% change in oxygen consumption. This is easily represented by the following expression relating actual to nominal oxygen consumption:

$$CONSO * .081 * (TEMP - 26.) ** 1.05$$

At a body temperature of 37 °C, the multiplier '.081 * (TEMP − 26.) ** 1.05' becomes unity and the effective tissue oxygen consumption becomes equal to CONSO (the nominal resting oxygen consumption of the body). Parameter C7 (see subroutine CONST) also incorporates the manual control of metabolic rate (PD).

The description of cardiac output has been considered already in Chapter 16; readers will recall that the cardiac output is incremented or decremented from its nominal value by the difference between actual and nominal oxygen consumption, by means of a function of factor C9 which was the difference between C7 and CONSO (see subroutine CONST). This gives a good match between the behaviour of MacPuf during simulated exercise and observed data from normal exercising subjects. It seems reasonable to imagine, as a first approximation at least, that a similar relationship might hold for reduced oxygen consumption consequent upon reduction of body temperature. Lacking exact data, but encouraged by the body's ability in a large variety of conditions to match cardiac output with body needs, I have simply used this same statement for O_2 consumption (C7—Appendix IV—subroutine CONST). If later data indicate that cardiac output is relatively more or less affected by changes in body temperature the statement can be appropriately modified.

A more difficult question is that of ventilatory control. By the nature of the ventilatory stimuli already discussed fully in Chapter 12 it is obvious that changes in metabolic rate will affect total ventilation by two mechanisms:

1. The production of carbon dioxide will alter and thus the potential stimulus from it will alter;
2. The 'central neurogenic drive' to ventilation, which is given the property of behaving *as if* it was matched with whole body oxygen consumption, will also proportionately change.

The effects of these two factors should be to change ventilation in proportion to metabolism without the need to specify any direct depressant of stimulant effects of changed body temperature. However, it is a common clinical observation that arterial PCO_2 tends to be lowered slightly in fever, and raised in hypothermia. Therefore I have incorporated a small additional term in the description of summated stimuli to total ventilation (U). This was described in Chapter 12 (p. 80) and appears in the main programme (Appendix IV) between statements 1220 and 1230 as part of parameter C47 (see subroutine CONST).

The final consideration is that of H^+ / OH^- ratios. The temperature dependence of pH could be allowed for in the pH function by the following description of pK:

$$pK = 6.086 + .042(7.4 - pH) + (38 - TEMP).(.0047 + .0014.(7.4 - pH)).$$

The inaccuracy in using a value of 6.1 for pK is slight, and I have therefore not used the complex expression, but it would be possible to incorporate it into subroutine GASES if desired.

SUMMARY

The effects of temperature changes on water vapour pressure, solubility of gases, dissociation curves of oxygen and carbon dioxide in blood, metabolic rate, cardiac output, ventilation, and acid-base balance are considered. The simple means to describe temperature effects in the model are mostly derived from well-known published data.

19
Representation of Artificial Ventilation

Earlier in Chapter 10 I described how gas exchange was determined by alveolar ventilation and pulmonary blood flow, and in Chapter 12 how some of the main controlling influences upon natural ventilation could be quantified and represented. It is obvious that an accurate model of gas exchange and transport has potential clinical value to anaesthetists and to other clinicians using machines to provide artificial ventilation. In MacPuf an index (NARTI) specifies either that ventilation should be NATURAL, i.e. determined by known natural stimuli, or ARTIFICIAL. When using artificial ventilation (NARTI = 0) the sets of statements which determine tidal volume and respiratory rate at each iteration interval are by-passed. The operator can directly specify the ventilation rate and tidal volume. A test is incorporated so that if the index NARTI is 0 (instead of its normal value of 1), the specified values for respiratory rate (RRATE) and tidal volume (TIDVL) are used to calculate total ventilation. The previously derived expressions for total dead space (Chapter 11, p. 68) are used as before to determine how much the total ventilation is alveolar and how much is dead space ventilation.

The opportunity to change the type of ventilation is obtainable any time after a run has stopped, by means of the 'CHANGE' options, discussed in Chapter 24. If artificial ventilation is specified, the operator is asked first for a value for respiratory rate, which is stored as a parameter RRATE, and for a value for tidal volume, in cc, stored as TIDVL.

Since positive end-expiratory pressure is nowadays often used to improve arterial oxygenation, especially in neonatal practice, I have incorporated a way of specifying the changes likely to be brought about by this technique. The interactive dialogue provides a question asking the operator to specify end-expiratory pressure as some value (in cm water) from zero (normal) to + 15 (the maximum commonly used in practice). This is stored as another parameter (PEEP). The effects of PEEP are known to be: (1) improvement in the oxygenation of the blood probably due to the opening up of collapsed alveoli—this can be represented by reduction in the apparent venous admixture effect (see Chapter 9); and (2) a reduction in cardiac output. The latter is brought about by a reduction in venous return because of an increase in mean right atrial pressure.

113

The statements in the main programme and subroutine CONST (Appendix IV) describing effective venous admixture are as follows:

$$[C18 = VADM * 80.]$$
$$[C19 = (PD - 90.) * RVADM * .05]$$
$$[C21 = (40. - PEEP) * .025]$$
360      $$PW = (C18 / X + C19) * C21 + FADM$$

All the other components of the above equation were discussed fully in Chapter 9, with the exception of the expression '(40. − PEEP)', which has a normal value of 40 with zero value for PEEP. When maximum PEEP is used (i.e. 15 cm H_2O) the effective venous admixture is reduced to 25/40, i.e. five eighths of its previously computed value, though any specified *fixed* right-to-left shunt (FADM) is still added to the whole expression, as already discussed. The values for arithmetical constants in the above expression, when used in the whole model, create changes which correspond to the general experience of anaesthetists with whom I have discussed this aspect of model simulation. I have not found any very helpful published quantitative studies.

The change in cardiac output is similarly empirical. Clearly if the heart is overfilled to start with, and operating on the flat portion of the Starling function curve a moderate increase of the average intrathoracic pressure will have no effect on cardiac output. The formulation in MacPuf appears in the main programme as statement 240, as follows:

240          $$COADJ = DAMP((C8 / Y + C9) * C16, COADJ, C61)$$

The rest of this expression was described in Chapter 16, p. 103. This function depresses cardiac output, when using maximum PEEP, to a value which is some fraction of the previously computed value. The expression for C8 (see subroutine CONST) includes a term describing elastance. If the lungs are very stiff (elastance high) PEEP has little effect on cardiac output. If the lungs are compliant cardiac pumping is brought virtually to zero with maximum PEEP. This effect will of course underestimate the ill-effects of PEEP on cardiac filling if filling is already inadequate, and overestimate them if cardiac filling is adequate.

The user of the artificial ventilation option has a choice: either he accepts the empirical formulation of the effects of PEEP as a reasonably realistic package correct for average conditions; or he fixes PEEP at zero, and uses the manually-changeable controls to make his own more appropriate changes in dead space, venous admixture, and cardiac output.

Whether or not artificial ventilation is used, the known ventilatory stimuli are summed together in the way previously described in Chapter 12 to describe the total ventilatory drive—(U). The effective stimuli to ventilation, taking account of the limit for tidal volume and some degree of damping of the rate of exchange of ventilation are expressed as another index (SVENT). The value of SVENT is stored as a COMMON variable, so that when artifical ventilation is removed, breathing will be at once restored to its appropriate rate and depth. In addition, discrepancies between actual ventilation, and ventilatory stimuli are made to produce 'symptoms' (Chapter 26). Thereafter the following statements appear (see main programme between statements 1230 and 1400):

```
1290        IF (NARTI .EQ. 0) GO TO 1320
1300        DVENT = SVENT
            RRATE = ...
1320        ......
1340        DSPAC = expression described for 'dead space' in chapter 11
1350        TIDVL = DVENT * 1000. / RRATE
1360        AVENT = (TIDVL − DSPAC) * RRATE * FT
```

The use of the artificial ventilation option defines exactly the total ventilation in terms of respiratory rate and tidal volume. Thereafter the effective dead space and the resultant alveolar ventilation are determined as they would have been during natural ventilation, except that no limit is set to tidal volume.

There is one additional statement in the programme not mentioned in this account so far. This appears at the start of subroutine CONST (statement 120) which specifies that if artificial ventilation is in use—NARTI (N95) equal to zero—and that if either tidal volume or respiratory rate are very small (less than one cc or breath/min) the alveolar ventilation (AVENT) will be effectively zero. This statement is necessary so that if zero artificial ventilation is specified alveolar ventilation will fall to zero at once, without the time delay created by the ventilatory damping function (p. 81).

SUMMARY

Artificial ventilation is represented in the model by the disconnection of normal ventilatory stimuli, thus allowing values for respiratory rate and tidal volume to be specified. Allowance for the addition of positive end-expiratory pressure is made by an index which appropriately reduces both venous admixture and cardiac output. An operator can specify his own more appropriate changes when using PEEP if he so desires. The values for effective dead space, venous admixture and cardiac output are unchanged by artificial ventilation, unless PEEP is used.

20

Representation of Tracheal Obstruction and the Collection and Rebreathing of Expired Gases in Bags

In this chapter I shall discuss ways in which MacPuf can be made to allow an operator to simulate and study the effects of certain manoeuvres commonly performed in clinical and physiological respiratory practice. The most important of these comprise bag experiments such as the collection of expired gases in a bag and their subsequent analysis, and the rebreathing of specified gas mixtures from small bags, as a means of determining mixed venous gas tensions and the ventilatory response to carbon dioxide. I shall also discuss means to simulate tracheal obstruction.

These options are available to an operator by interactive dialogue which will be described in Chapter 24. All of them are made possible by a single subroutine (BAGER). This is written separate from the main programme so that someone wishing to run MacPuf on a computer with limited storage capacity can simply omit the subroutine and the calls to it, or substitute a dummy subroutine, thus shortening the main programme without any effect on other computations.

On entering the subroutine for the first time, the operator is given a set of options, as follows (see subroutine BAGER in Appendix IV):

1. Closure of the glottis;
2. Collection of expired air in a bag;
3. Rebreathing from a bag;
4. Rebreathing from a bag, with a CO_2 absorber attached;
5. Restoration of the *status quo*: glottis open, bag disconnected.

The specification of the option chosen alters an index (PL) which has a value between -1. (glottis closed), and $+3$. (option 4 above). This index is located in the main COMMON store of variables as factor 100. PL has a normal value of 0. (specifying option 5 above); $+1$. specifies collection of expired air, and $+2$. specifies simple rebreathing from a bag. When options 2 to 4 are asked for the operator can specify the initial bag volume in cc (BTPS), which is stored as a variable called BAG. This can be filled with

BAGO cc of oxygen, and BAGC cc of carbon dioxide (both STPD) by specifying percentages of O_2 and CO_2. Any residual volume is assumed to be nitrogen. When option 1 above is requested, changes will obviously occur in lung volume (VLUNG). The nominal resting lung volume with the airway unobstructed, at normal atmospheric pressure, is stored as another parameter (REFLV). Both are in cc BTPS. Under normal conditions they are equal.

Changes in lung volume and other variables during tracheal obstruction

Reference to the main programme (Appendix IV, subroutine CONST) will show that the presence of tracheal obstruction is tested for early in this sub-routine. If PL is less than zero this test is satisfied, and alveolar ventilation (AVENT) is thereafter made .001. Subsequently, total ventilation (DVENT) and respiratory rate (RRATE) are also made effectively zero (main programme between statements 1240 and 1290). At statement 790, subroutine BAGER is called with the first argument=5, which executes statement 500 in the subroutine, specifying that the operative lung volume (VLUNG) becomes equal to the volume remaining in the lung after alveolar gas exchanges have occurred (CA). The correction factor CC(= C12) is used, as an argument in the subroutine call, to correct STPD to BTPS. The lung volume continues to diminish, under normal conditions when oxygen uptake exceeds carbon dioxide output; or if a full INSPECT table is printed (see Chapter 24) sub-routine BAGER automatically ensures that the current lung volume is printed (statement 510). The lung volume can also be continually monitored by other types of display described in Chapter 25. When the *status quo* is restored, and the glottis opened again, the lung volume is immediately allowed to return to the normal specified resting value (REFLV—statement 170) and any ventila-tory stimuli still present can act again.

This option, as described in the technical section above, sounds more complicated than it is. In practice it can simply be used to examine the net change in lung volume with glottis closure. This allows simulation of changes in a whole-body plethysmograph during tracheal obstruction, for example, and certain other physiological manoeuvres.

Collection of expired gases in a bag

This procedure is commonly used to determine metabolic rate, especially in exercise. It is also easy to simulate in MacPuf.

At the end of the statements describing alveolar gas exchanges, a variable (XVENT) represents the volume of gases exhaled in time FT (see Chapter 10, p. 60, and the main programme—statement 800). If the index PL is greater than zero, so that collection or rebreathing of expired gases is specified, sub-routine BAGER is called with the first argument=4 (statement 820), which transfers to statement 440 in the subroutine (see Appendix IV). The dead space volume per unit time interval (see Chapter 11) is then computed (X) and augments the bag volume, bag oxygen and bag carbon dioxide by the amounts of each gas present in inspired air. The bag volume is also appropriately incremented by XVENT and the individual gas volumes by a function of it which represents the proportion of O_2 and CO_2 in the alveolar air after gas exchange has taken place. Appropriate BTPS / STPD corrections are applied.

When bag collection (PL = 1.) or rebreathing (PL = 2. or 3.) is in action, the values for bag volume, bag CO_2 volume, and bag PCO_2 are automatically displayed (by statements 530 to 540) in the INSPECT table previously referred to, and described in greater detail in Chapter 24. Although the description is in highly compressed Fortran notation, it should be clear on careful inspection. The reader who is considering altering this part of the programme might well be warned that it took me a great deal of time and many discussions with colleagues before I was satisfied that the conversion factors were used in the correct way. I now believe that the description in the programme is correct, and advise against making any radical changes in it!

Rebreathing of expired gases

Rebreathing of gas mixtures from a small bag is a most convenient way of supplying a rapidly increasing stimulus from carbon dioxide accumulation in the inspired air (Read, 1966). Measurement of the ventilatory response at different values of inspired PCO_2 and of arterial PCO_2 has become a standard test of ventilatory function in clinical and physiological practice. It is now well known also that if the bag volume is small, and the initial bag PCO_2 reasonably close to mixed venous PCO_2, there is a plateau during rebreathing, lasting half a minute or so, during which the PCO_2 in the bag, at the mouth and in the alveoli will be almost the same as that in mixed venous blood. This is a simple way of estimating mixed venous PCO_2 without having to withdraw blood. More sophisticated uses of bags are also possible: e.g. the use of a nitrogen-filled bag to determine mixed venous oxygen tensions during certain special conditions with very short rebreathing periods.

All these experiments and many more can be simulated extremely easily in the model. Once again subroutine BAGER is used for the purpose.

If bag rebreathing is in action the percentages of oxygen and carbon dioxide in the inspired air are no longer fixed, but change with each iteration of the programme, according to the gas concentrations in the bag. This is performed with the call to subroutine BAGER with the first argument = 2, which occurs at statement 200 (see main programme, Appendix IV). Later, during the computation of alveolar ventilation, a further call to the subroutine with the first argument = 4 transfers control to statement 450 in subroutine BAGER, providing that index PL is greater than unity. This then so arranges matters that bag volume, bag oxygen and bag carbon dioxide are changed appropriately to take account of the net gas volume changes during the ventilation *in* and ventilation *out* procedures. The dead space term can in this case be ignored, since it is small compared with the volumes of the bag and of the lungs. A test is made at this point (statement 450) to ensure that the tidal is not greater than the bag volume.

A simple refinement allows carbon dioxide to be removed from the bag (PL = 3.), thus allowing simulation of the (highly dangerous) experiment of rebreathing air in such a way that the ventilatory stimulus from rapidly progressive hypoxia is measured without concomitant hypercapnia. The way in which this is accomplished and the effective inspired gas concentrations adjusted will be clear from inspection of the again highly compressed equations in the subroutine (around statement 470). As in the previous section, the logical analysis and choice of the ideal as well as the correct places to apply BTPS/STPD corrections is very difficult. At least it proved so for me. I believe that the description as it stands is now correct, since it matches physiological experiments (see Chapter 23). The correctness of this part of the programme could be most crucially tested by experiments on bag rebreathing performed at different barometric pressures. I have not yet performed such experiments myself, nor am I aware of data in the literature with which the predictions of MacPuf can be compared. This is one of the many areas opened up to experimental analysis by the use of a holistic model (see also Chapter 28).

SUMMARY

Reasons are given for including in the model simple ways of representing the changes expected in closure of the glottis, in bag collection of expired gases, and in bag rebreathing experiments. Such simulations allow a large variety of interesting clinical and physiological experiments to be logically analysed. The simulation methods, which involve careful consideration of the correct use of BTPS/STPD conversion factors, are described in detail. The specification of these options is made possible by a subroutine called from the main programme when it is needed.

21
Adjustment of Model Parameters to Sex, Age, Height and Weight

In the preceding chapters I have shown how a working model can be built up using data appropriate for a typical normal subject—e.g. a 70 kg, 180 cm male of 25 years. When describing the size of the venous blood pool, the cardiac output, the maximum tidal volume, the tissue store of carbon dioxide, or the tissue oxygen consumption I have used figures suitable for this young normal subject.

Nothing more is needed for most simulated physiological experiments. The model can serve its original purpose and act as a convenient and flexible resource allowing a student to teach himself how each part of the complex system reacts with every other part. Only very recently, when my colleagues at McMaster and I began to appreciate the possible clinical uses of an accurate model, did the limitation of a standard subject begin to prove frustrating. There are many clinical problems capable of formulation in quantitative terms which MacPuf can in principle solve. For example: (1) can a man with a known and quantified restriction of breathing capacity and response to ventilatory stimuli safely travel in an aircraft pressurised to 7000 feet? (2) what is the P_aCO_2 likely to be in a short fat girl of 15 with normal lungs, ventilated artificially 15 times per minute at 800 cc tidal volume?

An experienced chest physician can take in the clinical data from the first patient, weigh it against his clinical experience and process the data in his personal analogue computer, i.e. his brain, and come up with a reasonably accurate answer. An experienced anaesthetist or intensive care physician can give an equally good answer to the second question. But if they both had access to a model in which every relevant aspect of ventilation, gas transport and metabolism could be quantitatively simulated, they would be able to give considerably more accurate answers than those derived from the product of their intelligence and experience. Furthermore, such a model could provide even an inexperienced person with the means of giving expert answers to difficult questions.

Since few patients conform to the shape and size of the typical normal subject, MacPuf in its original form could only answer such questions semi-quantitatively. For clinical purposes this is largely useless. In this chapter I shall describe the means used to give MacPuf the capability of simulating subjects with widely differing body shapes and sizes, so that physiological experiments and clinically important functional disorders may subsequently be correctly simulated and studied.

The use of a special PRESET subroutine

Incorporation of such a facility as I have justified above uses up some storage space in the computer, and might place a barrier to the effective running of the model in a small computer. Therefore I have placed all the statements and data constants necessary for the facility in a separate subroutine (CLIN2) which is brought into action from the main programme, via subroutines DEADY and CLIN1, in response to a request for PRESETS: (DO YOU WANT) 1. CHANGED VALUES, 2. NAT/ART VENT, 3. STORE/ BKTRK, 4. RUN CHANGE, 5. PRESETS? (the interactive dialogue is explained more fully in Chapter 24).

In the next paragraph I shall explain the preliminary manoeuvres necessary before using subroutine CLIN2. These are of no interest except to a programmer.

When the PRESETS option is requested a test is first made to see whether the simulated subject is intact or not, i.e. whether any changes have been made in any of the model parameters which may give trouble in later parts of the simulation process. This is done by testing an index 'NW' which is initialised at unity whenever the model is first run, or whenever a new subject is created (see Chapter 24). When any change is made in the model parameters, NW is thenceforward set at zero. If changes have already been made (NW = 0) in any parameter the values for the old subject are rubbed out and a new subject is automatically created by a logical operation, difficult to describe briefly, but evident upon inspecting the early part of subroutine DEADY between statements 430 and 470. If NW is zero, an alphanumeric array of 72 digits (ITRIG) which stores a sequence of operation instructions is changed in such a way that before subroutine CLIN2 is called, an extra set of instructions calling for the creation of a new, average subject (through subroutine MINIT) is inserted before the first instruction in the array ITRIG. This operation inserts the characters '1/5/' before the next instruction. As I shall mention in chapter 24, '1' specifies a CHANGE option, and the slash '/' says, in effect, 'proceed to the next numerical instruction in array ITRIG without printing any more interactive dialogue'. Therefore, under all circumstances, regardless of what may have gone before, when the option 'PRESETS' is specified a new subject is created with values appropriate for an average young man. Once this has been done, control eventually returns to statement 430 in subroutine DEADY, and the subroutine CLIN1 is called by the instruction '5'. Unless preset patients are requested (see next chapter) this subroutine calls another one (CLIN2), which holds the instructions for the creation of specified special patients or subjects. CLIN2 modifies certain key parameters to change the average normal young man into any other specified subject (see below).

Specification of a particular normal subject

It would be theoretically possible but practically cumbersome to store huge tables of data giving every parameter and variable appropriate for every imaginable shape and size of person. I have therefore used tables of normal data in standard textbooks (e.g. Briscoe, 1965) to provide sliding scales allowing the specification of a small number of key parameters from sex, height, weight and age. These values are first entered through an interactive dialogue which provides values for XMALE (= 1. for a male, = 0. for a female), HT, WT, and AGE. Two functions are specified to save storage space in the programme:

$$FUNC1(HT,AGE,X,Y,Z) = X * HT - Y * AGE - Z$$
$$FUNC2(HT,X,Y) = X + (HT * .01) ** 3 * Y$$

Resting lung volume (VLUNG) in litres is given by the formulation

$$VLUNG = FUNC1(HT,AGE,X,Y,Z)$$

in which X, Y, Z are constants derived from tables of normal data, stored in a 2-dimensional array (ARRAY) which contains separate values for men and women. This is later converted to units of cc.

Oxygen consumption at rest ('CONSO') is taken to be a simple exponential function of weight:

$$CONSO = WT ** .75 * 10.33$$

where WT is in kg and CONSO in cc/min.

Nominal cardiac output at rest (CONOM) in l/min is correlated with oxygen consumption in normal people, so that we can write

$$CONOM = CONSO * .0195$$

In the case of women a slightly lower cardiac output is used:

$$IF (XMALE .LT. .5) CONOM = CONOM * .9$$

Maximum cardiac output (COMAX) in l/min is also taken from normal data tables, and formulated as follows:

$$COMAX = (210. - .65 * AGE) * .0008 * HT$$

  Two commonly used respiratory function tests are the forced expired volume in one second (FEV_1), the forced vital capacity (FVC), and the steady state carbon monoxide diffusing capacity or transfer factor. Readers of preceding chapters will appreciate that all functional statements in the model are in terms of ventilatory response to stimuli rather than of FEV as such, and in terms of effective venous admixture rather than of 'diffusing capacity' as such. (There is no reliable way of distinguishing a barrier to diffusion of gases from mismatching of ventilation and blood flow.) However, it is possible to make use of our knowledge of the functional disorders expected in patients with different degrees of impairment of ventilatory and 'diffusing' or 'transfer' function to allow the specification of FEV_1, FVC and diffusing capacity to change the more fundamental model parameters in an appropriate way, thus making it possible for an operator familiar only with clinical data from routine tests to be able to create a good simulation of any particular patient. In the next chapter I shall discuss ways in which data from function tests can be made to modify model parameters. In this chapter I shall briefly mention the formulae used to obtain normal, i.e. predicted values, for people of any given sex, height, weight and age.

Predicted vital capacity (PVC) and predicted forced expired volume in 1 sec (PFEV) in litres are derived from the following functions:

$$PVC = FUNC1(HT,AGE,X,Y,Z)$$
$$PFEV = FUNC1(HT,AGE,X,Y,Z)$$

in which, as before, X, Y and Z are stored in ARRAY as data constants from which predicted values can be derived. X, Y and Z are different for men and women. If the age is less than 17, different formulations are used:

$$PVC = FUNC2(HT,X,Y)$$
$$PFEV = FUNC2(HT,X,Y)$$

Predicted diffusing capacity (PDCO) in cc/mmHg/min is obtained from VLUNG by

$$X = ABS(20. - AGE)$$
$$PDCO = (7.6 * VLUNG + 5.) * (100. - X) * .01$$

In this case a value of VLUNG previously calculated in litres, not cc, is used; then VLUNG is converted into cc for use elsewhere in the programme.

Elastance (ELAST) in cm water/litre has an influence on respiratory rate (see p. 81) and is empirically related to FEV in such a way as to give reasonable respiratory rates when FEV is low, e.g.;

$$ELAST = FEV + 96. / (FEV + 4.) - 11.$$

Venous blood volume (VBLVL) in ml is empirically related to nominal cardiac output (in litres/min) as an approximation accurate enough for gas transport simulations:

$$VBLVL = CONOM * 600.$$

Extracellular fluid volume (TVOL), in litres, is empirically related to weight to give approximately correct values for extracellular fluid volume:

$$TVOL = (WT ** .6 * .456) + 6.$$

Haemoglobin (HB) and packed cell volume (PCV) are reduced from the standard initial values of 14.8 (g/100 ml) and 45 (%) for men, to 13.5 and 43, respectively, for women, to give approximate average figures.

Running in to obtain a steady state

Once these relatively few parameters have been specified by the values given for a subject's sex, height, weight and age a minimum number of repetitions is necessary to obtain a steady state. Except with minor deviations from the average normal subject the internal values are changing up to at least the 30th repetition of the main programme, i.e. 5 minutes of simulated time, when using a 10 s iteration interval. In particular, CO_2 stores change only slowly. Some approximate preliminary guesses about CO_2 and bicarbonate stores are made to speed operation (see subroutine CLIN2 between statements 230 and 240.) Empirically I have found it best to allow 72 successive computations to be performed when setting up a new specified subject, to ensure that a truly steady state has been achieved. During the course of computation various other values will have been automatically derived. For example, the dead space will be recalculated on the basis of lung volume and total ventilation; the respiratory rate will be computed from total ventilation and elastance; all gas amounts, contents and tensions in every compartment will be recalculated. While this computation is going on the normal graphical or other output obtained during running of the main programme is suppressed by an index NB until the steady state is reached. If ludicrously low values are specified for FEV and/or diffusing capacity MacPuf may fail to create a simulated living subject, in which case a necropsy report will be issued instead, and the operator will have to try again with more reasonable values.

It should be obvious that many of the values given are simply reasonable guesses; and if an exact value is available for any subject (e.g. for resting

```
DO YOU WANT TO..1.CHANGE, 2.CONTINUE, 3.RESTART, 4.INSPECT, 5.STOP

? (1)
1.CHANGE VALUES, 2.NAT/ART VENT, 3.STORE/BKTRK, 4.RUN CHANGE, 5.PRESETS
? (5)


---- NEW SUBJECT ----

DO YOU WANT..1.PRESET PATIENTS OR  SUBJECTS
2.TO SPECIFY YOUR OWN PATIENTS  OR SUBJECTS
? (2)
70 KG AVERAGE MAN. DO YOU WANT TO SPECIFY SOMEONE ELSE..1.YES, 2.NO
? (1)
PLEASE SPECIFY..1.MALE, 2.FEMALE
? (2)
GIVE ME THE HEIGHT IN CM (183 CM=6 FT)
? (166)
NOW WEIGHT IN KG
? (52)
AND AGE IN YEARS
? (34)
            LITRES      CC/MM/MIN    CC/MIN      LITRES/MIN      % IDEAL
PREDICTED  FEV1    VC   DIFF.CAP.   O2 CONSN.   CARD.OUTPUT      WEIGHT
           3.0   3.8      16.3        200.          3.5           91.

DO YOU WANT TO ENTER SPIROMETRY RESULTS..1.YES, 2.NO
?_
```

Figure 21.1 Typical example of printout of predicted values for respiratory function tests for a specified subject, created by user interaction. Later entry of different respiratory function test results will appropriately modify estimates of gas exchange and ventilatory responses

cardiac output) then, for example, factor 3 (controlling cardiac output as a percentage of average resting subjects) could be changed appropriately and further running continued until the state was again steady. I shall give an example of such a procedure in Chapter 28.

Printing a table of predicted values

A useful additional feature, easy to provide, is to make the computer print a short table of values predicted for the specified subject (see Figure 21.1). This has nothing to do with the operation of the model, as such, but is a simple check each time that the values with which the model is to work are reasonable and that patient parameters have been correctly entered. 'Per cent ideal weight' is obtained simply from a ratio (RAT):

$$RAT = WT * 5880. / HT ** 1.6$$
$$IF (XMALE .LT. .5) RAT = RAT * 1.064$$

SUMMARY

Reasons are given for providing the model with the ability to simulate subjects of any size, shape, age or sex. This is accomplished by an optional subroutine (CLIN2) which contains data tables allowing predictions to be made for certain key parameters. After appropriate changes have been made in these, the model is run for 72 iterations while its output is suppressed, during which time it achieves a steady state, representing the expected conditions of the specified subject.

22

Adjustment of Model Parameters by Insertion of the Results of Pulmonary Function Testing; Preset Patients

The method of providing predicted values for FEV_1, FVC, diffusing capacity and other respiratory function tests was described in the last chapter. In this chapter I shall describe how these are used to change the model parameters to give realistically appropriate values in steady state conditions.

Figure 22.1 shows in schematic form the processes involved in the creation of an individually simulated patient from body dimensions and respiratory function test results. The operator is asked whether he wishes to enter spirometry results. If the answer is negative, the predicted values for FEV and VC are used without modification. Otherwise, the measured values are entered and stored as FEV and VC. The FEV/VC ratio (RATIO) is computed and printed. A value less than 0.65 prints a message confirming airways obstruction, and thereafter alters the essential parameters in a somewhat different way from that in which they are altered in the absence of obstruction. Another ratio (RAT) is computed by dividing predicted FEV by measured FEV. Its reciprocal (TAR) is also computed for later use. After some more dialogue, the operator is asked if diffusing capacity has been measured. If no measured result is available, the predicted value is used. This is based not only on the subject's sex, height, weight and age but also on the observed value entered for FEV. This is called GUESS and is computed as follows:

$$GUESS = PDCO * (1. + TAR) * .5$$

(see between statements 490 and 500 in subroutine CLIN2, Appendix IV). Values entered at each part of the dialogue are checked as reasonable before being used; unreasonable values are refused. Another ratio (TEST) is computed by dividing the measured diffusing capacity by the predicted diffusing capacity:

$$TEST = XXX / GUESS$$

where 'XXX' is the value entered by an operator.

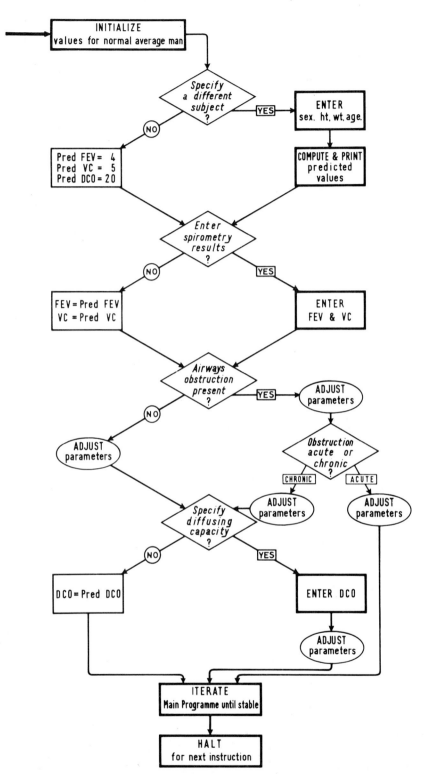

Figure 22.1 Possible sequences of interactive dialogue by which the operator is interrogated by subroutine CLIN2 and first creates a subject, then modifies him or her by insertion of any available routine pulmonary function tests

The logic of changes in model parameters which follows as a result of these entries is designed to identify different possibilities:

1. Airways obstruction or no airways obstruction?
2. Acute breathlessness or no recent change in respiratory state?

Question (2) is not posed unless airways obstruction has been previously diagnosed.

The whole logical sequence in subroutine CLIN2 is shown in Figure 22.1

Airways obstruction present

The question about acute or chronic airways obstruction allows MacPuf to simulate both asthma and chronic ventilatory failure due to airways obstruction. In both cases the following changes are made:

$$VLUNG = VLUNG * (.5 + .43 / RATIO)$$
$$BO2MT = 30.$$
$$TO2MT = 700.$$

Later changes are mostly self-explanatory. Lung volume (VLUNG) is increased by airways obstruction; venous admixture (VADM) is also increased in proportion to the excess of predicted over measured FEV. The parameter 'CZ' was described in Chapter 12, and determines the intrinsic neurogenic drive to ventilation. This is increased as actual FEV is reduced, to simulate increased ventilatory drive from lung reflexes which is made to be greater in acute airways obstruction (i.e. asthma).

If chronic airways obstruction is specified, statements from 450 in CLIN2 are executed. These allow for the renal retention of bicarbonate (by increase of TC3MT) appropriate to the degree of reduction of FEV and consequent elevation of P_aCO_2. The first (statement 450) adjusts brain bicarbonate in the same direction. (BC3AJ is added to brain bicarbonate—see Chapter 13). Extra dead space and venous admixture may be added. Finally, an appropriate guess is made for the variable TC2MT (the tissue store of carbon dioxide) so as to speed up the attainment of a steady state under conditions where there is considerable ventilatory failure.

After this a value is requested for diffusing capacity. If none is available the predicted value is quoted, no further change is made, and control returned to the calling programme (subroutine CLIN1). Otherwise, a change is made in venous admixture as follows:

570             $$RVADM = GUESS / XXX - 1.$$

Reference to Chapter 9 will show that the variable RVADM specifies an addition to effective venous admixture arising only during exercise, when metabolic rate is increased. This index gets increased when the diffusing capacity is reduced below that expected in an obstructed subject, i.e. when the functional disturbance is that characteristic of emphysema.

Airways obstructions absent

If the FEV/VC ratio exceeds 0.65 a different set of statements is executed.

460             $VADM = VADM * RAT ** 1.6$
                 $IF (FEV .LT. 1) VADM = 7. * RAT$
                 $ELAST = FEV + 72. (FEV + 2.) - 11.$
                 $CZ = 20. * RAT + 80.$

The predicted venous admixture is adjusted so as to rise as FEV falls. Elastance is appropriately increased, and central neurogenic drive to breathe (CZ) increased to simulate nervous reflexes from the lungs in severe restrictive defects. The extra dead-space term (XDSPA), previously added if the FEV is less than the predicted value, is later adjusted to increase the mismatching of ventilation and perfusion if diffusing capacity is below the expected value:

570             $RVADM = GUESS / XXX - 1.$
                 $XDSPA = XDSPA * 2. / (1. + TEST)$

These alternative paths converge finally at statement 580 in subroutine CLIN2, and 72 iterations with output suppression are specified (by 'NA' and 'NB'). Control is returned to subroutine CLIN1, and thence to the main interactive subroutine (DEADY).

Limitations in the construction and use of specified computer 'patients'

An obvious limitation to the accuracy of specified computer patients is that the model is built up strictly *as if* it had three compartments for gas exchange, and three components to ventilatory drive. The relationship of FEV, vital capacity and diffusing capacity to the model parameters is entirely empirical, except obviously in so far as the coupling of ventilatory stimuli to their response is likely to be impaired if FEV is low, and apparent venous admixture is likely to be increased if 'diffusing capacity' is low.

A second limitation is that although the adjustment of model parameters is made to give average results, subjects with the same structural disease may have different patterns of disordered function (e.g. 'pink puffers' and 'blue bloaters'). Therefore, the exact simulation of an individual patient requires much more than entering respiratory function test results, and needs careful further adjustments (especially to CO_2 sensitivity) to obtain, for example, the measured values for blood gases.

Construction of PRESET patients

The individually tailored subjects, which can be created for study by means of the changes specified by instructions described in this chapter and the last, are likely to be preferred over normal subjects for clinical work. It is time-consuming and difficult for inexperienced students to produce simulated patients for class exercises. In some situations, e.g. Cheyne–Stokes respiration, there is no combination of body size and standard respiratory function tests which specify the initiation and maintenance of periodic breathing. If one is asking a student to examine the amount of extra oxygen delivered to a patient with chronic respiratory failure by, say, 24, 28 and 35% inspired oxygen concentrations, there is an obvious advantage in being able to call for a specified patient by a single instruction without having to enter a lot of function test results.

The facility is provided in MacPuf by subroutine CLIN1, which is called from the main interactive subroutine DEADY as described in Chapter 21, after all values have been initialised for an average subject. The first question posed is then: 'DO YOU WANT 1. PRESET PATIENTS OR SUBJECTS, 2. TO SPECIFY YOUR OWN PATIENTS OR SUBJECTS?' The second response calls subroutine CLIN2 with the results which have already been described. The first response, asking for PRESET patients brings up a list of stored patients. These can be created with little difficulty, and subroutine CLIN1 in Appendix IV is self-contained and easily changeable by altering a few lines to specify physiological or clinical disturbances other than those listed. The PRESET patients and conditions in CLIN1 are simply examples of what can be done. Muscular exercise involves specifying an increase in metabolic rate and tissue R.Q.: all the rest is done automatically during the steady state running-in period. Cheyne–Stokes breathing can be brought into action by removing the central neurogenic drive to ventilation (see Chapter 12) by making CZ = 0., decreasing cardiac output, adding some venous admixture, altering hypoxic and hypercapnic sensitivity ('BZ' and 'AZ') and reducing whole body bicarbonate. The time scale and number of repetitions can be chosen separately for each example, in accordance with the likely needs.

For example, specification of either of the two patients with chronic airways obstruction and ventilatory failure changes the time scale by supressing five out of every six output results, thus giving blood gas results at one-minute intervals. The run time is also extended to 10 min. This is a suitable time scale for the examination of the effects of, say long term oxygen therapy. The time scale is specified by FT, the number of repetitions for running in to a steady state by NA. Index NB = 2 prevents display of intermediate values during running in, and index ISPAR suppresses 5 out of 6 lines of output in subsequent experiments. I shall not describe this subroutine in any greater detail because its function and arrangement will be obvious on inspection of the whole programme in Appendix IV, and because in any case different operators or owners of MacPuf might want different things. A school of diving instruction, for example, might have a number of preset patients acclimatised for different periods at different depths, so that the physiological principles of safe ascent could be investigated or practised.

SUMMARY

A further development stemming from the techniques used to construct simulated normal subjects of any specified sex, height, weight and age allows, in the same part of the programme, the specification of the results of pulmonary function testing, the resultant and appropriate modifications of the model parameters, and then the creating of preset patients by a running-in period during which a steady state is achieved. It is also possible to specify virtually any set of conditions by a few appropriate instructions which specify certain preset changes to be produced, prior to running the model into a steady state. By these means both normal and diseased subjects can be simulated.

23
Dynamic Testing of the Model

The author of a scientific paper describing a physiological model character-istically concludes by comparing the behaviour of his model with the real system. The representation invariably proves well-nigh perfect. Otherwise, the author would have modified the model until it did fit the experimental observations; or the referees would have rejected the paper; or (to be less charitable) the inaccurate or damaging comparison would have been con-veniently overlooked.

I hope not to disappoint the expectations of those who wish to see how closely MacPuf can simulate real life situations. Since I am not a masochist the reader may take it that I am reasonably happy about the accuracy of the simulations. However, as I pointed out in Chapter 3, 10^{30} discretely different experiments are possible on a model in which each or all of 30 parameters can take up one of only 10 different values. The possible experiments are therefore virtually unlimited, and I can only present a small sample of them.

As the accuracy of each part of the model has been improved during the last five years or so, its power to predict the results of experiments for which it had not previously been specially programmed has also increased. This has not so far been my experience in another field. Alongside MacPuf I have also been trying to develop a comprehensive simulation on similar lines ('MacPee') comprising the heart, blood vessels, intracellular and interstitial fluid com-partments, certain hormones and the kidneys. Despite much work I remain dissatisfied with certain aspects of this simulation, particularly because of difficulties in representing the compliance of the interstitial fluid compartment and of the body cells, and in quantifying the excretory behaviour of the kidney. I have so far failed to find a synthesis of the whole system which is simultaneously correct for primary hyperaldosteronism, low salt diet, chronic renal failure, excretion of a water load, diabetes insipidus, renovascular hypertension, nephrotic syndrome, haemorrhage and heart failure (to take a few of the more important clinical syndromes affecting the whole system studied). Any one of these phenomena, or even several of them, can be accurately simulated by a single set of functions and constants; but I have been unable so far to simulate all of them at once to an acceptable degree of accuracy. I have not experienced the same frustrations with MacPuf—which encourages me to take the step of publishing the model at this stage of its evolution, even though I recognise that it is far from perfect. One justification for publishing it now is that I have gone almost as far as the data I have for specification of functions and constants allow me to go: I hope now to benefit from the experience of those of my readers who are interested enough to set up the programme, to run it in a teaching, clinical or research environment, and to send me back corrections and adjustments which can be used to improve the model further.

The few examples that follow have been chosen to cover as wide a field as possible. I have tried to select situations in which the computed values are derived through several stages from the supplied parameters. For example, my descriptions of ventilatory responses to altered arterial PCO_2 and PO_2 are relatively simple, and obviously the functions and constants used have been carefully chosen to match human data from the literature. There is thus no point at all in making any formal comparison between computer predictions and experimental data here because one variable is directly derived from another. Instead I shall take situations such as inhalation of carbon dioxide, in which almost all the components of the system are tested simultaneously. Other simulations examined will be transients in response to atmospheric pressure changes, effects of O_2 on Cheyne–Stokes breathing, the bag re-breathing method for determining mixed venous PCO_2, nitrogen washout curves, and changes during extremely strenuous muscular exercise.

Steady state ventilatory responses to carbon dioxide inhalation

Figure 23.1 compares some published results of steady state ventilatory responses to CO_2 inhalation in man, and shows the steady states obtained in

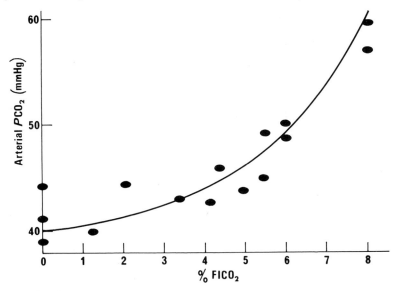

Figure 23.1   Data points from the literature (cited by Grodins, Gray, Schroeder, Norins and Jones, 1954) showing the relationship between inspired $FICO_2$ (abscissae) and steady state P_aO_2 (ordinate). The performance of a standard MacPuf is given by the continuous line. Alteration of the CO_2 sensitivity of the model (Factor 10) allows it to embrace all recorded data

a standard normal MacPuf in terms of alveolar or arterial PCO_2. The carbon dioxide sensitivity of MacPuf can be altered by an operator. If this is varied through a sixteen-fold range (e.g. from 0.5 to 8.0 l/min total ventilation per mmHg rise in arterial PCO_2), corresponding to one quarter to four times the standard average sensitivity curve, the performance of the model easily embraces all recorded observations.

Transients in response to carbon dioxide inhalation

A wide range of responses has been recorded by different authors (Padget, 1927; review by Grodins, Gray, Schroeder, Norins and Jones, 1954; Gelfand

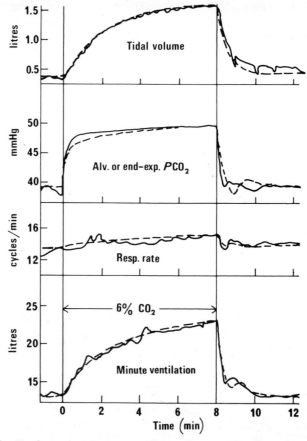

Figure 23.2   The four traces shown as continuous lines recording (from above down) tidal volume, end-expired PCO_2, respiratory rate and minute volume are taken from a typical experiment by Gelfand and Lambertsen (1973) (modified from Figure 2 of their paper) in which a normal subject breathed 6% CO_2 for eight minutes. During this time arterial PO_2 was kept constant by progressively diminishing inspired FIO_2 as ventilation increased. The interrupted lines show the performance of MacPuf in respect of its on-and-off transients under the same conditions. CO_2 sensitivity (factor 10) was adjusted so that the steady state ventilation at the end of eight minutes was the same as in the actual experiment, but no other changes were made in the standard model. As in the actual experiment inspired FIO_2 in MacPuf was progressively reduced to keep P_aO_2 between 90 and 100 mmHg

and Lambertsen, 1973), but in general these show a relatively slow asymptotic rise, and a more rapid fall. The more rapid fall than rise presumably results from CO_2 being washed out faster at the prevailing high ventilation rates when air breathing is resumed than it is washed in immediately after switching from air to carbon dioxide. Again, the normal performance of MacPuf is well within the range of experimental findings, though it fails to correspond entirely with some observations quoted by Grodins and his colleagues of a ventilatory response to inhaled carbon dioxide which continues to increase for up to 20 minutes or so after starting the inhalation. Such a phenomenon has not been invariably found, remains inexplicable by all authors, and is not possible to simulate in MacPuf without the imposition of a rather improbable function to describe central CO_2 chemosensitivity. Figure 23.2 compares the response of MacPuf (with slightly reduced CO_2 sensitivity) in terms of the time course of increase of tidal volume, end-tidal PCO_2, respiratory frequency and total ventilation to a steady state inhalation of 6% CO_2, with the findings of Gelfand and Lambertsen (1973) on normal subjects. It is obvious that there is no important respect in which the performance of the model differs from the observations on the normal subject.

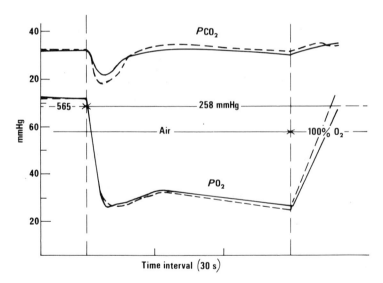

Time interval $\left(30\ s\right)$

Figure 23.3   Solid lines are records of alveolar PCO_2* (upper trace) and PO_2* (lower trace) recorded at four-second intervals before and during decompression of a human subject from 565 to 258 mmHg (data kindly supplied by Dr. D. Denison). At 90 s after decompression 100% oxygen was substituted for air, with a consequent rapid rise of PO_2. During the whole run the subject tried to maintain respiratory rate and depth constant.

The interrupted lines represent the same manoeuvres carried out on a simulated normal MacPuf subject. Artificial ventilation at 12 cycles/min and 580 cc tidal volume gave initial values for PCO_2 (32 mmHg) and PO_2 (72 mmHg) which exactly matched the human subject's initial gas tensions. In both cases the decompression was acute, and maintained for 90 s before 100% oxygen was substituted for air

* Alveolar PCO_2 was derived from measured end-tidal PCO_2 by the method of Jones, McHardy, Naimark and Campbell (1966) and alveolar PO_2 was derived using the Riley–Cohn correction

Transients in response to atmospheric pressure change

Figure 23.3 compares the response of MacPuf to a sudden decompression from a simulated altitude (corresponding to 565 mmHg) to a pressure of 258 mmHg (such as would result from the blowing out of a partially-pressurised aircraft window at 27,000 feet). The figures for alveolar gas tensions during this manoeuvre were kindly supplied me by Dr. David Denison from experiments on himself. Note that not only do the transients match closely, but so also do the later curves, showing the rise in end-tidal PO_2 when 100% oxygen was inhaled. The curious time course of alveolar PO_2, showing an abrupt fall, then a slow rise, and then a late fall, are very exactly mirrored by the behaviour of the model. Incidentally, I have not so far investigated exactly what produces this shape of the alveolar PO_2 curve; but the behaviour of the model suggests that it can be explained in terms of present physiological knowledge, without the necessity for constructing any new hypotheses. This is a good example of the way in which the complex behaviour of a living system is rendered amenable to exact analysis by using a holistic model.

Interaction of oxygen and carbon dioxide inhalation on Cheyne–Stokes breathing

Figure 23.4 shows established Cheyne–Stokes breathing, created in MacPuf by eliminating the central neurogenic drive to breathe (see Chapter 12), increasing central CO_2 and hypoxic drives to breathe, increasing venous admixture and decreasing cardiac output. Note the phase relations of ventilation and the (presumably) causal changes in arterial gas tensions, and the slight phase lead of P_aCO_2 rise and P_aO_2 fall on total ventilation. These correspond closely with what has been observed in man during Cheyne–Stokes respiration. It is known that either oxygen inhalation or inhalation of low percentages of carbon dioxide can abolish Cheyne–Stokes breathing and MacPuf demonstrates the same behaviour. The lower section of Figure 23.4 shows an example. The effects of oxygen are consequences of the high hypoxic drive in Cheyne–Stokes breathing, and of the multiplicative interaction of hypoxic and hypercapnic stimuli, which emerge clearly from the observations of Rebuck and his colleagues (Rebuck and Campbell, 1973), and which are incorporated in the ventilation controller expressions described in Chapter 12. Incidentally, it is interesting to find that a potentially 'Cheyne–Stoking' MacPuf has two possible steady states during inhalation of room air: one is typical Cheyne–Stokes breathing; the other is regular non-periodic breathing. In the steady state, Cheyne–Stokes breathing can be induced under suitable circumstances by a sharp transient applied to the system (see Figure 23.5). I have myself witnessed such behaviour in patients, and others to whom I have spoken confirm that oscillation may sometimes be started by transients and stopped by giving and then withdrawing O_2 or CO_2.

```
MINS 0        20        40        60        80        100       120
+SECS  .    .      .     .     .     .     .     .     .     .     .     .     .
P
 25.40.   V   F            C         O
 25.45.   V   F            C         O
 25.50.   V   F            C         O
 25.55.   V   F            C         O
 26. 0.   V   F            C         O
 26. 5.   V   F            C         O
 26.10.   V   F            C         O
 26.15.   V   F            C         O
 26.20.   V   F            C         O
 26.25.   V   F            C         O
 26.30.   V   F            C         O
 26.35.   V   F            C         O
*
 26.40.          V         C         O
 26.45.          V         C         O
 26.50.          V      C             O
 26.55.          V   C                O
DO YOU WANT TO..1.CHANGE, 2.CONTINUE, 3.RESTART, 4.INSPECT, 5.STOP
 (1/2/2/2/2/2/2/2/2/2/2/2/2)
 27. 0V              C                O
 27. 5V              C                O
 27.10V              C                O
 27.15V                C              O
 27.20V                   C           O
 27.25. V      F              C       O
 27.30.     VF                  C     O
 27.35.      F V                  C   O
 27.40.       F  V                 C    O
 27.45.       FV               C         O
 27.50.     V F       C                  O
 27.55.V      F       C                O
 28. 0V              C                O
 28. 5V              C                O
 28.10V                C              O
 28.15.V       F             C        O
 28.20.   V   F               C       O
 28.25.        V                 C    O
 28.30.      F V                  C   O
 28.35.      FV               C       O
 28.40.     VF          C             O
 28.45. V      F       C              O
 28.50V              C                O
 28.55V              C                O
 29. 0V                C              O
 29. 5V                 C             O
 29.10.   V   F              C        O
 29.15.     VF                C       O
 29.20.      F V                C   O
 29.25.      F V              C       O
 29.30.        V        C             O
 29.35.  V   F        C               O
 29.40.V     F       C                O
 29.45V              C                O
 29.50V                C              O
 29.55V              C                O
DO YOU WANT TO..1.CHANGE, 2.CONTINUE, 3.RESTART, 4.INSPECT, 5.STOP
```

Figure 23.4 Cheyne–Stokes breathing simulated by MacPuf by diminishing cardiac output, reducing central neurogenic drive for ventilation, increasing chemosensitivity to PCO_2 and PO_2, and increasing venous admixture. The time interval of the vertical graph is five seconds; P_aO_2 is represented by the symbols 'O', P_aCO_2 by 'C' (both in mmHg across the top scale), ventilation by 'V' (l/min) and frequency of breathing per minute by 'F'. Note that, as in documented human cases, there is a slight phase lead of rising PCO_2 on resultant ventilation, and that cycle time is about 50 s. Inhalation of 100% O_2 instead of air (see the 'Factor 1 = 100.0' change line) results in P_aO_2 disappearing off scale. The resultant reduction in chemoreceptor gain damps and eliminates the oscillation

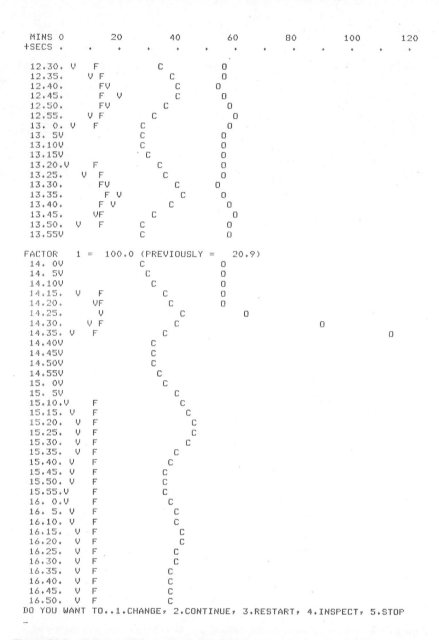

```
MINS 0        20           40          60        80        100       120
+SECS .    .      .      .      .      .      .      .      .      .      .      .

12.30. V     F            C            0
12.35.    V F            C            0
12.40.      FV            C          0
12.45.      F   V            C          0
12.50.      FV            C            0
12.55.    V F            C              0
13. 0. V     F        C              0
13. 5V                C          0
13.10V                C          0
13.15V              C          0
13.20.V     F            C          0
13.25.    V F            C          0
13.30.      FV            C        0
13.35.       F V            C        0
13.40.       F V          C          0
13.45.      VF        C            0
13.50.    V     F     C            0
13.55V              C            0

FACTOR    1  =   100.0 (PREVIOUSLY =    20.9)
14. 0V                C            0
14. 5V              C            0
14.10V                C            0
14.15.    V     F        C            0
14.20.      VF          C            0
14.25.       V              C          0
14.30.    V F          C                0
14.35. V     F        C                              0
14.40V            C
14.45V            C
14.50V            C
14.55V              C
15. 0V              C
15. 5V                C
15.10.V     F          C
15.15. V     F            C
15.20.   V F              C
15.25.   V F              C
15.30.   V F            C
15.35. V     F              C
15.40. V     F          C
15.45. V     F        C
15.50. V     F        C
15.55.V     F        C
16. 0.V     F          C
16. 5. V     F          C
16.10. V     F              C
16.15.   V F                C
16.20.   V F                C
16.25.   V F          C
16.30.   V F          C
16.35.   V F        C
16.40.   V F        C
16.45.   V F        C
16.50.   V F      C
DO YOU WANT TO..1.CHANGE, 2.CONTINUE, 3.RESTART, 4.INSPECT, 5.STOP
```

Figure 23.5 Follows on Figure 23.4, after putting the simulated subject back on room air. Note that at this stage a stable state of mild hyperventilation is present. At the asterisk (time 26.35) artificial ventilation of 20 cycles/min at 1000 cc tidal volume was applied for 20 s with a resultant fall of P_aCO_2. On resumption of normal breathing the imposed transient started MacPuf into Cheyne–Stokes breathing again

Plateau of mixed venous PCO₂ achieved during rebreathing procedures

Figure 23.6 shows the well-known pattern of continuous PCO_2 change at the mouth when a normal subject rebreathes from a small bag containing 100% oxygen. The PCO_2 rapidly climbs to a mixed venous value, then remains at the equilibrium plateau until recirculation of blood with increased PCO_2

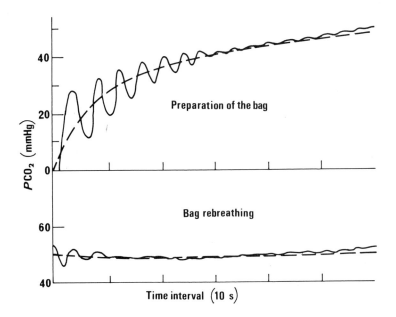

Figure 23.6 In the upper panel the solid line indicates the PCO_2 at the mouth of a normal subject rebreathing from a bag slightly less than twice the tidal volume, and containing 100% oxygen (after Campbell in Campbell, Dickinson and Slater, 1974). The interrupted line indicates the value for bag PCO_2 given by a normal MacPuf subject during the same simulated manoeuvre. In the lower trace the previous bag mixture is rebreathed for a further period. Note that the plateau reaches the same value at about the same time in a normal subject and in MacPuf, and that it is within 1 mmHg of the mixed venous value (in this case 46.5 mmHg). The rate of rise of bag PCO_2 in the steady state in MacPuf is slightly slower than in the experimental subject, indicating that the effective fast tissue CO_2 store in MacPuf is slightly larger than in this subject

causes the PCO_2 in the lungs (or bag) to rise gradually. If the bag is rebreathed subsequently (lower panel) a plateau is reached at 20 s. The performance of MacPuf is virtually identical, except that no respiratory fluctuations are shown (since the standard programme only computes mean alveolar and bag gas tensions). The bag collection and rebreathing options are available in the 'special experiment' option, obtainable by asking to change Factor 100 (see Chapter 20). It is possible to specify any size of bag, with any gas mixture.

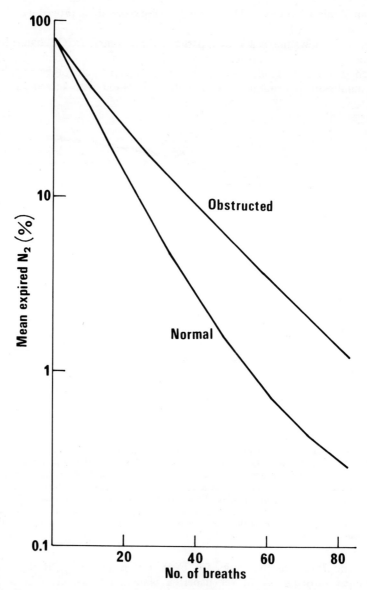

Figure 23.7 The solid lines indicate the percentage of nitrogen in the expired air of a normal subject in relation to the number of breaths after switching inspired gas from room air to 100% oxygen. Note the slight upward concavity of the curves (normally taken to signify inadequacy of gas mixing in the lungs). This is discussed in the text. Mean expired N_2 percentage was computed for this example by an extra line inserted in the main programme (between statements 810 and 820) making one of the dummy COMMON variables (e.g. X109) equal to the mean expired N_2 percentage

Nitrogen washout curves

Figure 23.7 shows two nitrogen washout curves plotted on semi-log paper, obtained from a MacPuf normal subject, and from a severely chronically obstructed simulated subject (85 Kg 60 year old male with FEV = 0.7, FVC = 1.5). Tidal volume in each case was maintained at the resting level throughout (441 cc for the normal subject, and 524 cc for the obstructed one) and respiratory rate likewise (12.8 for the normal, and 14.5 for the obstructed subject). In both cases the washout curves are very close to perfect exponentials, but it is interesting that both show some evidence of apparent 'maldistribution'. Analysis shows this to result from inhomogeneity of tissue nitrogen storage (specified of necessity in the model), not of gas mixing in the lungs. This is another example of the insight given by a holistic model.

Studies on exercise

The parameters chosen for MacPuf ensure that with metabolic rates from 300 to 1500% of normal (corresponding to oxygen uptakes from 750 to 3750 cc/min, and to work loads of 400 to 1500 kpm/min) the changes in cardiac output, minute ventilation and rate of lactic acid generation match average published values. An example of a test of maximal performance by the model is that of a simulated sprint in which it has been estimated that metabolic rate is equivalent to the consumption of 7 litres O_2 per minute (about 2800% resting value). Figure 23.8 suggests that after about 22 s at this work load the lactic acidosis of the tissues becomes intolerable. This estimate seems to correspond approximately to the experience of athletes.

Many other examples could be given, but I hope this brief survey of a few widely different examples will serve to show that MacPuf is a versatile and reasonably accurate holistic model. I have no doubt that as it is applied to many other situations, various problems and inaccuracies will be discovered. I reiterate that I should be pleased to hear of any such problems, so that the model may continue to evolve.

SUMMARY

Much so-called 'testing' of models is tautologous, since the tests recreate the processes by which the necessary functions and constants were derived. More searching tests take relations between variables which are not direct, but which involve many or all the functions and constants comprised by the system.

Examples chosen for comparison between computer simulation and real experimental or clinical data include: steady state and transient responses to inhaled carbon dioxide, transients during acute high altitude decompression, effects of oxygen inhalation on ventilation and blood gases during Cheyne–

Stokes breathing, the bag rebreathing method for determining mixed venous PCO_2, nitrogen washout curves, and studies on strenuous exercise.

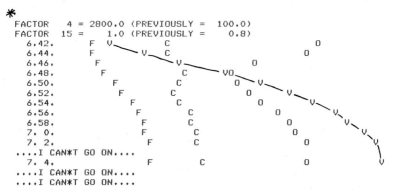

```
(FOR KPA,     P.PRESSURES        CONTENTS CC%    AMOUNTS IN CC    PH      HCO3-
X  0.1332)      O2     CO2          O2     CO2      O2     CO2

ARTERIAL       93.7    40.3        19.5    47.6    195.    476.    7.396   23.9
ALV./LUNG     101.7    40.2 (SAT= 97.)             346.    146.
(PULM.CAP)    101.7    40.2        19.7    47.5
BRAIN/CSF      31.8    55.6        10.8    56.1     20.    712.    7.321   22.7
TISSUE/ECF     40.6  ( 45.8)       14.6    51.6    180.  13403.    7.370
MIXED VEN. ( 40.6)    45.8         14.6    51.6    437.   1549.    7.370   25.6
PLASMA LACTATE CONC.= 1.0 MMOL/L

O2 UPTAKE=    249.   CO2 OUTPUT=    201. CC/MIN(STPD) EXPIRED R.Q.= 0.81
TOT.VENT.=   5.9   ALV.VENT(BTPS)= 4.2 R.RATE=12.8   VEN.ADMX.= 2.4
DEAD SPACE(BTPS)= 129.   TIDAL VOL.= 458. D.SP./TID.VL.RATIO=0.28
CARDIAC OUTPUT=  5.0   CEREBRAL BLOOD FLOW= 54.5 ML/100G/MIN
```

```
*
FACTOR   4 = 2800.0 (PREVIOUSLY =  100.0)
FACTOR  15 =    1.0 (PREVIOUSLY =    0.8)
   6.42.        F  V.      C                            O
   6.44.        F      V   C                         O
   6.46.         F         V               O
   6.48.          F         C        VO
   6.50.           F        C          O  V
   6.52.            F       C          O     V
   6.54.             F      C          O    V  V
   6.56.              F     C              O      V  V
   6.58.               F    C            O            V  V
   7. 0.               F     C          O               V  V
   7. 2.                F    C            O               V  V
....I CAN*T GO ON....                                       V
   7. 4.                F    C                O               V
....I CAN*T GO ON....
....I CAN*T GO ON....

      I AM VERY SHORT OF BREATH

YOUR PATIENT IS TWITCHING
(FOR KPA,     P.PRESSURES        CONTENTS CC%    AMOUNTS IN CC    PH      HCO3-
X  0.1332)      O2     CO2          O2     CO2      O2     CO2

ARTERIAL       89.2    52.1        18.8    34.7    188.    342.    7.122   16.2
ALV./LUNG     102.9    52.0 (SAT= 94.)             324.    220.
(PULM.CAP)    102.9    52.0        19.2    33.0
BRAIN/CSF      43.1    51.8        14.7    53.3     27.    664.    7.267   22.7
TISSUE/ECF     15.1  ( 87.2)        2.1    54.4     67.  14331.    7.081
MIXED VEN. ( 15.1)    87.2          2.2    54.8     66.   1645.    7.101   26.2
PLASMA LACTATE CONC.= 8.5 MMOL/L

O2 UPTAKE=   5985.   CO2 OUTPUT=   7044. CC/MIN(STPD) EXPIRED R.Q.= 1.18
TOT.VENT.=115.1   ALV.VENT(BTPS)=97.0 R.RATE=35.4   VEN.ADMX.= 2.4
DEAD SPACE(BTPS)= 511.   TIDAL VOL.=3250. D.SP./TID.VL.RATIO=0.16
CARDIAC OUTPUT= 35.0   CEREBRAL BLOOD FLOW=159.4 ML/100G/MIN
```

Figure 23.8 Simulation of the 200 metre dash. In the control period the iteration interval has been set to 2 s. During the race it is assumed that the metabolism of muscles corresponds to an oxygen uptake of 7 l/min (2800% of resting value) and that carbohydrate is consumed (RQ = 1.0). (These changes were made at the asterisk acutely in the model, which was then run for 24 s.) The symptoms and end-of-run values indicate the intensity of tissue acidosis resulting from anaerobic metabolism. (The 'INSPECT' table of values at the start of the run can be compared with those at the end.) Note the rapid rise of total ventilation (symbols V–V)—the scales across the paper are as in Figure 23.4

Part II
Communication with the Model and Consideration of the use of Models in Teaching, Clinical Practice and Research

24
Principles of Interactive Dialogue; Changing Model Parameters

The evil of dictionaries

In perhaps twenty years or so, when the principles of English grammar are better understood and fast computer storage more highly developed, the computer dictionary may be a commonplace peripheral attachment to a computer. By 'dictionary' I imply that, given an English word, phrase or sentence typed in by an operator, the computer can interpret it and take appropriate action. The simplest possible dictionary recognises 'YES' and distinguishes it from 'NO', rejecting attempts to enter other words. This sort of recognition is unobjectionable. It is easy to combine with the possibility of entering digits expressing choices from a set of numbered alternatives, and of entering floating point numbers such as '20.93' when specifying the value of a parameter such as inspired oxygen percentage. Alas, this is only the beginning. Once the programmer of an interactive system gets really hooked on 'YES' and 'NO' his feet sometimes come right off the ground. He embarks on a dictionary. First comes the recognition of 'HELP' or '?' (to ask the computer to explain a question more fully). This is reasonable in itself, though more letters need now to be checked in the dictionary for correct action. Then comes, perhaps, 'WHATS' (Miller and Walters, 1974)—which is a request to print the current value of some variable: e.g. 'WHATS RO2PR?' where RO2PR stands for arterial oxygen partial pressure. This means that the dictionary has to contain a list of the abbreviations or symbolic representations of variables used in the programme, and that the user must now have a handbook, and refer to it each time. Such an instruction can be a very useful and powerful tool, but the provision of such a facility complicates and expands the programme, and makes it more time-consuming and extravagant to run. To avoid this extravagance I have in MacPuf preferred to use a single, global, INSPECT option, which spells out the values of virtually everything that one might wish to check up on. This uses more space and time in execution, but much less in the programme.

It is tempting to advance a dictionary still further and perhaps insert words such as 'OXYGEN', 'PO2', 'PRESSURE' and 'ARTERIAL' and arrange things so that when an operator types in:

WHATS THE PARTIAL PRESSURE OF OXYGEN IN ARTERIAL
BLOOD?

or

WHATS THE ARTERIAL PO2?

or

WHATS THE PO2 IN ARTERIAL BLOOD?

certain combinations of key words are interpreted and the right answer given.

When applied to the rest of the variables even in the relatively small simulation programme described in this book, the dictionary is getting bigger. Soon the designer will find it occupying a large file on its own. Unless the grammatical structure is extraordinarily well thought out, the programmer will find himself making the computer search the entire dictionary to identify each word. Much time may be lost if one word is misspelt by the operator, who then has to look back at the dialogue to see where he went wrong.

In the time it takes an operator who is not used to a typewriter keyboard to type 'WHATS THE PARTIAL PRESSURE OF OXYGEN IN ARTERIAL BLOOD?' and perhaps correcting his mistyping he could, in MacPuf have typed '4' to specify 'INSPECT', and at 30 characters/s a table such as that illustrated in Figure 24.1 would have given him the answer in about 20 s.

```
DO YOU WANT TO..1.CHANGE, 2.CONTINUE, 3.RESTART, 4.INSPECT, 5.STOP

?(4)            P.PRESSURES      CONTENTS CC%    AMOUNTS IN CC   PH    HCO3-
                 02     CO2       02     CO2      02     CO2

ARTERIAL        92.7   40.5      17.8    49.8    178.    498.    7.407  24.6
ALV./LUNG      101.1   40.3 (SAT= 97.)   210.     89.
(PULM.CAP)     101.1   40.3      18.0    49.7
BRAIN/CSF       30.1   56.9       9.3    58.1     19.    730.    7.320  22.8
TISSUE/ECF      38.8 ( 46.2)     12.9    53.8    158.  12367.    7.376
MIXED VEN. ( 38.8)     46.2      12.9    53.8    328.   1373.    7.376  26.2
PLASMA LACTATE CONC.= 1.2 MMOL/L

02 UPTAKE=     208.   CO2 OUTPUT=    166.  CC/MIN(STPD) EXPIRED R.Q.= 0.80
TOT.VENT.=     4.6   ALV.VENT(BTPS)= 3.5  R.RATE=13.7   VEN.ADMX.= 2.4
DEAD SPACE(BTPS)=    83.   TIDAL VOL.= 336.  D.SP./TID.VL.RATIO=0.25
CARDIAC OUTPUT=    4.2   CEREBRAL BLOOD FLOW= 55.3 ML/100G/MIN

DO YOU WANT TO..1.CHANGE, 2.CONTINUE, 3.RESTART, 4.INSPECT, 5.STOP

?_
```

Figure 24.1 Typical example of an 'INSPECT' table displaying current values of all important computed values

At the same time the computer would have given him everything else he was likely to think of or want.

I am therefore against even the apparently innocuous 'YES' and 'NO', even when abbreviated to 'Y' and 'N'. Why not phrase all questions in numerical alternatives, and get every operator familiar with this approach? For example, the computer can ask:

DO YOU WANT TO . . . 1. GO ON, 2. STOP?

If you make it ask

DO YOU WANT TO GO ON?

and invite 'Y' or 'N' then it may not necessarily be clear what will happen if you type in 'N' or 'NO'. You may get the programme designer's favourite rude message. In all that follows, therefore, I shall stick to numerical answering only, retaining the use of the typed letter 'Q' or 'QUERY' to ask the computer for extra help in interpreting a question.

The design of interactive dialogue

There is more to the design of economical and easy-to-use dialogue than meets the eye. The analysis which follows is naive but it is based on much personal experience in designing interactive dialogue for the self-instructional models which have been used by medical students at McMaster University, University College Hospital and St. Bartholomew's Hospital. This has given me experience of what is convenient and acceptable and what is obscure and confusing.

I shall start by considering an interactive system which provides an operator, seated at the keyboard of a computer console, Teletype or visual display unit with 16 possibilities of action: A B C D E F G H I J K L M N O and P. One may envisage two extreme possibilities. The first is a series of questions such as:

DO YOU WANT TO DO A . . . . 1. YES, 2. NO? — ②
DO YOU WANT TO DO B . . . . 1. YES, 2. NO? — ①
DO YOU WANT TO DO C . . . . 1. YES, 2. NO? — etc.
     etc.

The other extreme is to have the computer type out its complete list of options, then ask for a selection from the list:

AVAILABLE OPTIONS ARE:
1. A . . . .,
2. B . . . .,
3. C . . . .,
    etc.
16.P . . . . ,
TYPE THE ONE OR ONES YOU WANT TO SELECT __

In the first example the questions have to be posed singly, they must be on successive lines, and time-consuming transfers of control from reading to writing devices will make the operation slow and cumbersome. In the second example the list could be compressed into fewer than 16 lines, but at the expense of easy legibility, e.g.

AVAILABLE OPTIONS ARE: 1. A . . . . . ., 2. B . . . . . ., 3. C . . . . . .,
4. D . . . . . ., 5. E . . . . . ., 6. F etc.
TYPE THE ONE OR ONES YOU WANT TO SELECT __

Yet another approach is to rely entirely on the operator having an instruction manual. This saves a lot of space in storing text, allowing the programme to be much shorter, e.g.:

WHICH OPTION(S) DO YOU WANT (REFER TO HANDBOOK)? __

A handbook is always necessary to help students and others to use this or any large model effectively, but on the other hand it seems a pity to force the operator to be continually turning the pages. I have tried in designing MacPuf to keep the handbook in the background, so that most work can be conducted without an operator having to refer to the handbook at all. The use of a handbook is obviously necessary for complex experiments in which an operator may wish to change the value of many different parameters of the model. Examples from the handbook are given at the extreme end of this book in Appendix VII. This contains a list of all the COMMON specified variables whose values can be changed, and of the computed variables whose values may be printed on request.

What is the best and most economical design of interactive dialogue? I believe that it is a compromise—to divide the questions up into groups of 4 or 5. This allows the questions, if brief, to be put along a single line of text, and the whole interactive dialogue for 16 different options consumes only 4 lines of question and answer, e.g.:

DO YOU WANT 1. A . . . . . ., 2. B . . . . . ., 3. C . . . . . ., 4. D . . . . . .? __ ③
DO YOU WANT 5. E . . . . . ., 6. F . . . . . ., 7. G . . . . . ., 8. H . . . . . .? __
    etc.

Lacking expert psychological knowledge I am forced to give my unverified and pontifical opinion that most people engaging in interactive dialogue with a computer can easily and reliably take in four of five questions or alternatives and choose from them, but that deciding between more than about five takes much longer. Perhaps experimental psychologists have already established the truth of the matter; but until I hear evidence to the contrary I shall be guided by my own experience.

The method I have chosen, after much trial and error, is as follows: when presenting any set of alternatives, make option (1) that of passing to the next section (which will probably be the most commonly used option) and then to string the other options out in descending order of probable use. An example will make things clearer. At the end of each particular operative run of MacPuf, computation halts, and the following question is asked:

DO YOU WANT TO . . 1. CHANGE, 2. CONTINUE, 3. RESTART,
4. INSPECT, 5. STOP? __

These 5 possibilities have been placed in descending order of probability of use. The '2. CONTINUE' instruction starts off another run; but before that several things may have to be changed, so that the '1. CHANGE' option may have to be used two or three times successively. '3. RESTART' will be less commonly used, and '4. INSPECT' (which produces a complete table laid out to show nearly all useful computed values) will not be needed except by those who are using the model in a sophisticated way, or for research purposes. '5. STOP' will presumably only be used once, on leaving the console or terminal. Use of any options other than STOP brings about a sequence of events which always leads back again to this single question. (See Figure 24.2.)

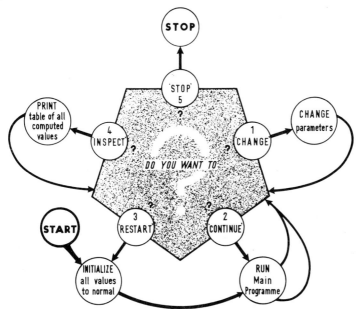

Figure 24.2   Schematic diagram of the central interactive dialogue (in subroutine DEADY) which is the starting and finishing point of every operation

It is worth trying to abbreviate the possibilities so as to put all the options on the same line. This economises slightly on time (and paper, when using a printer rather than a visual display unit) and is easier for the eye and brain to take in than:

DO YOU WANT TO
1. CHANGE VARIOUS DIFFERENT THINGS?
2. CONTINUE FOR ANOTHER RUN?
3. START AGAIN WITH A NEW SUBJECT?
4. PRINT A COMPLETE TABLE OF ALL STORED IMPORTANT
VALUES?
5. STOP THE PROGRAMME?
TYPE YOUR CHOICE FROM THE FIVE ABOVE __

Such a table may be helpful to the user coming to the programme for the first or second time, but becomes irksome to an experienced user. I have preferred to retain an option for help at any question by typing 'Q' (for QUERY). A few lines of explanatory text can then be stored in a subroutine (in MacPuf this is subroutine QUERY which is given in full in the complete programme in Appendix IV). To give an example from the programme:

DO YOU WANT TO .. 1. CHANGE, 2. CONTINUE, 3. RESTART, 4. INSPECT, 5. STOP? __ ⓪

1 IS OBVIOUS, 2 STARTS ANOTHER RUN OF STANDARD 3 MIN, 3 STARTS AGAIN WITH A NEW SUBJECT, 4 PRINTS A TABLE OF MOST USEFUL VALUES, 5 STOPS THE PROGRAMME PLEASE TRY AGAIN

When the user selects option 1 (to 'CHANGE') he is offered 5 more choices:

1. CHANGE VALUES, 2. NAT/ART VENT, 3. STORE/BKTRK, 4. RUN CHANGE, 5. PRESETS? __

Once again these are presented in the order of frequency in which they are likely to be used by the average operator. He is most likely to want to change variable factors (e.g. inspired oxygen or cardiac output) and at first unlikely to want to change the type of run or display, still less to start using preset subjects and inserting the results of pulmonary function tests.

Working on the same principles, other parts of the interactive dialogue can be considered. Upon the 'death' of a simulated subject (when one of the computed variables moves outside the range compatible with life), post mortem reports are issued and MacPuf enquires:

... 1. BACKTRACK, 2. CONTINUE, 3. RESTART, 4. INSPECT, 5. STOP? __

which follows once again the principle of placing the alternative course of action on a single line in the most likely order of frequency of use.

Factor changing

Somewhat different principles need to be considered when it comes to changing primary variable values. Our first interactive teaching model limited to the systemic circulation (Dickinson, Goldsmith and Sackett, 1974) had only a few parameters, each or all of which could be changed prior to a run (e.g. systemic arterial resistance, cardiac contractility, blood volume). MacPuf has many more parameters which an operator might wish to change, but I have selected the first six of them as having the greatest physiological interest, and have arranged for them to be initially printed in abbreviated form, as a list, at the end of each run, e.g.

1. INSP. O2 = 20.9, 2. CO2 = 0.0 PER CENT, 3. CARD. CONT. = 100 PER CENT, 4. TISS. METAB. = 100. PER CENT, 5. VENOUS ADMXT. = 2. PER CENT, 6. D. SPACE = 0. ML

In this list, the INSPired O2, and the inspired CO2 are in per cent, CARDiac CONTractility is given as per cent normal value, TISSue METABolic rate is per cent resting value, VENOUS ADMIXture is its normal low value (about 2%), and there is no added Dead SPACE. In response to the question:

1. CHANGE VALUES, 2. NAT/ART VENT, 3. STORE/BKTRK, 4. RUN CHANGE, 5. PRESETS? __

an operator wishing to change one of the above factors requests option '1' and is then asked to

TYPE NUMBER OF FACTORS (1–30) TO CHANGE, OR 100 FOR SPECIAL EXPERIMENTS __

If he now wishes to change, say, inspired CO_2 from zero to 5 (per cent) he responds '2' (for factor 2, which is the inspired CO_2 percentage), and gets told

FACTOR 2 (CURRENT VALUE = 0.0), SPECIFY NEW VALUE __

This reminds him of the present value and invites the response '5' or '5.0' to specify that the new value for factor 2 will now change to 5. After confirming the instruction control then returns again to home base, e.g.

DO YOU WANT TO . . 1. CHANGE, 2. CONTINUE, 3. RESTART, 4. INSPECT, 5. STOP? __

Reference to the handbook (Appendix VII) shows that it is possible to change more than one factor at once by placing blanks between each factor number, in which case the programme will request each successive new value for each factor specified. The computational techniques are straightforward and appear in subroutines DEADY and NXTWD (see Appendix IV).

Storage of factors in the computer

The six factors given above, and another 24 other factors can be changed in the same way. To economise on space and on the time taken to print output, the latter 24 factor numbers and their current values are not spelt out after each run. An operator wishing to change barometric pressure, for example, has to consult the handbook, discover that barometric pressure is factor 13, and then change it by the technique described above. On the way he will always be reminded of the current value for the factor he is about to change. A list of the changeable parameters of the model is given at the end of the handbook for the model which appears in Appendix VII at the end of this book. It is also available on comment cards in the (magnetic tape) complete programme available from McMaster University. McMaster can also supply student handbooks for the model at nominal cost.

All these changeable factors make up a COMMON storage block, or array, which is common to both the main line programme and the interactive subroutine DEADY—and indeed to all other parts of the programme as well. These factors are all given Fortran symbolic names, which have already been described in the preceding text. For example, factor 2, the inspired CO_2 percentage, is called 'FIC2'; but a Fortran programmer will appreciate that in subroutine DEADY (see Appendix IV) the COMMON block which begins 'FIO2, FIC2, CO, PD' etc. is made equivalent to an array (T) which stores not only the 30 or so changeable parameters but also another 90 or so computed variables. These can also be changed by the 'CHANGE' option just described; but there is no point in an operator changing them since after a single iteration of the programme they will be recomputed anyway. A warning to this effect is issued to the operator if he tries to change them. Most of the first 30 factors are fixed and unchangeable during any particular run of the programme, e.g. inspired CO_2 percentage, barometric pressure, nominal cardiac contractility. Some, however, have characteristics both of supplied parameters and computed variables, because they change extremely slowly. Examples are the tissue CO_2 store (TC2MT) which is of the order of 14 litres, and the brain bicarbonate concentration (BC3CT) which is eventually influenced by the prevailing level of brain PCO_2. To assist in achieving a steady state after a large change in model parameters it is an advantage to be able to create a comparatively large, acute (and quite unrealistic) change in some slowly changing values so that a steady state can be achieved without undue expenditure of computer time. It was for this reason that I decided to hold both basic model parameters and computed variables in the one COMMON array, or block. This has certain other advantages for display of the state of the model at any moment (see Chapter 25), when the whole array can be written out on demand, and also for a store/backtrack option allowing the present state of simulated subjects to be stored, so that the same subject can be exactly recreated later when needed.

Time-saving devices for interactive dialogue

A reader who has read the earlier chapters will realise that I favour the use for instructional purposes of a reasonably large holistic model in which the user will be continually reminded of Haldane's dictum that 'a living organism is constantly showing itself to be a co-ordinated and self-maintaining whole'. Therefore I have striven to create a general purpose model which will be as useful to clinicians as to physiologists, and to the advanced student or researcher as well as to the novice. In accordance with these principles the model should be largely self-explanatory and usable by a beginner without need for a personal instructor; but it should also be convenient for an experienced operator to use without wasting time. I have therefore copied a device which was shown to me by Professor R. D. Cohen on the well-designed interactive medical record keeping system installed at the London Hospital. In this system, a string of numerical instructions to the computer can be made to act in succession, with all the interactive dialogue suppressed, by the use of 'slash' separators; e.g. 1/1/1/100 (These make index NW2 greater than 19, which skips all text material).

We might instruct the computer to make inspired oxygen $=100\%$ as follows:

DO YOU WANT TO 1. CHANGE, 2. CONTINUE, 3. RESTART,
4. INSPECT, 5. STOP? __ ①
.. 1. CHANGE VALUES, 2. NAT/ART. VENT., 3. STORE/BKTRK,
4. RUN CHANGE, 5. PRESETS __ ①
TYPE NUMBER OF FACTORS (1–30) TO CHANGE, OR 100 FOR
SPECIAL EXPTS __ ①
FACTOR 1 (CURRENT VALUE 20.93), SPECIFY NEW VALUE __ ⑩⓪
DO YOU WANT TO 1. CHANGE, 2. CONTINUE, 3. RESTART,
4. INSPECT, 5. STOP __

These four separate instructions can be reduced to one, as follows:

DO YOU WANT TO 1. CHANGE, 2. CONTINUE, 3. RESTART,
4. INSPECT, 5. STOP? __ (1/1/1/100)
FACTOR 1 = 100 (PREVIOUSLY 20.93)
DO YOU WANT TO 1. CHANGE, 2. CONTINUE, 3. RESTART,
4. INSPECT, 5. STOP? __

Since on most teleprinter or visual display unit keyboards, at least 72 characters are available in each line, an enormous string of instructions can be given economically. This saves a great deal of time, not only during model development, but also in practical and research use.

SUMMARY

The seductive evils of computer dictionaries are described, and reasons given for preferring simple numerical alternatives, even for the simplest questions. The logic of interactive dialogue suggests that the most satisfactory way of conducting a dialogue is by means of successive questions presenting four or five alternative courses of action, preferably as a single line across a screen or teleprinter, in an abbreviated form if necessary, keeping an explanatory text available for use on request.

The techniques for storing and changing variables are discussed, and means described whereby speeding-up of operations can be obtained by devices which remove much or all of the interactive dialogue.

25
Types of Display: Storage and Retrieval of Previously Stored States

Graphical display

Everyone with a scientific training is familiar with graphs, and it is simple to programme a computer to produce graphs coming out vertically from a Teletype or visual display unit. Usually 72, sometimes 80 spaces are available across the whole width of the paper. In a lineprinter there are usually 120. Since few biological measurements are made to much more than 2% accuracy a digitally produced graph is usually adequate, and has the advantage of needing no special graphics terminal to produce it. It is worth considering carefully what a respiratory model can most profitably display.

Clearly there is little point for the computer to present a graph of something which a student or doctor cannot measure or is ever likely to want to measure in clinical practice. There may be research value in watching the cerebral venous oxygen content, for example; and since this value needs to be computed at each iteration interval anyway, its value is available and it can easily be plotted. But it is obviously of much more practical use to plot the arterial PO_2 or the total ventilation, both of which are easily measured. One needs also to consider how many things to plot. A graph which has more than about four overlapping lines is confusing to look at. There are certain problems about presenting data on ordinary output devices routinely available with computer systems. It is not practicable to present four or more independent graphs representing variable values on the same time scale, one above another, except when using a graphics terminal. Such a display demands a great deal of storage space during execution of the programme, unless a storage oscilloscope is available. All the values computed during a long run—say of a simulated period of twenty minutes or longer—must be stored as successive iterations are being performed, so that they can be fed to the graphics plotting system for presentation after each run. There is an advantage in plotting graphs somewhat less accurately on a lineprinter or even on a simple console typewriter in vertical form, so that as each iteration is performed the computed values are printed, then discarded or overwritten by new values. In this way the size of storage space necessary to run the programme is kept within reasonable bounds. I do not propose to go in detail into the graphical plotting routines by which numerical floating point values can be converted into integer form and displayed upon a vertical graph on successive lines. The techniques involve standard Fortran, familiar to any programmer, and can be seen anyway by inspecting the full programme listing in Appendix IV (subroutine BRETH).

```
1.INSP.O2=  21., 2.CO2=    0. PERCENT, 3.NOM.CARD.OUTP.= 100.PER CENT
4.TISS.METAB.= 100. , 5.VENOUS ADMXT.=   0. ,  6.D.SPACE+=    0. ML

(THE FACTOR LIST ABOVE WILL NOW DISAPPEAR - REFER TO HANDBOOK)
DO YOU WANT TO..1.CHANGE, 2.CONTINUE, 3.RESTART, 4.INSPECT, 5.STOP

?_(1)
1.CHANGE VALUES, 2.NAT/ART VENT, 3.STORE/BKTRK, 4.RUN CHANGE, 5.PRESETS
?_(1)
TYPE NUMBER OF FACTORS (1-30) TO CHANGE, OR 100 FOR SPECIAL EXPTS
?_(1)
FACTOR   1 (CURRENT VALUE=   20.9), SPECIFY NEW VALUE
?_(5)
FACTOR   1 =   5.0 (PREVIOUSLY =   20.9)
DO YOU WANT TO..1.CHANGE, 2.CONTINUE, 3.RESTART, 4.INSPECT, 5.STOP

?_(2)
MINS 0         20        40        60        80        100       120
+SECS .     .     .     .     .     .     .     .     .     .     .     .
  3.10. V  F         C                         0
  3.20. V  F         C                0
  3.30. V  F         C           0
  3.40.  V  F        C      0
  3.50.    VF       C 0
  4. 0.     V       C
  4.10.    VF      C
  4.20.   V F     C
  4.30.    V    0 C
  4.40.    FV 0   C
  4.50.    V  0   C
  5. 0.   VF   0  C
  5.10.   VF  0   C
  5.20.   VF  0   C
  5.30.   V F 0   C
  5.40.   V F 0   C
  5.50.   V F 0   C
  6. 0.   V F 0   C

FINAL VALUES FOR THIS RUN WERE...

ARTERIAL PO2 =   23.1 (  3.1 KPA), O2 CONT =   8.6, O2 SAT=  43.
ARTERIAL PCO2=   33.2 (  4.4 KPA), CO2 CONT=  41.9
ARTERIAL PH  = 7.42( 38.NM), ARTERIAL BICARBONATE= 20.6

RESPIRATORY RATE = 18.1, TIDAL VOL.=  814. ML
TOTAL VENTILATION=  14.7 L/MIN, ACTUAL CARD.OUTPUT=  11.4 L/MIN
TOTAL DEAD SPACE= 159. CC, ACTUAL VENOUS ADMIXTURE=   4.4 PERCENT


    MY EYES ARE GOING DIM

YOUR PATIENT IS VERY BLUE

DO YOU WANT TO..1.CHANGE, 2.CONTINUE, 3.RESTART, 4.INSPECT, 5.STOP

?_
```

Figure 25.1 Typical printout of interactive dialogue leading to a graph showing changes in arterial gas tensions and values expected at the end of a three-minute run at the start of which inspired O_2 concentration was reduced acutely to 5%. Note anoxic hyperventilation, which lowers P_aCO_2 and raises arterial pH, and also the production of appropriate symptoms and signs

The limitations of this display are of course chiefly that the plotting can only be performed to the nearest integer value. Any display must be confined between predetermined limits, which means that the scale must be carefully chosen so that the values spread out across the paper, can be read accurately, and are intelligible. In the final scheme of presentation I chose to restrict the display to four computed variables—arterial PO_2 and PCO_2, total ventilation and frequency of breathing—and to allow them to move across a scale of 72 spaces including a time scale in minutes and seconds. Each individual value is coded by an appropriate symbol, and allowed to overlap. The presentation is more easily illustrated than described. Figure 25.1 shows an example of a graphical display at 10 s intervals of arterial PO_2 (symbol 'O'), arterial PCO_2 (symbol 'C'), total ventilation (symbol 'V'), and frequency of breathing (symbol 'F') during the 3 minutes immediately after inspired oxygen was reduced from 21 to 5%. Note that the same numerical scale, extending from 0 to 120, is used for all variables. Arterial PO_2 and PCO_2 are shown in mmHg. Total ventilation is shown in l/min. Normally this is well down at the base of the graph, but can of course increase to the limit of maximum ventilation, which is normally about 100 l/min (see p. 80). Frequency of breathing is less well shown, since this rarely exceeds 40 breaths/min and the scale is not fully used; but it seems simpler to use the same number scale for all values.

The graph emerges vertically from the lineprinter, Teletype, typewriter or visual display unit, one line at a time. It needs to be turned, mentally at least, through 90° to give it the conventional axes of numerial values of variables, plotted against time. The graph of Figure 25.1 can be turned in this fashion. It is easy to join up the discrete points to form reasonably smooth curves. Figure 25.1 was obtained from a fast console printer across 72 columns, but a more accurate display could be brought out from a lineprinter, using all available 120 columns, if the multiplication factors in the display routine (subroutine BRETH) were increased appropriately.

In an early version of MacPuf I used a lineprinter to display the graphs and some numerical output, and used a console typewriter to accept and print the interactive dialogue. This possibility is retained by having separate integer codes or logical numbers for the input device ('INI') from which instructions are read, and the two output devices ('KT' and 'KL') on which output is printed. 'INI' would normally be the console or Teletype; 'KT' would be the same device, used for output printing; 'KL' is used for those WRITE statements in the model whose output would best be directed to a lineprinter, if available. Probably in most installations, and in time-sharing, KT and KL would be given the same logical number. Since these integers are in the array COMMON to all parts of the programme, it is only necessary to specify the device number once, at the beginning of the programme, to change the device numbers everywhere (see main programme, Appendix IV, just before statement 100).

Routine output of important computed values

At the end of each graphical run, usually lasting three simulated minutes, with results being plotted at simulated 10 s intervals, it is desirable to display numerical values for a few of the more commonly measured computed variables. The standard ones in MacPuf are shown in Figure 25.1 and are, in order: arterial PO_2 (in mmHg or KPa), O_2 content (cc/100 ml), saturation (%); arterial PCO_2, CO_2 content; arterial pH and nmol/l H^+ activity; arterial bicarbonate (mmol/l); respiratory rate (per min), tidal volume (cc BTPS), total ventilation (l/min BTPS); cardiac output (l/min); total dead space (cc BTPS); venous admixture (% cardiac output). After this a reminder is issued of the current values of the six most commonly changed factors (see Chapter 24) and control returned to the operator.

Use of the 'INSPECT' option

MacPuf needs to compute many more values than are represented by the simple graphical display or by the short table of certain selected values, shown in Figure 25.1. It is convenient to be able to get at these and display them when necessary. For this reason at the end of every run the operator is offered the opportunity of 'inspection':

DO YOU WANT TO 1. CHANGE, 2. CONTINUE, 3. RESTART,
4. INSPECT, 5. STOP? __

The use of option '4' prints a large table of the main important values—all computed values rather than preset parameters (see Figure 24.1, p. 146). Most of these are self-explanatory.

Display of values for special and research use

A complete but much less easily read display is available by typing '6' (an option not offered in the list) in response to the request:

DO YOU WANT TO 1. CHANGE, 2. CONTINUE, 3. RESTART,
4. INSPECT, 5.STOP? __

```
DO YOU WANT TO..1.CHANGE, 2.CONTINUE, 3.RESTART, 4.INSPECT, 5.STOP

? (6)
    5.00     0.03 100.00 100.00     0.00   0.003000.00     5.00     3.00 100.00
  100.00 100.00 760.00   37.00     0.80  12.75   12.00   14.80   45.003000.00
    0.00  -0.06   3.96 100.00   29.00   0.40   35.00     0.00     5.00     0.00
    7.33   1.00   7.42   7.37   11.83   7.35     0.00     0.00   81.20 121.22
   23.84  33.00   7.40   11.82   13.41  48.44 813.51   18.07     8.561387.75
   14.70  14.70  41.42   8.90     7.52  45.99   2.94   52.20     7.37   20.64
   46.26  88.99 417.91   11.982276.06   8.38 620.98   82.49     3.14 158.75
 3000.00  23.06 240.00   33.16     0.00  42.88     0.00   41.93   82.64     4.36
    0.17   4.60   0.00   40.18 539.05  67.65   22.49   22.60 113.87     3.23
   22.70   1.00  11.44   8.69 105.15  22.13   40.18 219.981971.74     0.00
   41.85  85.50 641.25   4.00 563.00   0.83     0.00     8.32     0.00 570.00
    0.00 965.15  26.34   0.00     0.00   0.00     1.00 178.00   70.00   40.00
DO YOU WANT TO..1.CHANGE, 2.CONTINUE, 3.RESTART, 4.INSPECT, 5.STOP

? _
```

Figure 25.2 Typical printout of the 120 computed and preset values stored in the COMMON block. This option displays every current stored value in the model, excluding the values of local variables and those in the DELAY line

This executes a simple statement in subroutine DEADY (statement no. 610) which simply prints the entire COMMON array of values as a table of 10 columns and 12 lines (Figure 25.2). These read from left to right, and down the page; but the user obviously needs to know the order of the variables in the COMMON store to interpret the tables.

Sequential display of every value in the model can be made to occur at each iteration interval by replying '4' (again, an option not offered in the list) to the question in the 'RUN CHANGE' section which reads:

DO YOU WANT . . . 1. GRAPHS + TEXT, 2. GRAPHS ONLY, 3. SELECTED VALUES? __

In this event the full table of 120 values will be printed at each computation interval, thus consuming many yards of paper even for a short run.

Option 2 in the list above has the fairly obvious effect of preserving the standard graphical display, but suppressing the normal write-out of important values, thus allowing an operator to run quickly through a set of operations, asking for the full '4. INSPECT' option whenever he wants more information.

Option '3. SELECTED VALUES' allows an operator to choose up to eight different computed values from the COMMON store, and have these printed across the screen in eight columns, preceded by the time in minutes and seconds. In response to a choice of option '3. SELECTED VALUES' above, the operator is asked:

TYPE UP TO 8 NOS. — 69 is STANDARD __

Reference to the full list of values shows that factor 69 is the expired respiratory quotient, i.e. respiratory exchange ratio. The preset factors in this type of display are as follows: expired RQ; arterial pH; total ventilation; alveolar ventilation; arterial bicarbonate; alveolar PO_2; arterial PO_2; arterial PCO_2. (An example of this type of display is shown in the handbook, Appendix VII.) However, if different chosen values were needed, e.g. tissue PO_2 (96), tissue PCO_2 (97), tissue O_2 amount (95), tissue CO_2 amount (16), brain PO_2 (45), brain PCO_2 (46), tidal volume (47), respiratory rate (48), the operator would simply type the corresponding factor numbers as a string, separated by blanks, to have the display changed to give just those values in which he was interested (refer again to handbook examples, Appendix VII).

Length of run; iteration interval; output suppression

Subroutine 'DEADY', between statements 670 and 810, allows changes to be made in the length of each run (in seconds) and in the iteration interval (between 1 s minimum and 10 s maximum). These change the run repetition index (NA) and the fractional time interval (FT). Then there is a choice of suppressing 5 out of 6 or 29 out of 30 lines of output, so that if a 10 s iteration interval is used the output values or graphs are displayed only once each minute or once each 5 minutes. This saves output space and printing time, but has no effect on the internal computations of the model, which proceed just as if all the output was being displayed.

The techniques for doing this involve the use of an index (ISPAR) whose mode of action will be clear on inspecting the main programme (Appendix IV, between statements 1470 to 1590).

Storage and retrieval of newly created conditions

The model as described already allows the creation of complex states simulating a variety of clinical disorders. Some of these may have taken considerable time, trouble and computing time to assemble. A student or doctor might have spent a lot of time gradually matching the clinical situation of his patient to the simulation by the computer. Then he might wish to perform a variety of different experiments on this particular simulated patient, e.g. to observe the effects of giving different percentages of inspired oxygen, different types of artificial ventilation, different atmospheric pressures, and so on. It is inconvenient and inefficient to have to recreate the same complex series of conditions by juggling with the large number of variable preset factors, and it would be an obvious advantage to be able to freeze or store the state of the simulated subject and to be able to recreate it on demand.

I have therefore incorporated another COMMON area of 160 storage compartments. These are stored in the main COMMON block (array T holds the first 120), and the next 40 values are held in the venous DELAY system (p. 45) (array TDLAY). By means of a 'STORE' instruction the values of the 160 variables present at any one time in the model are copied into the store, and can be retrieved by a 'BACKTRACK' instruction at any later time. After the creation of any subject through a 'PRESETS' manoeuvre (Chapters 21 and 22) the current state is automatically STORED. The technique of doing this is simple. It appears in subroutine DUMP in the complete programme in Appendix IV. The two arrays are combined as array 'T'; the storage area is another COMMON array (TDUMP). Storage in the COMMON block prevents overwriting when an overlaid programme structure is used.

According to the principles of good interactive dialogue outlined in the last chapter, the option of storage appears as follows:

1. CHANGE VALUES, 2. NAT/ART VENT, 3. STORE/BKTRK, 4. RUN CHANGE, 5. PRESETS? __

After a request to '3. STORE/BKTRK' the operator gets asked:

DO YOU WANT TO 1. STORE PRESENT STATE, 2. BACKTRACK TO LAST STORED STATE? __

An example of this facility in use is shown in the handbook, Appendix VII.

There is an incidental advantage to the designer of a model in including a facility of this kind. Most of the fine adjustment of parameter values can only be made by operation of the whole model. For example, the way in which apparent dead space changes in the face of changes in ventilation and blood flow is known in only very approximate quantitative terms, but by incorporation of extra changeable variables during the course of programme development, it is possible to change the actual arithmetic involved in the computation, i.e. effectively change the programme itself, without the need for recompiling it. One can insert dummy variables in the model as multipliers having a default value of 1, or added factors, having a default value of zero, and make changes in such factors during a large variety of tests. It is then a great convenience to be able to create a simulated subject, make some change, run for a few minutes to enable a stable state to be reached, and then store the steady state so that the same simulated subject can be put through a large variety of different tests. Much of the adjustment of parameters in MacPuf was accomplished by such means.

SUMMARY

Reasons are given for making the basic display system a vertical graph of arterial PO_2 and PCO_2, total ventilation and frequency of breathing, with the output of a few selected important computed values at the end of each run. Further examination of the model is made possible by a global inspection option which prints a large table of all the computed values which an operator is likely to want. Display of even more extensive tables is possible by different instructions. Methods for changing the length of run and the iteration interval are described; and the facility of suppressing 5 out of 6 lines of output is useful to save printing space and time. Storage and retrieval of previously stored states gives added flexibility to the model, and prevents waste of time in repeatedly recreating the same complex functional disturbance in a simulated patient. It is also an advantage to the designer of the model.

26
Generation of Symptoms, Signs and Necropsy Reports

I have explained earlier my motives for including appropriate symptoms and signs, with the idea of improving the realism of the model, and making it more entertaining and lively for a student. The subroutine controlling the appearance of symptoms and signs is not essential to the operation of the programme, and could simply be omitted if storage space was scarce or if the model was being used for research purposes. The subroutine SYMPT (Appendix IV) is largely self-explanatory. I have tried to bring in particular symptoms and nursing observations with approximately realistic deviations from normal conditions. For example, at a brain oxygen pressure less than 13.9 mmHg 'MY EYES ARE GOING DIM' is issued; at a brain PCO_2 greater than 80 the simulated subject complains of drowsiness; at a tissue pH above 7.59 he complains of tingling and cramps in the hands; at a tissue pH less than 7.09 he is observed to be twitching. If the brain oxygenation is inadequate (PO_2 less than 13) or brain PCO_2 greater than 91 mmHg, or tissue PN_2 greater than 6000 the subject is reported to be 'UNROUSABLE', and other symptoms are suppresssed. The amount of reduced haemoglobin is computed, and if this exceeds 5 g/100 ml the patient is reported as being 'BLUE' and over 7 g/100 ml as 'VERY BLUE'. Since this index is triggered by reduced haemoglobin the sign will not appear in the presence of gross anaemia. The symptoms of nitrogen narcosis are adjusted to correspond with average expectations of this event (Curtis, 1973) and those of decompression sickness to correspond approximately to an average subject's expectation of 'bends' and other symptoms (Fulton, 1951; Fryer, 1969).

The reader may be surprised by the absence of breathlessness as a symptom of anything other than tachypnoea, since dyspnoea is so common in chest diseases. The reason is the difficulty of assigning the generation of this symptom to one or even to several indices. There are several types of breathlessness. Some patients with gross carbon dioxide retention and obstructive airways disease will not complain spontaneously of breathlessness, yet those with asthma and normal blood gas tensions may complain very severely. Pending some suggestions by others of appropriate indices to use, therefore, I have simply derived breathlessness from tachypnoea. It would be a nice exercise in logic and applied physiology to write a section of programme here which triggered or suppressed this symptom appropriately and realistically.

Symptoms of improvement

Many years ago, when I showed an early clinical simulation model to Dr. Arnold Naimark, now Dean of the Medical School in Winnipeg, he commented that it was a pity than an operator obtained nothing but complaints and alarming signs from his simulated patient, and was never rewarded by any expression of gratitude! I therefore arranged that symptoms should be in two categories, mild and severe. For mild symptoms an index (K1) stored in the common block (and therefore retained during calls to subroutines) is changed from its normal value of zero in the subroutine to be equal to 1. A severe symptom specifies another index (K3) as unity instead of zero. At the end of the execution of the subroutine, the current value of K1 is copied into K2 and that of K3 into K4. During the next operation of the subroutine, the new value of K1 is compared with its old value. In the event of removal of a minor symptom, with no major symptoms present, the message

'THATS BETTER DOCTOR . . . BUT ARE YOU GOING TO DO ANY OTHER NASTY THINGS TO ME?'

is issued. In the event of a severe symptom being removed, without the intermediate creation of a mild symptom, the message

'GOD BLESS YOU DOCTOR. I FEEL REALLY WELL AGAIN. ITS LIKE A MIRACLE!'

is issued; and in the event of a partial improvement the intermediate message is generated:

'I FEEL BETTER BUT NOT RIGHT YET. CANT YOU DO ANYTHING MORE FOR ME?'

I realise that to many physiologists and clinicians these messages, and indeed the whole SYMPT subroutine may appear extremely childish; but in several respects it has proved useful. It keeps users entertained, and also forces them to ask 'why is this symptom appearing?' or 'what's gone wrong now?' and perhaps makes the operator notice some change, e.g. an unduly alkaline pH, which he might otherwise have overlooked.

It would obviously be a waste of computing time and output paper or screen space to have these symptoms appearing after each iteration. I have therefore confined the generation of symptoms to the moment that any specified run has come to a stop and the current values of variables have been printed. Then subroutine DEADY is called from the main programme, and symptoms issued, before control is returned to the operator after the question

'DO YOU WANT TO 1. CHANGE, 2. CONTINUE, 3. RESTART, 4. INSPECT, 5. STOP?' __

An exception is made for the combination of increased metabolic rate, i.e. strenuous muscular exercise, which, if combined with extremely low tissue pH, produces the symptom (subroutine DEATH, statements 300 to 360)

... I CAN'T GO ON ...

at each iteration of the programme—which gives the operator a warning that he is stressing his simulated subject beyond the limits of human endurance, and that death is likely to follow soon afterwards.

Detection of 'death' and issue of necropsy reports

The possibility of 'death', i.e. the transgression of important values outside the range compatible with life, is tested after each iteration of the main programme loop, by a call to subroutine DEATH. (The reason for this arrangement is that in the event of 'death' occurring, control can be passed at once to options of backtracking, restarting and inspecting: further iterations of the main programme cease.) An index operated by time and severity of brain anoxia ('PG') is started when brain oxygenation is inadequate (BO2AD less than 1—statements 1400 to 1420). Index PG has been made to function in such a way that irreversible anoxia occurs at about the right time interval that it is known to do in clinical practice after such catastrophes as unrelieved asphyxia, breathing nitrogen and cardiac arrest. PG is therefore tested, and if it exceeds a predetermined value, the message 'ANOXAEMIA HAS BEEN SEVERE AND IRRECOVERABLE' is issued. Recovery of brain oxygenation brings PG slowly back again (see main programme, Appendix IV, between statements 1400 and 1420). Limits are also set on tissue pH, from 6.63 to 7.8—which again seem reasonably in accord with clinical findings (subroutine DEATH, statements 160 to 280). These also lead to explanatory messages, followed by the general message:

'YOUR PATIENT HAS DIED.'

If the terminal has a 'bell' this may be made to sound a death knell at this point by a suitable format character!

Again I recognise that these facilities may appear to be simply ludicrous, and wasteful of space in an already large computer programme. However, regular testing for lethal values performs a number of useful functions. One is to prevent silly experiments being done or continued. Also, it is salutary to remind students and doctors that certain situations and clinical experiments are dangerous. For example, the administration of 100% oxygen to a simulated patient with severe ventilatory failure leads to cessation of respiration, and to eventual death from hypercapnia and acidosis, despite an arterial oxygen tension which may be normal. This situation is one which has often occurred in clinical practice. I hope that no student nowadays will see it; but if he can be reminded of its possibility he may be cautious with unrestrained oxygen therapy in such conditions, and understand better the merits of controlled oxygen therapy.

Once 'death' has occurred, the final values of the main variables are printed, and various choices offered:

... 1. BACKTRACK, 2. CONTINUE, 3. RESTART, 4. INSPECT, 5. STOP? __

These options include all the things one might wish to do.

SUMMARY

The justification for having the model produce symptoms and signs, and detect lethal derangements of its internal chemistry is that it becomes more realistic and interesting to a student operator. He is reminded of the limits of normal values, and of the deviations in normal values likely to produce symptoms, signs and death of a real subject; and he is prevented from carrying out silly experiments. The methods for the generation of such messages are described.

27
General Consideration of the use of Interactive Simulation Models in Teaching and in Evaluation of Physiological and Clinical Competence; Suggested Physiological and Clinical Problems

The reader who has already come this far will have some idea of the potential ways in which a model such as MacPuf can be used for teaching medical students and post-graduates. I am far from sure how to use this educational resource to the best advantage. Some of the ways in which computer simulation models have been used at McMaster University and at University College Hospital and at St. Bartholomew's Hospital Medical Colleges are as follows:

(1) Simulation models can simply be supplied as an educational resource on an existing Medical School computer system, being made available with an explanatory brochure, so that students can call up a model and play about with it in any way that takes their fancy, to get the feel of quantitative aspects of respiratory physiology and clinical respiratory problems. Some students have been entertained by this, and some may even have learnt something, but I doubt whether it is worth the trouble and expense of making models available only in this way. Models are totally different from programmed texts, in which the student's sequence of operations is planned in outline right from the starting line to the finishing post. Without guidance students are likely to waste their own as well as the computer's time.

(2) A model can be offered as an educational resource for a specific course, with some attempt by the class or small group instructor to introduce the model at the start of the course. Undoubtedly, as I have seen both in Canada and in Great Britain, a good introductory talk preferably accompanied by a demonstration well-planned in advance can excite the interest of many students. However, unless they are given some properly defined objectives most students quickly lose interest, after they have amused them-

selves making the model produce a mass of semi-humorous symptoms.

(3) Given enough resources the computer terminal (Teletype or visual display unit) can be treated as if it were a flexible piece of apparatus in a physiology practical class (such as a spirometer, Douglas bag, smoked drum, muscle lever, nerve stimulator or manometer) and MacPuf can be supplied in place of the animal or experimental subject. In the Department of Physiology of New York State University at Buffalo Dr. L. H. Farhi recently showed me a practical classroom equipped with a number of 10 character/second Teletypes around the sides of a room, each connected to a small flexible time-sharing computer in the department. Before the class the technician (as for an animal class) switches on the apparatus, logs in and loads the appropriate model for each terminal. The students enter, each armed with a simple instruction book and a set of practical exercises. With two students at each terminal, ten terminals will support a class of 20. Demonstrators can walk around, answering questions and giving help just as they do in a conventional animal class.

As I have already mentioned, the models the students use at Buffalo are quite small, of limited scope, but economical and practical to run. The criticism of offering a large holistic model such as MacPuf to such a class is that students do not usually know enough to take advantage of a holistic model and that they will waste large amounts of computer time to no purpose.

As a junior demonstrator in the Department of Physiology at Oxford I once had the job of anaesthetising, then decerebrating, decapitating or otherwise irreversibly mangling a dozen or so cats each week for the mammalian class. It is true that students learnt in this class how to handle living tissues, surgical instruments and apparatus, but they would have learnt these things anyway in the operating theatre and elsewhere. Such a class exercise is exceedingly extravagant in resources of all kinds, and, to say the very least, is far less aesthetic than a physiology practical class using computer terminals. Furthermore a well-planned and accurate holistic model is capable of interesting and surprising even a sophisticated researcher and instructor, as I shall attempt to show in Chapter 28. A student mammalian class very rarely, if ever does this. When they occur, the surprises are seldom of a scientifically valuable kind.

A time-sharing system large enough to contain MacPuf can usually support ten student users without embarrassing other simultaneous users of the system, because students spend most of their time thinking, arguing and writing, and relatively little actually operating the computer—which is as it should be. It would also be possible to keep the model in core and allow each user a small store compartment for the COMMON store integer and floating-point values, which would be processed by the stored programme on a time-sharing basis.

I shall mention the cost of this type of exercise in Appendix V, but it is still possible to make use of MacPuf in a department having only a single small dedicated computer, or only one time-sharing terminal avilable at any one time. There are several techniques which allow one or two students working in their own time to use a small dedicated computer or a single terminal. Many keen students are quite prepared to work at night and enjoy having the computer to themselves. Given around-the-clock operation, even a large class can be given the opportunity to do several simulated experiments each during, say, a two-month course. The only disadvantage of elective use of this kind is that the student himself must usually physically switch on and enter the few necessary keyboard instructions to start the model off. However, students not well enough motivated to find out how to do this are unlikely to get much out of any practical class, of any kind.

(4) A course can be designed around a problem-solving approach and a certain number of illustrative problems handed out. Students can be asked either to bring back solutions to one or more problems to their tutor, to a small group tutorial or even, if the students are extrovert enough, to a large class. The model is again demonstrated to the whole class; but it is presented not as a resource which has to be used but as one which can help a student to start sizing up a problem and to get to grips with it by doing experiments which will give him a feel for the quantities and time scales involved. I have tried to encourage students to regard the model as an extremely obliging subject who will patiently offer himself for any experiment, even a lethal one, and who will arrange all the necessary internal changes or external apparatus almost immediately, in whatever way an operator wishes to specify them.

An example of a problem suitable and relevant for a first year student of medicine is: 'What happens to a patient on the operating table, during anaesthesia with a 80% nitrous oxide and 20% oxygen gas mixture, when the oxygen cylinder runs out?' The instructor may supply the hint that nitrous oxide can be treated as an inert gas in the model, and the problem can be studied simply by acutely reducing inspired oxygen concentration to zero. Operation of MacPuf over the succeeding six minutes or so (until 'death' occurs) will quickly give the operator an impression of the frighteningly small stores of oxygen in the body and especially in the brain, and the relatively enormous stores of CO_2, and will remind him how dependent breathing is on cerebral oxygenation. If he follows out the problem, and perhaps restores the inspired oxygen to normal after brain depression by hypoxia, he will of course have to specify some artificial ventilation. This will take him to a consideration of the optimal rate and depth to produce normal alveolar gas tensions. If he is perceptive he may also notice evidence of long-persisting metabolic acidosis generated during the period of systemic hypoxia. The ramifications of even such a simple problem are very considerable, and I have seen very keen students spend many hours getting completely to grips with such a problem, and emerge at the end with a quantitative knowledge of body oxygen consumption and carbon dioxide output at rest, cardiac output and tissue gas stores, and realising how rapidly lack of oxygen switches on anaerobic respiration, thus producing organic acids which take time to be metabolised.

Another problem, perhaps more suitable to a senior or clinical student might be: 'What is the lowest haemoglobin compatible with life?' This can be studied in considerable depth using MacPuf. It involves consideration of oxygen consumption, haemoglobin dissociation curve changes with pH and 2,3-diphosphoglycerate concentration, cardiac output, alveolar ventilation, and the effects of exercise. A study of this problem in depth would, for example, prevent the newly-qualified doctor from getting too much alarmed by a chronically anaemic patient with a haemoglobin of 7 g/100 ml. (I have seen bank blood for transfusion ordered as an emergency measure in such a situation.)

This individual problem-solving approach, which is a keystone of the McMaster philosphy works very well in small groups. I have also used it with some success for two consecutive student years at University College Hospital in London and also at St. Bartholomew's Hospital, more recently. We have had a course on Applied Physiology of Respiration in which discrete problems have been studied by individual students who have reported back to the class with a short (10 minute) prepared lecture. This then becomes the basis for a discussion between students and staff. This technique is economical in Faculty time, does not go stale, and usually holds the interest of those students who are minded to come to the first session or two. Necessarily it leans on extrovert students to make it work.

The disadvantage of small groups is that each small group instructor has to be familiar with the model to be able to use it effectively.

(5) As an occasional entertainment a problem can be set as a class experiment, and all interested students invited to study it and to bring back solutions, with perhaps a prize offered for the best solution (e.g. to the problem about the lowest haemoglobin compatible with life, or to the problem of bringing back to normal ambient pressure a preset subject, previously compressed to 10 atmospheres, without the production of symptoms).

(6) Individual students who show the necessary aptitude and interest can be invited to use the model intensively during a short elective period, and perhaps use it to design experiments in, for example, collection of expired air in different circumstances, comparing theoretical predictions of the model with data collected from himself or a colleague.

It is unrealistic to suppose that more than perhaps half an average class of medical students will get much out of a model like MacPuf, however it is presented. Although no mathematics to speak of, and no knowledge at all about computers is needed to operate the model, some medical students are psychologically antagonistic to any attempt to bring quantitative applied physiology to medicine. This attitude is irrational if it is adopted consistently by a doctor working in a hospital or any environment in which he has to use powerful and potentially dangerous therapeutic agents (such as artificial ventilators, oxygen, sodium bicarbonate, hyperbaric chambers, tracheostomy, ventilatory stimulants and depressants). Any such doctor needs to understand his subject to be able to handle these things safely. But knowledge of lung physiology is largely irrelevant for a psychiatrist, a dermatologist, a morbid anatomist, or a community physician. Anyone who brings this or other similar models into a medical curriculum therefore should not expect to interest or excite more than half the class, and he may only 'switch on' a quarter. Many students anyway are unfamiliar with the typewriter keyboard —incidentally another reason for avoiding text material having to be typed in by the operator.

However, the approach using simulation models for self-instruction has one considerable merit: it excites and stimulates the minds of the academically more gifted students of a group, who will generally select themselves by probing subjects in depth, asking difficult questions. Successful stimulation of such students, whose minds so often lie fallow during their student years, especially in the ambling British medical course, also has the effect of gingering up the Faculty, who have to keep finding answers to difficult questions.

This argument is my main justification for claiming some instructional value for MacPuf, even though my colleagues and I have not yet formally evaluated it by assessing student performance and understanding of some problem in two randomised groups, one being given and one being denied access to it. No doubt this needs to be done, but I do not want to do it myself. It seems enough if a student's interest is aroused, providing that he is not being taught or teaching himself knowledge or habits which are wrong or undesirable.

I hope that readers of this book who acquire the model, use it in an educational context, and run into problems or inaccuracies will write to me direct, or inform the Software Supervisor at the Computation Services Unit, McMaster, who has kindly offered to provide the services of a clearing house. Models of the size and complexity of the one I have described cannot be wholly accurate, but they are capable of being indefinitely improved and refined. We need to hear of difficulties and failures before we can correct them.

Potential use of models in evaluation of competence in physiology and clinical medicine

Most courses in biology incorporate a practical examination involving dissection of a dead animal. Many courses in physiology culminate with a practical examination in which a physiological experiment is performed on an anaesthetised animal. Almost all medical schools attempt to assess their students' clinical competence by an examination carried out on a real patient. Since I have claimed that the respiratory model described in this book is accurate and realistic enough to simulate physiological and clinical problems, there is obviously a potential use of such a model to assess competence in physiological and clinical understanding, and in medical problem management. I have no experience whatever of such applications, but some of the problems involved in using simulation models and other computer devices for testing competence of physicians have recently been admirably summarised by Senior (1976). The chief bar to the use of any computer model for an exercise in evaluation is that at least half an average class of students of physiology or medicine will be unfamiliar with the typewriter keyboard, visual display unit and computer interaction. When such familiarity is truly universal in a particular course or class, then it becomes entirely logical to consider the use of computer models in evaluation exercises. Recently Dr. K. Ahmed and I have devised a simple system ('McAid') in which a short Fortran driver programme controls the output of text and questions, from a text file which is not itself compiled. We have been able to arrange a question and answer sequence and then allow the user to branch into the model, which is treated as a subroutine of the Fortran driver programme. Control can then return to the question-and-answer sequence in a completely flexible way. Such a system allows one to envisage the possibility of a student or physician sitting at a terminal and being presented with an interactive dialogue in the course of which a variety of physiological or clinical simulations might be produced, and the examinee's efforts scored in some appropriate manner. Some initial progress along these lines, and a discussion of the difficulties involved is given in Senior's helpful review.

Suggested problems, suitable for examination in depth using MacPuf

Since, as I pointed out in Chapter 1, there is virtually an infinite number of problems which can be examined by MacPuf it is only possible to list a minute proportion of them here; but these may suffice to give some idea of the range of problems which can be studied. The problems embrace virtually the whole of clinical respiratory physiology apart from detailed consideration of lung mechanics, which are only sketchily simulated in the model. The problems which follow have already been tried out on students, who have had no difficulty in running the model so as to produce sensible answers. I have divided up the problems into mainly 'physiological' ones suitable for first or second year students, and to more clinically relevant problems which are more likely to interest third or fourth year clinical students and postgraduates. In each case I have supplied in brackets hints to the student how the model can be used to examine the problem.

Physiological problems

1. Examine the effects of increased venous admixture on blood gases, keeping total ventilation fixed (using the artificial ventilation option). Plot P_aO_2 and P_aCO_2 against the percentage shunt. What happens if you do the same with natural ventilation? (Use factor 5 to specify a fixed shunt added to the small natural shunt, and allow time in each case for a steady state to be reached.) What can you deduce from your results about the shapes of the oxygen and carbon dioxide dissociation curves of blood?

2. Examine the effects of increased dead space on blood gases, first with fixed artificial ventilation (e.g. 15 l/min, tidal volume 500 cc) and then with natural ventilation. (Use factor 6 to add extra dead space.) How much improvement in alveolar ventilation might be expected from tracheostomy (reducing dead space by 70 cc—make factor 6 equal to -70 for this).

3. What is the highest altitude compatible with life (a) at rest, (b) with minimal exercise? (Factor 13 specifies barometric pressure in mmHg; minimal exercise such as walking on the flat increases metabolic rate—factor 4—to about 300% resting value.) What changes occur with acclimatisation which help survival at low barometric pressures?

4. Investigate the limitation of exercise tolerance with progressive reduction of (a) cardiac output (progressively reduce cardiac performance—factor 3) and/or (b) ventilatory capacity (factor 24). (Probably best first to make a normal subject exercise moderately: factor $4 = 600\%$ resting value corresponds roughly to a work load of 600 kpm/min.) What limits the exercise

tolerance of patients with (a) heart disease and (b) lung disease in practice?

5. Examine the effects of breathing 5% carbon dioxide (factor 2 is inspired CO_2 concentration). In a steady state what is the relation between the rise of arterial PCO_2 and the rise of total ventilation (expressed as a ratio of mmHg/l/min)? Perform a dynamic CO_2 response curve by making MacPuf rebreathe from a small bag (e.g. 6 litres) filled initially with oxygen. Is the steady state sensitivity to CO_2 different from the dynamic response? If so, why? (Bag rebreathing is available by asking to change factor 100—for so-called 'SPECIAL EXPERIMENTS'; this allows specification of the volume and composition of a bag.)

6. What happens if the body becomes acutely acid, e.g. through the development of lactic acidosis? (Use factor 21 to specify the addition of acid: making this − 100 will have the same effect as acutely adding 100 mmol of HCl to the body). How closely does the end result mimic chronic metabolic acidosis? (Allow time for each 100 mmol or so of acid to circulate and for the resultant changes to settle.)

7. During the 200 metre dash it is estimated that total metabolic rate (factor 4) rises to the *equivalent* of 7 litres oxygen consumed per minute (about 2800% normal resting value), and cardiac output rises to about 30 l/min. Examine the sequence of events, in short (e.g. 4 s) runs at a short iteration interval (e.g. 2 s) (use the '4. RUN CHANGE' option to change length and type of run; change factor 4 alone since the heart will respond automatically—though you can modify the cardiac response by changing factor 3; RQ (factor 15) should also presumably be 1.0 since carbohydrate will be metabolised). Compare the possible maximum oxygen delivery to this demand. How does the body meet the demand during and after the dash? What is the maximum oxygen consumption which could be sustained, e.g. for a 5-mile run, at 25–30 l/min cardiac output? (It is advisable to use the '4. INSPECT' table frequently to examine the oxygen stores and acid–base state of the blood and tissues.)

8. The respiratory neurones in the brain stem have some intrinsic activity independent of chemical stimuli (this function is represented in 'MacPuf' by factor 12). There is also a potential stimulus from hypoxia (factor 11) and from a rise of PCO_2 (factor 10). Try eliminating each of these factors separately and in various combinations (i.e. by making their value equal to zero). What happens to ventilation and blood gases? What clinical conditions have you simulated?

9. What are the effects of a prolonged period of hyperventilation? (Use the artificial ventilation option to give an excessive total ventilation, e.g. 15/min; tidal volume 1000–1500 cc. Run for 3–6 minutes, then return acutely to natural ventilation.) What can you infer about the central control of respiration by CO_2 and about the time course of the response?

10. Examine the most economical way to breathe by looking at the steady state gas tensions with a total ventilation 7.2 l/min produced by 6 breaths/min of 1200 cc, 9 breaths/min of 800 cc, 12 breaths/min of 600 cc, 18 breaths/min of 400 cc, and 36 breaths/min of 200 cc (use the artificial ventilation option). Why is tachypnoea in pneumonia disadvantageous? What causes it? What are the probable (teleological) disadvantages of breathing only, say, once per minute?

11. Devise a means to measure the oxygen consumption of the respiratory muscles, and by extrapolating from results at about 20, 40 and 60 l/min total ventilation determine the probable resting O_2 consumption of the respiratory muscles. Do the same for preset subject No. 5 with airways obstruction and ventilatory failure. Is the oxygen consumption the same? If not, why not? (This exercise requires stimulation of ventilation, either by CO_2 inhalation or by increasing central neurogenic drive simulating voluntary hyperventilation.)

12. Exercise a normal subject (e.g. at 400, 600 and 800% resting metabolic rate), and collect the expired gas in a bag (use factor 100 to specify bag collection). If you also determined mixed venous PCO_2 at each level of exercise, what could you deduce by this bloodless technique which might be helpful in the clinical assessment of a patient?

'Clinical' problems

13. Examine cardiac arrest (factor 3 = zero), such as might occur through ventricular fibrillation after a myocardial infarct. What happens if the heart is restarted at, say, half normal contractile function after a 3 to 6 minute arrest? (The iteration interval is reduced to prevent the model having to compute impossibly large swings of gas tensions.) Why is the administration of bicarbonate desirable and sometimes lifesaving? (Use the 'INSPECT' table to look at the tissue acid–base status and oxygen stores; examine particularly the content and partial pressure of CO_2 in the tissues.)

14. A surgeon during a banquet becomes suddenly blue in the face, stops breathing and loses consciousness. Necropsy shows a lump of steak wedged in his larynx. What events follow acute asphyxia? (You can simulate asphyxia by using zero artificial ventilation, or, more realistically, by obstructing the glottis—an option available if you change factor 100 for 'SPECIAL' experiments.) Would you have time to fetch a scalpel or forceps from your car?

15. What is the lowest haemoglobin compatible with life? (Change factor 18—haemoglobin—and factor 19—packed cell volume appropriately.) What adaptive changes take place (*a*) at once (as shown in 'MacPuf') and (*b*) in a few days? (The effects of increased levels of 2,3-diphosphoglycerate can be simulated by changing factor 23.)

16. An endo-tracheal tube slips into the right main bronchus, blocking off the whole left lung (not all that uncommon an accident). What happens? (Consider the likely effects on dead space (factor 6), effective lung volume (factor 7), venous admixture (factor 5) and lung stiffness (elastance) (factor 8).)

17. A patient throws off a large pulmonary embolus which blocks the right main pulmonary artery. What happens? (Consider cardiac output, dead space, lung elastance.) In practice, arterial PO_2 is commonly low and respiratory rate increased. What additional factors may play a part in the clinical syndrome? (When local PCO_2 in part of the lung falls, its elastance increases.)

18. Take one or two ready-made subjects with airways obstruction, chronic CO_2 retention and hypoxaemia (ask for 'PRESETS' and 'PRESET PATIENTS' 5 or 6). Calculate for each the possible maximum tissue oxygen delivery with (1) room air, (2) 24%, (3) 28%, (4) 60%, (5) 100% oxygen in the

inspired air. Why is a high inspired oxygen concentration dangerous in patients with severe ventilatory failure?

19. Try to explain periodic (Cheyne–Stokes) breathing in terms of altered respiratory control mechanisms. (PRESET PATIENT No. 7.) (Consider central neurogenic drive to breathing (factor 12); central CO_2 sensitivity (factor 10), cardiac output (factor 3) and venous admixture (factor 9).) Can you reproduce this effect by making changes in a normal subject, and what effects do the following have and why: (1) inhalation of CO_2, (2) inhalation of oxygen, and (3) altered cardiac output?

20. Hyperbaric oxygen (e.g. 100% oxygen at two atmospheres pressure) has been used in medical treatment. How much extra oxygen is potentially supplied to the tissues by this means? In what circumstances could this teatment be beneficial? What are its dangers?

21. What happens, and how fast does it happen, when an anaesthetist's oxygen cylinder runs out and a patient is breathing, for example, pure nitrous oxide? (Change factor 1—inspired O_2—to zero.)

22. What proportion of one's airways can be blocked, compatible with life? (Consider first breathing capacity (factor 24) and elastance (factor 8) and then what you might expect to happen in terms of venous admixture (factor 9).)

23. In status asthmaticus there is hypersecretion of mucus. This blocks the airways. What effect will this have? (Consider elastance and venous admixture; perhaps try successive increments of 10% in venous admixture and of 5 in elastance.) If we tell you that in moderately severe asthma (e.g. FEV_1 about 0.8) the P_aCO_2 is often *below* normal, what additional factors must be operating?

24. Consider a man with severe acute myocardial infarction with a cardiac output of, say, 2.5 l/min (reduce factor 3 to about 50%). What would happen if he developed pulmonary oedema (which increases both venous admixture (factor 9) and lung elastance (factor 8))? How could the disorder be treated?

25. Examine the effects of progressive reduction of body temperature to, say, 30 to 33 °C on respiration and body gases. (Factor 14 is body temperature. Use the 'INSPECT' table frequently to report on oxygen consumption, cardiac output, ventilation, and blood gases.) What are the effects on the partial pressure and oxygen content of arterial blood? Compare the effects of asphyxia in a normal and a severely hypothermic subject. Should the acid–base disturbance be corrected?

25. Take a normal subject breathing air and simulate a deep dive (e.g. to 4 atmospheres) for different lengths of time (e.g. 15 minutes, 30 minutes, 1 hour) with different kinds of decompression. Draw up schemes for safe ascent to the surface under these conditions. (This is a difficult and time-consuming problem, involving careful use of 'RUN CHANGE' options for length of run, the INSPECT table and other special display options to find out continually the amount of free nitrogen in the tissues. It uses a lot of computer time and should only be attempted by experienced 'MacPuf' operators!) What causes death in acute 'decompression sickness'?

27. What are the effects of a left-to-right intracardiac shunt? (Factor 28, normal value zero, will create a 1:1 shunt if it is made equal to 1.0, and a 2:1 shunt if it is made 2.0, and so on.) Using the 'INSPECT' table examine the

values of tissue blood and arterial blood oxygen and CO_2 contents in comparison with mixed venous blood contents (from the right heart): in the steady state work out how to calculate the percentage shunt from the measured content values. Do your calculations agree with your specified shunt?

SUMMARY

Models can be used in teaching in different ways. Probably the best context is a small group meeting with a tutor to discuss a problem, and (better still) with students taking away individual problems for study in depth using the model. Not all students take to using models; but about half an average class will find them interesting and learn from them.

Twelve preliminary 'physiological' and 15 'clinical' experiments are listed and described. All have been tried with student classes, and all can be examined in quantitative detail using the model.

28
Clinical and Research Applications

Insofar as MacPuf has already increased the understanding of some doctors and students treating patients with acute respiratory diseases it may have already been of some clinical use; but I cannot truthfully claim that it has yet brought any tangible direct clinical benefit to an individual patient. It may be worth speculating briefly about the possible ways in which such a model could do so in future.

First, as I mentioned in Chapter 21, it is possible to make use of the model's ability to work itself into a steady state after any moderate change in its parameters. Since changes can be indirectly specified in terms of sex, height, weight and age and in terms of measured values for respiratory function tests, it is possible to build up in the model a simulation of almost any individual patient. (At present MacPuf has a lower age limit of 8 years, since I have not yet been able to find reliable data tables of all the predicted values needed for the unknown parameters for smaller children.) Having created the patient, further changes can be made. If, for example, the operator has measured values for haemoglobin, packed cell volume, cardiac function and ventilatory response to CO_2 he can make his simulated subject even more closely resemble the real-life patient. Venous admixture (factor 9) and dead space (factor 6) can be adjusted to give precisely the observed arterial gas tensions. Bicarbonate or acid can be added and brain bicarbonate similarly changed to create chronic metabolic alkalosis or acidosis. It is then possible to give a quantitative answer to such clinically relevant questions as:

Could this person safely travel in an aircraft pressurised to 7000 feet? Should he be able to perform moderate exercise (e.g. 600 kpm/min)? If the model says he should be able to do so, and he says he cannot, the way would be open to planning further clinical observations which could be compared with model predictions to find whether the limitation of exercise was due, for example, to limited cardiac performance or to inadequate psychological motivation.

Could he safely be given a general anaesthetic, assuming known changes resulting therefrom in, say, metabolic rate, cardiac performance, dead space and increased venous admixture? How much margin of safety would there be?

What blood gases could be expected if such a person was ventilated 14 times/min at 600 cc tidal volume, and 5 cm H₂O positive end-expiratory pressure, using 35% oxygen?

Could he spend 20 minutes in a diving bell at 3 atmospheres pressure, and safely ascend to the surface at once?

Would he be able to survive an acute haemorrhage bringing haemoglobin down to 6 g/100 ml?

A second way in which a model such as MacPuf can be used is in quantifying the functional disorder of a patient, e.g. in terms of effective venous admixture and effective dead space. In a steady state, given a known rate of production of carbon dioxide (which can be readily measured) there is only one value of effective dead space which gives the correct PCO_2 for the measured total ventilation. Simple arithmetical formulae are, of course, available which do not necessitate the use of a complex computer model; and the same applies to effective venous admixture, which can be computed and adjusted to match blood gas findings, if haemoglobin and acid–base status are known. However, a holistic model allows every possible interfering factor to be taken into account.

A third more elaborate way of quantitative assessment and prediction is being explored at present by some of my colleagues who have made a further computer programme capable of searching in one or more 'dimensions' to match a computer patient to the real one. Having created a good initial match in terms of body size, sex and age, the computer can be instructed to run through MacPuf computations until a steady state is reached, then progressively to change, for example, dead space and venous admixture until the unique match is found which gives the correct value for that subject. Such a technique requires a larger computer than the relatively small one on which MacPuf can be run; and the programme of the model is then a part of the whole system, rather than comprising the whole system.

A fourth development along the same lines is also conceivable. We are trying to use it in a Premature Baby Unit to predict the ideal percentage of inspired oxygen to bring the arterial oxygenation of the baby to a safe value between damaging hypoxia and damaging hyperoxia, and to predict in advance the likely course of respiratory changes perhaps 10 minutes ahead of real time. (This will obviously involve considerable further research to adjust model parameters and dissociation curves to conditions in the new-born; but in principle it should not be difficult.)

Many other clinical applications are possible. Especially if the model parameters can be crucially tested against actual observations (e.g. see Chapter 23) and can be adjusted if necessary to give accurate matches of observation to computer prediction, MacPuf could be used to design the best techniques for administration of oxygen, for example, in states of acute decompression in aircraft; or to draw up tables for individual subjects of the safe limits for staged decompression after deep dives. Minor additions to the model could easily be made to include the representation of other gases (e.g. helium).

Despite this (I hope) impressive catalogue, the clinical value of MacPuf is likely to be greatest in its educational role, even for the dedicated professional clinician. It is instructive, for example, to be able to follow the speed and phasic relations of changes, e.g. in brain and body gas stores, in metabolic or respiratory acidosis, in impending asphyxia, impaired cardiac performance or after changes in inspired gas concentrations. It is salutary to appreciate the difference between the less important things one can easily measure (such as the arterial PO_2) and the vital things that one cannot measure (e.g. the brain oxygen store). A few sessions with a holistic model can lessen the arrogant confidence of those who hope to practise acute respiratory medicine on measurements rather than on understanding.

Potential research value of the model

Many people, usually justly, scorn the research uses of models of all kinds. However the fact may be disguised, any discovery that is made through using a model will be essentially tautologous, i.e. it can only tell you what you could work out anyway from the premises, quantitative relationships and experimental data which are incorporated in the model. But sometimes the intellectual or mathematical sophistication needed to do this is of a much higher order than most of us possess, because of the reaction of each part of a complex system with every other part of the system, at different rates. To return to my introductory example: Watson and Crick's physical model of the DNA molecule could have been checked for internal consistency by purely mathematical geometric techniques, but it would have been a formidable undertaking. It was far simpler, and much more convincing for the less mathematically sophisticated, to fashion a physical model of the structure to see whether hydrogen bonds could be formed at the appropriate places, and whether the molecule could assume and maintain the proposed double helix structure. The use of a holistic model of gas exchange and gas transport is, on a much lower intellectual plane, exactly analogous. I believe that MacPuf is in most of its essential structures and relationships internally consistent and accurate enough for us to be able to build upon it, and argue from it. I can best illustrate the potential research value or insights available from such a model by a few examples.

Why is the administration of bicarbonate sometimes life-saving after cardiac arrest? The simple answer is that anaerobic respiration generates metabolic acids and extra carbon dioxide in the tissues. Severe tissue acidosis is bad for you, and may irreversibly damage vital functions such as co-ordinated cardiac contraction. Having examined cardiac arrest and recovery from cardiac arrest using MacPuf (in the first place as part of a small-group exercise with students) it now appears to me that the persistent tissue acidosis is probably importantly a function of the high tissue PCO_2, and that because of the metabolic acid and low bicarbonate in the tissues the amount of CO_2 which can be carried away by the blood is much reduced. It is possible for the tissue PCO_2 to be 100 mmHg despite a subnormal concentration of carbon dioxide in the effluent venous blood, e.g. only 50 volumes per cent. This means that until the metabolic acidosis is corrected by the administration of bicarbonate, or by the very slow metabolism of lactic acid by the anoxic liver, it is not possible for the excess carbon dioxide to be carried away by the blood, so that the acidosis in the tissues will persist for a very long time. Administration of bicarbonate prevents the works (of tissue gas exchange) getting gummed up, although relatively small quantities are usually enough to improve matters. Perhaps this way of looking at the effect of bicarbonate is well known; it certainly was not to me before I began to investigate it in the model.

Why are hypothermic patients often not cyanosed despite a low P_aO_2? It is obvious, like so many things, when one thinks about it carefully. I realised the answer when examining hypothermia in another student exercise. The blood can have a normal content of oxygen at a much lower than normal PO_2 if the temperature is, say, 30 °C; the empirical equations of Kelman embedded in MacPuf show that the reduction of PO_2 may be very considerable. Use of MacPuf in simulated hypothermia reminds one that what appears to be a dangerously reduced total ventilation may be entirely adequate for a state in which the metabolic production of CO_2 is perhaps only 80 cc/minute. This sort of insight can be clinically helpful in demonstrating the pitfall of rushing into unnecessary or excessive artificial ventilation.

Would it be possible to estimate the arterial PO_2 approximately by a blood-less technique in which a subject breathed first from air and then from 100% oxygen in a closed system whose volume was continuously monitored? According to my calculations from MacPuf such a technique could give an acceptably accurate answer to the question, 'Does this patient need oxygen?'

Can all the phenomena known to occur with acute decompression after long exposure to high barometric pressures be adequately simulated by a model in which there are assumed to be only two tissue compartments for nitrogen, a slow one and a fast-exchanging one? I believe that the answer is probably 'yes'—in which case MacPuf could be used to predict the probable outcome of different decompression regimes as a basis for experimental and (eventually) human studies.

What is the optimum length of time at different respiratory rates for a rebreathing procedure designed to determine mixed venous PCO_2, starting from a 1200 cc bag containing 7% CO_2 in oxygen?

Given a known degree of adaptation in terms of a known increase of red cell 2,3-diphosphoglycerate concentration and a known decrease of brain and whole body bicarbonate concentration, what percentage oxygen enrichment would be necessary to enable a 25 year old man of 175 cm and 62 kg to perform continuously a work-load of 900 kpm/min at 10000 feet altitude?

What is the effect of a change in lung volume, *per se*, on the nitrogen washout curve?

Can the apparently paradoxical observation of an arterial, and even some-times a mixed venous PCO_2 *lower* than the alveolar PCO_2 during certain rebreathing manoeuvres in man (Jones, McHardy, Naimark and Campbell, 1966) and in dog (Jennings and Chen, 1975), be explained by known physio-logical relationships, or must a new hitherto unsuspected mechanism be invoked to explain it? Under certain conditions MacPuf appears to show this anomalous behaviour. I am still investigating the reason for it, but its interest lies in the possibility of being able to explain the phenomenon by some simple means.

What is the explanation for the clinical observation that return to air-breathing of a patient with severe chronic ventilatory failure previously breathing high concentrations of oxygen may result in fatal hypoxaemia?

Before examining this problem on MacPuf I believed, following the suggestions of Dr. E. J. M. Campbell, that this was due to the relentless effect of the alveolar air equation, so that the large excess of accumulated CO_2 being blown off through the lungs would not allow enough room for an adequate alveolar oxygen tension to be achieved, so that the original steady state on air breathing could not be regained before hypoxia became fatal. When examining the problem in MacPuf I was able artificially to create conditions in which this occurred; but if a reasonably realistic ventilatory response to hypoxia was assumed, this explanation was not adequate. The large amounts of oxygen stored in the lungs of such subjects after oxygen breathing provide a buffer against an unduly rapid fall of alveolar PO_2, and P_aO_2 is also stabilised by the small total ventilation at the time. It now appears to us that the sometimes fatal effect of return to air breathing in this situation is more likely due to the progressive shutting down of alveoli during the shallow breathing resulting from the initial relief of hypoxia. This could result in a considerable increase in effective venous admixture which is the more likely cause of clinical deterioration.

I do not know yet whether this interpretation is correct; but the insight gained by studying this problem in a holistic model has already pointed the way to designing further experiments to investigate the problem. Similarly, the insights that my colleagues and I have gained using the model in some of the other situations mentioned—and these could be indefinitely multiplied—have helped at least to clarify our thoughts. It is my hope, as well as the *raison d'être* of this book, that other users of MacPuf may find the model equally useful.

SUMMARY

A holistic model of respiration and gas transport can provide quantitative answers to clinically difficult questions. It can give a simple means of quantifying a respiratory disorder in terms of functional disorders. This analysis is in principle capable of being further automated by computer techniques. It is possible even to envisage the model being used on-line in a predictive capacity in a real clinical situation, although probably the main clinical use of the model will remain its educative role.

Its main use in research is in providing insights into the way a complex system works, thus allowing theoretical analysis of a problem to pave the way for crucial experiments. It must always be true that a model cannot itself generate new discoveries, but can help to point the way in which future observations and measurements can be most relevant and helpful.

References

Adair, G. S. (1925). The hemoglobin system VI. The oxygen dissociation curve of hemoglobin. *J. biol. Chem.*, **63**, 529–545

Barcroft, J. (1934). *Features in the Architecture of Physiological Function* (Cambridge: Cambridge University Press)

Briscoe, W. A. (1965). Lung volumes. In *Handbook of Physiology*, Sect. 3, II (ed. W. O. Fenn and H. Rahn), 1345–1379 (Washington, D.C.: Amer. Physiol. Soc.)

Butler, J. P. and Mohler, J. G. (1970). The alveolar-arterial difference for O_2 and CO_2 in an infinite alveolus lung model. *Math. Biosc.*, **9**, 195–203

Christiansen, J., Douglas, C. G. and Haldane, J. S. (1914). The absorption and dissociation of carbon-dioxide by blood. *J. Physiol. (Lond.)*, **48**, 244–271

Clegg, B. R., Goodman, L. and Fleming, D. G. (1964). A dynamic model of respiratory regulation with peripheral and medullary chemosensors. *Proc. 17th Ann. Conf. on Engineering in Med. and Biol.*, Cleveland, Ohio, 11

Cohen, R. D. and Yudkin, J. (1975). The contribution of the kidney to the removal of a lactic acid load under normal and acidotic conditions in the conscious rat. *Clin. Sci. and Mol. Med.*, **48**, 121–131

Cohen, R. D., Lloyd, M. H., Iles, R. A., Simpson, B. R., Strumm, J. M. and Layton, J. M. (1973). The effect of simulated metabolic acidosis on intracellular pH and lactate metabolism in the isolated perfused rat liver. *Clin. Sci. and Mol. Med.*, **45**, 543–549

Comroe, J. H., Jr., Forster, R. E., Dubois, A. B., Briscoe, W. A. and Carlsen, E. (1962). *The Lung* (2nd ed.) (Chicago: Year Book)

Cotes, J. E. (1966). The regulation of respiration during exercise in normal subjects. In *Breathlessness* (ed. J. B. L. Howell and E. J. M. Campbell), 93–113 (Oxford: Blackwell)

Curtis, A. S. G. (1974). *Decompression and narcosis*. N. D. C. Paper 1. (Glasgow: Scottish Sub-Aqua Club)

Defares, J. G. (1964). Principles of feedback control and their application to the respiratory control system. In *Handbook of Physiology*, Sect. 3, I (ed. W. O. Fenn and H. Rahn), 649–680 (Washington, D.C.: Amer. Physiol. Soc.)

Defares, J. G., Derksen, H. E. and Duyff, J. W. (1960). Cerebral blood flow in the regulation of respiration. *Acta Physiol. Pharmacol. Neerl.* **9**, 327–360

Dickinson, C. J. (1972). A digital computer model to teach and study gas transport and exchange between lungs, blood and tissues ('MacPuf'). *J. Physiol. (Lond.)*, **224**, 7–9P

Dickinson, C. J., Sackett, D. L. and Goldsmith, C. H. (1973). MacMan: A digital computer model for teaching some basic principles of haemodynamics. *J. clin. Computing*, **2**, 42–50

Eldridge, F. L. (1975). Relationship between turnover rate and blood concentration of lactate in exercising dogs. *J. appl. Physiol.*, **39**, 231–234

Farhi, L. E. (1964). Gas stores of the body. In *Handbook of Physiology*, Sect. 3, I (ed. W. O. Fenn and H. Rahn), 873–885 (Washington, D. C.: Amer. Physiol. Soc.)

Farhi, L. E. and Rahn, H. A. (1955). A theoretical analysis of the alveolo-arterial O_2 difference with special reference to the distribution effect. *J. appl. Physiol.*, **7**, 699–703

Farrell, E. J. and Siegel, J. H. (1973). Investigation of cardiorespiratory abnormalities through computer simulation. *Comput. Biomed. Res.*, **5**, 161–186

Fry, D. L. (1968). A preliminary lung model for simulating the aerodynamics of the bronchial tree. *Comput. Biomed. Res.*, **2**, 111–134

Fryer, D. I. (1969). *Subatmospheric Decompression Sickness in Man* (Slough: Technivision Services)

Fulton, J. F. (ed.) (1951). *Decompression Sickness* (Philadelphia and London: Saunders)

Geppert, J. and Zuntz, N. (1888). Ueber die Regulation der Athmung. *Pflug. Arch. ges. Physiol.*, **42**, 189–245

Gomez, D. (1963). A mathematical treatment of the distribution of tidal volume throughout the lung. *Proc. Nat. Acad. Sci. U.S.A.*, **49**, 312–319

Gray, J. S. (1945). *The Multiple Factor Theory of Respiratory Regulation*. U.S. Army Air Force School of Aviation Medicine Project Rept. 386 (1, 2, 3)

Gray, J. S. (1950). *Pulmonary Ventilation and its Physiological Regulation* (Springfield: Thomas)

Green, H. D. (1944). Circulation: physical principles. In *Medical Physics* (ed. O. Glasser), Vol. 1, 208–232 (Chicago: Year Book)

Grodins, F. S. (1963). *Control Theory and Biological Systems* (Columbia: Columbia Univ. Press)

Grodins, F. S., Buell, J. and Bart, A. J. (1967). A mathematical analysis and digital computer simulation of the respiratory control system. *J. appl. Physiol.*, **22**, 260–276

Grodins, F. S., Gray, J. S., Schroeder, K. R., Norins, A. L. and Jones, R. W. (1954). Respiratory responses to CO_2 inhalation. A theoretical study of a non-linear biological regulator. *J. appl. Physiol.*, **7**, 283–308

Grodins, F. S. and James, G. (1963). Mathematical models of respiratory regulation. *Ann. N.Y. Acad. Sci.*, **100**, 852–868

Haldane, J. S. (1922). *Respiration* (1st ed.) (Oxford: Oxf. Univ. Press)

Haldane, J. S. and Priestley, J. G. (1935). *Respiration* (2nd ed.) (Oxford: Clarendon Press)

Hermansen, L. and Stensvold, I. (1972). Production and removal of lactate during exercise in man. *Acta Physiol. Scand.*, **86**, 191–201

Hess, W. R. (1927). Die Gesetze der Hydrostatik und Hydrodynamik. In *Hndbch d. normalen u. path. Physiol.* (Ed. A. Bethe, G. V. Bergmann, G. Embden and A. Ellinger). Vol. VII ii, 888–903 (Berlin: Springer)

Hey, E. N., Lloyd, B. B., Cunningham, D. J. C., Jukes, M. G. M. and Bolton, D. P. G. (1966). Effects of various respiratory stimuli on the depth and frequency of breathing in man. *Resp. Physiol.*, **1**, 193–205

Hill, E. P., Power, G. G. and Longo, L. D. (1973). Mathematical simulation of pulmonary O_2 and CO_2 exchange. *Amer. J. Physiol.*, **224**, 904–917

Hill, R. (1936). Oxygen dissociation curve of muscle haemoglobin. *Proc. roy. Soc. B.*, **120**, 472–483

Horgan J. D. and Lange, R. L. (1965). Digital computer simulation of respiratory responses to cerebrospinal fluid PCO_2 in the cat. *Biophysical J.*, **6**, 935–945

Hubbard, J. L. (1973). The effect of exercise on lactate metabolism. *J. Physiol. (Lond.)*, **231**, 1–18

Jennings, D. B. and Chen, C. C. (1975). Negative arterial-mixed expired PCO_2 gradient during acute and chronic hypercapnia. *J. appl. Physiol.*, **38**, 382–388

Jones, N. L., McHardy, G. J. R., Naimark, A. and Campbell, E. J. M. (1966). Physiological dead space and alveolar–arterial gas pressure differences during exercise. *Clin. Sci.*, **31**, 19–29

Katsaros, B., Loeschcke, H. H., Lerche, D., Shönthal, H. and Hahn, N. (1960). Wirkung der Bicarbonat–Alkalose auf die Lungenbelüftung beim Menschen. Bestimmung der Teilwirkungen von pH und CO_2-Druck auf die Ventilation und Vergleich mit der Ergebnissen bei Acidose. *Arch. ges. Physiol.*, **271**, 732–747

Kellog, R. H. (1964). Central chemical regulation of respiration. In *Handbook of Physiology*, Sect. 3, I (ed. W. O. Fenn and H. Rahn), 507–534 (Washington, D.C.: Amer. Physiol. Soc.)

Kelman, G. R. (1966). Digital computer subroutine for the conversion of oxygen tension into saturation. *J. appl. Physiol.*, **21**, 1375–1376

Kelman, G. R. (1967). Digital computer procedure for the conversion of PCO_2 into blood CO_2 content. *Respir. Physiol.*, **3**, 111–115

Kelman, G. R. (1970). A new lung model: An investigation with the aid of a digital computer. *Comput. Biomed. Res.*, **3**, 241–248

King, T. K. C. and Briscoe, W. A. (1967). Bohr integral isopleths in the study of blood gas exchange in the lung. *J. appl. Physiol.*, **22**, 659–674

Kreisberg, R. A. (1972). Glucose–lactate inter-relations in man. *New Engl. J. Med.*, **287**, 132–137

Lanphier, E. H. (1958). Nitrogen–oxygen mixture physiology, phases 4 and 6. U.S. Naval Experimental Diving Unit, Research Rept., 7–58. Washington D.C.

Lassen, N. A. (1959). Cerebral blood flow and oxygen consumption in man. *Physiol. Rev.*, **39**, 183–238

Lerche, D., Katsaros, B., Lerche, G. and Loeschcke, H. H., (1960). Vergleich der Wirkung verschiedener Acidosen (NH₄Cl, CaCl₂, Acetazolamid) auf die Lungenbelüftung beim Menschen. *Arch. ges. Physiol.*, **270**, 450–460

Lloyd, B. B. and Cunningham, D. J. C. (1963). A quantitative approach to the regulation of human respiration. In *The Regulation of Human Respiration* (ed. D. J. C. Cunningham and B. B. Lloyd), 331–349 (Oxford: Blackwell)

Matthews, C. M. E., Laszlo, G., Campbell, E. J. M. and Read, D. J. C. (1968). A model for the distribution and transport of CO_2 in the body, and the ventilatory responses to CO_2. *Resp. Physiol.*, **6**, 45–87

Meyer, J. S., Ryu, T., Toyoda, M., Shinohara, Y., Wiederholt, I. and Guiraud, B. (1969). Evidence for a Pasteur effect regulating cerebral oxygen and carbohydrate metabolism in man. *Neurology*, **19**, 954–962

Milhorn, H. T., Jr., Benton, H., Ross, R. and Guyton, A. C. (1965). A mathematical model of the human respiratory control system. *Biophys. J.*, **5**, 27–46

Milhorn, H. T., Jr., and Brown, D. R. (1971). Steady-state summation of the human respiratory system. *Comput. Biomed. Res.*, **3**, 604–619

Milhorn, H. T., Jr., Reynolds, W. J. and Holloman, G. H., Jr. (1972). Digital simulation of the ventilatory response to CO_2 inhalation and CSF perfusion. *Comput. Biomed. Res.*, **5**, 301–314

Miller, N. C. and Walters, R. F. (1974). Interactive modelling as a forcing function for research in the physiology of human performance. *Simulation*, Jan. 1974, 1–13

Modell, M. I., Farhi, L. E. and Olszowka, A. J. (1974). Physiology teaching through computer simulations—problems and promise. *Physiology Teacher*, **3**, 14–16

Padget, P. (1927). The respiratory response to carbon dioxide. *Amer. J. Physiol.*, **83**, 384–394

Paiva, M. and Demeester, M. (1971). Gas transport in the air phase of the lung simulated by a digital computer. *Comput. Biomed. Res.*, **3**, 675–689

Patterson, J. L., Jr. (1965). Circulation through the brain. In *Physiology and Biophysics* (ed. T. R. Ruch and H. D. Patton), 950–958 (Philadelphia: Saunders)

Pernow, B., Wahren, J. and Zetterquist, S. (1965). Studies on the peripheral circulation and metabolism in man. IV. Oxygen utilization and lactate formation in the legs of healthy young men during strenuous exercise. *Acta Physiol. Scand.*, **64**, 284–298

Radford, E. P., Jr. (1964). The physics of gases. In *Handbook of Physiology*, Sect. III, 1 (ed. W. O. Fenn and H. Rahn), 125–152 (Washington, D.C.: Amer. Physiol. Soc.)

Read, D. J. C. (1966). A clinical method for assessing the ventilatory response to carbon dioxide. *Austral. Ann. Med.*, **16**, 20–32

Rebuck, A. S. and Campbell, E. J. M. (1973). A clinical method for assessing the ventilatory response to hypoxia. *Amer. Rev. resp. Dis.*, **109**, 345–350

Riley, R. L., and Cournand, A. (1949). 'Ideal' alveolar air and the analysis of ventilation–perfusion relationships in the lungs. *J. appl. Physiol.*, **1**, 825–847

Roughton, F. J. W. (1964). Transport of oxygen and carbon dioxide. In *Handbook of Physiology*, Sect. III, 1 (ed. W. O. Fenn and H. Rahn), 767–825 (Washington, D.C.: Amer. Physiol. Soc.)

Senior, J. R. (1976). *Toward the measurement of competence in medicine* (Philadelphia: National Board of Medical Examiners)

Severinghaus, J. W. (1966). The regulation of ventilation at rest. In *Breathlessness* (ed. J. B. L. Howell and E. J. M. Campbell), 85–92 (Oxford: Blackwell)

Shephard, R. J. (1966). The oxygen cost of breathing during vigorous exercise. *Quart. J. exp. Physiol.*, **51**, 336–350

Swanson, G. D. and Bellville, J. W. (1974). Hypoxic–hypercapnic interaction in human respiratory control. *J. appl. Physiol.*, **36**, 480–487

Tashkin, D. P., Goldstein, P. J. and Simmons, D. H. (1972). Hepatic uptake during decreased liver perfusion and hypoxaemia. *Amer. J. Physiol.*, **223**, 968–974

Warrell, D. A., Edwards, R. H. T., Godfrey, S. and Jones, N. L. (1970). Effect of controlled oxygen therapy on arterial blood gases in acute respiratory failure. *Brit. med. J.*, **1**, 452–455

Weibel, E. R. (1963). *Morphometry of the Human Lung* (New York: Acad. Press)

Weibel, E. R. (1964). Morphometrics of the lung. In *Handbook of Physiology*, Sect. III, 1 (ed. W. O. Fenn and H. Rahn), 285–307 (Washington, D.C.: Amer. Physiol. Soc.)

West, J. B. (1969). Ventilation–perfusion inequality and overall gas exchange in computer models of the lung. *Resp. Physiol.*, 7, 88–110

Yamamoto, W. and Hori, T. (1971). Phasic air movement model of respiratory regulation of carbon dioxide balance. *Comput. biomed., Res.*, 3, 699–717

Appendices

Appendix I

SHORT PROGRAMME DESCRIBING THE PASSAGE OF GASES THROUGH THE ARTERIAL COMPARTMENT ASSUMING COMPLETE MIXING

```
C ESTABLISH PLOTTING SYMBOLS
      INTEGER EX(1),DOT(1),BLANK(1),XLINE(72)
      DATA EX,DOT,BLANK/'X','.',' '/
2     WRITE(1,100)
100   FORMAT(' CO=')
C READ IN CARDIAC OUTPUT & FRACTIONAL TIME INTERVAL
      READ(2,200)CO
200   FORMAT(F4.1)
      WRITE(1,101)
101   FORMAT(' FT=')
      READ(2,201) FT
201   FORMAT(F6.5)
C INITIALIZE VALUES FOR ARTERIAL OXYGEN CONTENT & AMOUNT
C AND FOR INCOMING BLOOD CONTENT
      EO2CT=20.
      RO2MT=200.
      PO2CT=20.
C ITERATE TO PLOT VERTICAL GRAPH
      DO 1 I=1,20
C ADD INCOMING BLOOD TO POOL AND RECALCULATE NEW ARTERIAL
C O2 CONTENT
      RO2MT=RO2MT+FT*CO*10.*PO2CT
C COMPUTE NEW CONTENT, ASSUMING POOL VOLUME OF 1000 ML BLOOD
      EO2CT=RO2MT*100./(1000.+CO*FT*1000.)
C RELEASE BLOOD FROM POOL & RETURN TO INITIAL 1000 ML VOLUME
      RO2MT=RO2MT-FT*CO*10.*EO2CT
C CALCULATE NEW VALUE FOR EO2CT
C SPREAD PLOTTING VALUES PRIOR TO DISPLAY
      X=EO2CT*3.-15.
      KK=X
      DO 3 J=1,72
3     XLINE(J)=BLANK(1)
      XLINE(2)=DOT(1)
      XLINE(KK)=EX(1)
C AFTER INITIAL CONDITIONS DEFINED, ACUTELY CHANGE INCOMING
C BLOOD OXYGEN CONTENT(PO2CT)
      IF(I.GT.2)PO2CT=15.
C ADJUST TIME SCALING FOR 5 SEC INTERVALS OR 10 SECONDS BY INSERTING
C EXTRA SPACE FOR 10 SEC
      IF(FT.GT..085)WRITE(1,104)
1     WRITE(1,103)XLINE
      GO TO 2
103   FORMAT(72A1)
104   FORMAT(1X)
      END
```

Appendix II

ALTERNATIVE SHORT PROGRAMME GIVING AN IMPROVED DESCRIPTION ASSUMING PARTIAL MIXING

```
C ESTABLISH PLOTTING SYMBOLS
      INTEGER EX(1),DOT(1),BLANK(1),XLINE(72)
      DATA EX,DOT,BLANK/'X',',','','/
2     WRITE(1,100)
100   FORMAT(' CO=')
C READ IN CARDIAC OUTPUT & FRACTIONAL TIME INTERVAL
      READ(2,200)CO
200   FORMAT(F4.1)
      WRITE(1,101)
101   FORMAT(' FT=')
      READ(2,201) FT
201   FORMAT(F6.5)
C INITIALIZE VALUES FOR ARTERIAL OXYGEN CONTENT & AMOUNT
C AND FOR INCOMING BLOOD CONTENT
      EO2CT=20.
      RO2MT=200.
      PO2CT=20.
C ITERATE TO PLOT VERTICAL GRAPH
      DO 1 I=1,20
C CALCULATE NEW VALUE OF ART. O2 AMOUNT.  FACTOR OF 10 NEEDED
C TO CONVERT LITRES TO 100 ML QUANTITIES
      RO2MT=RO2MT+FT*CO*10.*(PO2CT-EO2CT)
C COMPUTE NEW CONTENT, ASSUMING POOL VOLUME OF 1000 ML BLOOD
      EO2CT=RO2MT*.1
C SPREAD PLOTTING VALUES PRIOR TO DISPLAY
      X=EO2CT*3.-15.
      KK=X
      DO 3 J=1,72
3     XLINE(J)=BLANK(1)
      XLINE(2)=DOT(1)
      XLINE(KK)=EX(1)
C AFTER INITIAL CONDITIONS DEFINED, ACUTELY CHANGE INCOMING
C BLOOD OXYGEN CONTENT(PO2CT)
      IF(I.GT.2)PO2CT=15.
C ADJUST TIME SCALING FOR 5 SEC INTERVALS OR 10 SECONDS BY INSERTING
C EXTRA SPACE FOR 10 SEC
      IF(FT.GT..085)WRITE(1,104)
1     WRITE(1,103)XLINE
      GO TO 2
103   FORMAT(72A1)
104   FORMAT(1X)
      END
```

Appendix III

ALTERNATIVE SHORT PROGRAMME (as in Appendix II), INCLUDING THE USE OF A DAMP FUNCTION

```
C ESTABLISH PLOTTING SYMBOLS
      INTEGER EX(1),DOT(1),BLANK(1),XLINE(72)
      DATA EX,DOT,BLANK/'X',',',' '/
C SET UP DAMPING FUNCTION
      DAMP(X,Y,Z)=(X*Z+Y)/(1.+Z)
2     WRITE(1,100)
100   FORMAT(' CO=')
C READ IN CARDIAC OUTPUT & FRACTIONAL TIME INTERVAL
      READ(2,200)CO
200   FORMAT(F4.1)
      WRITE(1,101)
101   FORMAT(' FT=')
      READ(2,201) FT
201   FORMAT(F6.5)
C INSERT DAMPING CONSTANT
      WRITE(1,107)
107   FORMAT(' DAMP CONST=')
      READ(2,202)Z
202   FORMAT(F4.1)
C INITIALIZE VALUES FOR ARTERIAL OXYGEN CONTENT & AMOUNT
C AND FOR INCOMING BLOOD CONTENT
      EO2CT=20.
      RO2MT=200.
      PO2CT=20.
C ITERATE TO PLOT VERTICAL GRAPH
      DO 1 I=1,20
C CALCULATE NEW VALUE OF ART. O2 AMOUNT.  FACTOR OF 10 NEEDED
C TO CONVERT LITRES TO 100 ML QUANTITIES
      RO2MT=RO2MT+FT*CO*10.*(PO2CT-EO2CT)
C INSERT DAMPING OF EFFLUENT ART. BLOOD O2 CONTENT BY TAKING
C VALUE PART-WAY BETWEEN INITIAL & FINAL VALUES
C COMPUTE NEW CONTENT, ASSUMING POOL VOLUME OF 1000 ML BLOOD
      EO2CT=DAMP(RO2MT*.1,EO2CT,Z)
C SPREAD PLOTTING VALUES PRIOR TO DISPLAY
      X=EO2CT*3.-15.
      KK=X
      DO 3 J=1,72
3     XLINE(J)=BLANK(1)
      XLINE(2)=DOT(1)
      XLINE(KK)=EX(1)
C AFTER INITIAL CONDITIONS DEFINED, ACUTELY CHANGE INCOMING
C BLOOD OXYGEN CONTENT(PO2CT)
      IF(I.GT.2)PO2CT=15.
C ADJUST TIME SCALING FOR 5 SEC INTERVALS OR 10 SECONDS BY INSERTING
C EXTRA SPACE FOR 10 SEC
      IF(FT.GT..085)WRITE(1,104)
1     WRITE(1,103)XLINE
      GO TO 2
103   FORMAT(72A1)
104   FORMAT(1X)
      END
```

Appendix IV

THE COMPLETE FORTRAN PROGRAMME OF 'MACPUF'

MACPUF MAIN PROGRAMME

```
        DIMENSION T(120),TJJ(8),NO(23),NTAB(23),C(70)
C INI,KT,KL = INPUT/OUTPUT NOS.; NW1,NW2,JKL,ITRIG AND NEOF USED IN
C INTERACTIVE DIALOGUE (S/R NXTWD). NW=1(NEW), NW=0(CHANGED SUBJECT)
        COMMON KT,KL,INI,NW1,NW2,JKL,ITRIG(73),NEOF,NW
C NFLAG IS SPARE (INIT.=1) FOR CODING ANY USER'S SPECIAL INSTRUCTIONS
C J3 + ND=TIME, ISPAR-NC, ALSO MT, CODE OUTPUT INSTRUCTIONS
        COMMON NFLAG,J3,ISPAR,NA,NB,NC,ND,NE(8)
C NARTI (1= NAT., 0= ARTIF.) VENTLN. K2+K4 CONCERN SYMPTOMS (S/R SYMPT)
C INDEX IS POINTER IN DELAY LINE, S/R DELAY.
        COMMON NARTI,MT,K2,K4,INDEX
        COMMON FIO2,FIC2,CO,PD,FADM,BULLA,VLUNG,ELAST,VADM,AZ,
     X    BZ,CZ,BARPR,TEMP,TRQ,TC2MT,TVOL,HB,PCV,VBLVL,
     X    ADDC3,BC3AJ,DPG,PR,FITNS,SPACE,COMAX,SHUNT,VC,PEEP,
     X    VO2CT,PA,RPH,VPH,FVENT,BPH,BAGO,BAGC,AO2MT,AC2MT,
     X    AO2PR,AC2PR,DPH,XLACT,BO2CT,BC2PR,TIDVL,RRATE,RO2CT,VC2MT,
     X    DVENT,SVENT,FC2CT,PO2CT,TO2CT,TC2CT,BO2CT,BC2CT,TPH,RC3CT,
     X    VC2CT,RO2MT,RC2MT,XRESP,AN2MT,BO2MT,BC2MT,CBF,PC,DSPAC,
     X    REFLV,RO2PR,CONSO,RC2PR,PG,PJ,TND,RC2CT,QB,PW,
     X    FT,CONOM,BUBBL,TC2RF,TC3MT,VC3MT,TC3CT,VC3CT,TLAMT,RLACT,
     X    BC3CT,BO2AD,COADJ,EO2CT,TO2MT,TO2PR,TC2PR,VO2MT,AVENT,PL,
     X    EC2CT,TN2MT,TN2PR,FEV,SN2PR,EN2CT,UN2MT,RN2MT,X109,X110,
     X    TC3AJ,SN2MT,QA,RVADM,XDSPA,BAG,XMALE,HT,WT,AGE
C COMMON TDLAY IS USED FOR GREATER ACCURACY, PROVIDING A DELAY IN VENOUS
C RETURN. IF S/R DELAY IS NOT USED THIS COMMON BLOCK CAN BE REMOVED
        COMMON TDLAY(40)
C COMMON NDUMP + TDUMP ARE ONLY USED FOR STORE/BACKTRACK (S/R DUMP)
        COMMON NDUMP(20),TDUMP(160)
C EQUIV.STATEMENT BELOW ECONOMISES ON LOCATIONS OF MULTI-USED LOCAL
C VARIABLES, AND MAKES LOCAL VARIABLES COMPUTED OUTSIDE MAIN 'DO' LOOP
C EQUIVALENT TO VALUES OF ARRAY C() PRECALCULATED BY S/R CONST
C*** THE WHOLE EQUIVALENCE OF C() CAN BE REMOVED AND VALUES FROM S/R
C*** CONST INSERTED IN THE PROGRAMME. THIS RUNS SLOWER, BUT SMALL STORE
C*** COMPUTERS MAY NOT ALLOW THE COMPLETE EQUIVALENCE STATEMENT BELOW
        EQUIVALENCE (C1,C(1)),(C2,C(2)),(C3,C(3)),(C4,C(4))
     X ,(C5,C(5)),(C6,C(6)),(C7,C(7)),(C8,C(8)),(C9,C(9))
     X ,(C10,C(10)),(C11,C(11)),(C12,C(12)),(C13,C(13)),(C14,C(14))
     X ,(C15,C(15)),(C16,C(16)),(C17,C(17)),(C18,C(18)),(C19,C(19))
     X ,(C20,C(20)),(C21,C(21)),(C22,C(22)),(C23,C(23)),(C24,C(24))
     X ,(C25,C(25)),(C26,C(26)),(C27,C(27)),(C28,C(28)),(C29,C(29))
     X ,(C30,C(30)),(C31,C(31)),(C32,C(32)),(C33,C(33)),(C34,C(34))
     X ,(C35,C(35)),(C36,C(36)),(C37,C(37)),(C38,C(38)),(C39,C(39))
     X ,(C40,C(40)),(C41,C(41)),(C42,C(42)),(C43,C(43)),(C44,C(44))
C    X ,(C45,C(45)),(C46,C(46)),(C47,C(47)),(C48,C(48)),(C49,C(49))
C    X ,(C50,C(50)),(C51,C(51)),(C52,C(52)),(C53,C(53)),(C54,C(54))
C    X ,(C55,C(55)),(C56,C(56)),(C57,C(57)),(C58,C(58)),(C59,C(59))
C    X ,(C60,C(60)),(C61,C(61)),(C62,C(62)),(C63,C(63)),(C64,C(64))
C    X ,(C65,C(65)),(C66,C(66)),(C67,C(67)),(C68,C(68)),(C69,C(69))
C    X ,(C70,C(70))
        EQUIVALENCE(ITRIG(73),NTAB(1)),(FIO2,T(1))
        DATA NO/0,1,1,1,0,1,18,0,1,0,69,33,51,35,60,41,72,74,1,1,0,0,1/
```

```
MACPUF MAIN PROGRAMME
CONTINUED

C LL1=1 IS NORMAL; 2 IS DEATH; 3 IS ARITH. ERROR
      DATA LL1,LL2,LL3/10,1,17/
C 'E' SPECIFIES V.SMALL QUANTITY TO AVOID ZERO DIVISIONS
      DATA E/.00000001/
C SET UP DAMPING AND PH FUNCTIONS FOR USE LATER
      DAMP(X,Y,Z)=(X*Z+Y)/(1.+Z)
      PHFNC(X,Y)=6.1+ALOG(X/(.03*Y))*.434294482
C***********************************************************************
C INI=INPUT, KT=OUTPUT DEVICE (TERMINAL), KL=OUTPUT DEVICE (FOR PLOTS)
      INI=2
      KT=1
      KL=1
C***********************************************************************
C INITIALISE ALL INDICES FOR STANDARD OUTPUT, ETC AND PRINT OPENING
      DO 100 I=1,23
  100 NTAB(I)=NO(I)
      WRITE (KT,110)
  110 FORMAT (' -- MACPUF -- VERSION 76.4 -- 1 NOVEMBER 1976 --',/)
C INITIALIZE ALL WORKING VALUES FOR A NEW SUBJECT
  170 CALL MINIT (LL1,LL3,LL4,NREPT,SIMLT)
C COMPUTE WORKING PARAMETERS UNCHANGED DURING THE RUN
  190 CALL CONST (C,NREPT,SIMLT)
C MAIN PROGRAMME LOOP OPERATES EVERY FT(FRACTIONAL TIME) MINUTE(S)
      DO 1590 MORAN=1,NREPT
C IF BAG REBREATHING IN ACTION MAKE INSPIRED GASES SAME AS IN BAG
      IF (PL-1.5) 210,210,200
  200 CALL BAGER (2,C12,C12,C12,SIMLT)
C INCREMENT LOOP COUNTER
  210 LL4=LL4+1
C NEXT AUTOMATICALLY INCREASES CARDIAC OUTPUT IF O2 SUPPLIED IS LOW
      Y=RO2CT*.056
  220 IF (Y-.35) 230,240,240
  230 Y=.35
C COADJ IS ADJUSTED CARD.OUTPUT,USED MAINLY AS INDEX FTCO
C WHICH TAKES ACCOUNT OF CARD.OUTPUT PER UNIT TIME.
C OUTPUT GOES UP AS TOTAL O2 CONSUMPTION INCREASES.
  240 COADJ=DAMP((C8/Y+C9/(Y**2))*C16,COADJ,C(61))
      IF (CO-3.) 250,260,260
C IF HEART STOPPED MAKE OUTPUT AT ONCE ZERO TO STOP ARTERIAL
C COMPOSITION CHANGING - 'E' IS A VERY SMALL NUMBER(DATA)
  250 COADJ=E
      GO TO 280
C LIMIT MAXIMUM CARDIAC OUTPUT
  260 IF (COADJ-COMAX) 280,280,270
  270 COADJ=COMAX
C FTCO IS NO. OF 100 ML PORTIONS OF BLOOD CIRCULATING PER FRACTIONAL
C TIME INTERVAL
  280 FTCO=C17*COADJ
      FTCOC=FTCO*(1.-C(69)*COADJ)
C O2 CONT.OR PRESS. INFLUENCES VEN. ADMIXTURE AND (V.SLOWLY) 2,3-DPG
      DPG=DPG+(23.3-RO2CT-DPG)*C10
      X=AO2PR
      IF (X-200.) 300,300,290
  290 X=200.
C INCREASE EFF.VEN.ADM.IF ALV.PO2 VERY HIGH
  300 Y=AO2PR
      IF (Y-600.) 320,320,310
  310 Y=600.
  320 IF (AO2PR-400.) 340,340,330
  330 X=X-(Y-400.)*.3
  340 IF (X-55.) 350,350,360
  350 X=55.
C PW=EFFECTIVE VENOUS ADMIXTURE, AFFECTED BY PEEP, ALV.PO2, ETC
C AND ALSO INCORPORATING A FIXED SHUNT COMPONENT, FADM
  360 PW=(C18/X+C19)*C21+FADM
C LIMIT RIDICULOUS ADMIXTURES EXCEEDING 100
      IF (PW-100.) 380,380,370
  370 PW=100.
  380 X=PW*.01
```

MACPUF MAIN PROGRAMME
CONTINUED

```
        PC=1.-X
C ART.CO2 + O2 AMOUNTS INCREMENTED BY MIXTURE OF PURE VENOUS
C AND PURE IDEALIZED PULM.CAP.BLOOD,DETERM.BY RATIOS X AND PC
C NITROGEN CONTENT IS DETERMINED IN TERMS OF PARTIAL PRESURES
        RN2MT=RN2MT+FTCO*((X*TN2PR+PC*(C11-AO2PR-AC2PR))*.00127-EN2CT)
        U=X*VC2CT+PC*PC2CT
        V=X*VO2CT+PC*PO2CT
        RC2MT=RC2MT+FTCO*(U-EC2CT)
        RO2MT=RO2MT+FTCO*(V-EO2CT)
C CONTENTS PASSING TO TISSUES AFFECTED BY RATES OF BLOOD FLOW
        W=C22/COADJ
C IF HEART STOPPED PREVENT CHANGES IN ART.BLOOD COMPOSITION
        IF (W-100.) 400,400,390
   390  W=0.
   400  EO2CT=DAMP(RO2MT*.1,EO2CT,W)
        EC2CT=DAMP(RC2MT*.1,EC2CT,W)
        EN2CT=DAMP(RN2MT*.1,EN2CT,W)
        Z=COADJ*C17
C R-2CT IS CONTENT OF BLOOD REACHING CHEMORECEPTORS
        RO2CT=DAMP(V,RO2CT,Z)
        RC2CT=DAMP(U,RC2CT,Z)
C O2CON AND C2CON ARE USED EVERY TIME FOR ENTERING S/R GASES. BEFORE
C ENTERING S/R GASES (DISSOC.CURVES) SET CONTENTS OF O2 + CO2 FOR ART.
C BLOOD, SAME FOR BICARB.(HCO3),WHICH HAS TO TAKE ACCOUNT OF IN VITRO
C INFLUENCE OF ART.PCO2 ON BICARB.CONC. SO THAT PH CAN BE CALCULATED.
        RC3CT=C3*(RC2PR-40.)+VC3MT*C1
        IF (RC3CT) 940,940,410
C ENTER ART.BICARB.,CALC.PH AND ENTER VALUE INTO RPH (ART. PH)
   410  RPH=PHFNC(RC3CT,RC2PR)
C*** (REPLACES ITERATIVE REVERSAL ROUTINE IN PREVIOUS VERSIONS)
        CALL GSINV (RO2PR,RC2PR,RO2CT,RC2CT,RPH,SAT)
C STORE ARTERIAL SATN. AS PERCENTAGE
        PJ=SAT*100.
C U IS ENERGY EXPENDITURE FROM 'METABOLIC RATE' SPECIFIED BY OPERATOR.
C 1ST=O2 CONSUMPTION OF RESP. MSMUSCLES, 2ND=O2 CONS. OF HEART, 3RD=REST
C OF BODY.  IN THE EVENT OF ANAEROBIC METAB., SAME ENERGY REQUIREMENTS
C INVOLVE 11X NO OF MOLES OF LACTATE PRODUCED WITH XLACT O2 SPARED
   490  U=FT*(ABS(SVENT)**C4*C5+COADJ+C7)
C COMPUTE NEW TISSUE GAS AMOUNTS(T-2MT)
   500  TO2MT=TO2MT+FTCOC*(EO2CT-TO2CT)-U+XLACT
        IF (TO2MT-E) 940,940,510
C COMPUTE TISS. PO2, DAMPING APPROPRIATELY
   510  TO2PR=DAMP(TO2MT*C31,TO2PR,C(55))
        X=TO2MT-250.
        IF (X) 530,530,520
C NEXT SECTION CONCERNS LACTIC ACID METABOLISM
   520  TO2PR=45.+.09*X
C LOCAL VARIABLE Y WILL BE USED LATER FOR CATABOLISM RELATED
C TO CARDIAC OUTPUT AND METABOLISM
   530  Y=RLACT*C29
C Z=CATABOLIC RATE FOR LACTATE
C X IS THRESHOLD - WHEN TPH LESS THAN 7.0 CATABOLISM IMPAIRED
C CEREB.BL.FLOW(CBF) IS USED AS DESCRIBED BELOW (EMPIRICALLY)
        W=CBF*.019
        IF (W-1.) 536,536,534
   534  W=1.
   536  X=TPH*10.-69.
        IF (X-W) 550,550,540
   540  X=W
C 1ST TERM IS HEPATIC REMOVAL, 2ND IS RENAL REMOVAL WITH PH INFLUENCE
C 3RD TERM IS BLOOD FLOW RELATED METABOLISM BY MUSCLES, MADE
C DEPENDENT ON CARDIAC OUTPUT (COADJ).  WHOLE EXPRESSION IS
C MULTIPLIED BY Y, A FUNCTION OF BLOOD LACTATE CONCENTRAION
   550  Z=Y*(X**.8612+.0232*2.**((8.-TPH)*3.33)+COADJ*.01)
C LOCAL VARIABLE W ABOVE MAKES SLIGHT ALLOWANCE FOR REDUCED
C LIVER BLOOD FLOW, WHICH CAUSES DECREASED METABOLISM AND
```

MACPUF MAIN PROGRAMME
CONTINUED

```
C INCREASED PRODUCTION WHEN THERE IS A LOW PCO2 OR ALKALOSIS.
C CEREBRAL BLOOD FLOW(CBF) IS USED FOR COMPUTATION SINCE IT
C IS COMPUTED ELSEWHERE AND CHANGES IN THE APPROPRIATE WAY
      W=C(70)/(W+.3)
C FITNS IS THRESHOLD FOR SWITCH TO ANAEROBIC METABOLISM
C RELATED TO FITNESS
      V=FITNS-TO2PR
      IF (V) 570,570,560
C NEXT STATEMENT PROVIDES VIRTUAL TRIGGER EFFECT AND
C RAPIDLY INCREASES LACTIC ACID PROD.IF TISS. PO2 LOW
  560 W=W+C42*(V+1.)**4
C CATABOLISM(Z) FALLS IF TISS. PO2 TOO LOW
      Z=Z*TO2PR*.04
C XLACT IS O2 SPARING EFFECT OF LACTIC ACID PRODUCTION
C (NOT ALLOWED TO EXCEED ACTUAL O2 CONSUMPTION)
  570 X=2.04*(W-C32)
      IF (X-U) 590,590,580
  580 X=U
  590 XLACT=DAMP(X,XLACT,C(53))
C LIMIT OF RATE OF LACTATE FORM DETERMINED BY METAB. DRIVE
C TO TISSUES (I.E. LEVEL OF EXERCISE),  AND TO BODY SIZE
      IF (W-C40) 610,610,600
  600 W=C40
C REDUCE LACTATE CATABOLISM IF CARD.OUTPUT LESS THAN 1/3 NORMAL
C TO TAKE ACCOUNT OF PROBABLE DIM.LIVER AND KIDNEY BL.FLOWS
  610 X=C24-COADJ
      IF (X) 630,630,620
  620 Z=Z*COADJ/C24
C INCR.TOTAL LACTIC ACID BY DIFFER.BETWEEN PROD. AND CATABOLISM
  630 V=W-Z
      TLAMT=TLAMT+V
      RLACT=DAMP(TLAMT*C15,RLACT,COADJ*C(55))
C NEXT IS FOR NITROGEN STORES IN TISSUES
C MOVE N2 BETWEEN FAST(T) AND SLOW(S) TISSUE COMPARTMENTS
C ACCORDING TO P.PRESS. DIFFS.
  640 X=(TN2PR-SN2PR)*C(60)
      TN2MT=TN2MT+FTCOC*(EN2CT-TN2PR*.00127)-X
      SN2MT=SN2MT+X
C TEST IF SLOW SPACE SUPERSATURATED
      Y=(SN2MT*C26-C11)*C27.
      IF (Y) 650,650,660
C IF SO, AUGMENT U AND DECREMENT S, OR VICE VERSA IF
C AMBIENT PRESSURE RELATIVELY HIGHER
  650 Y=Y*.3
      IF (UN2MT) 670,670,660
  660 SN2MT=SN2MT-Y
C BUBBL IS ARBIT.INDEX OF BUBBLE SYMPTS,TAKING INTO ACCOUNT
C BTPS VOLUME AND LOADING BY NUMBER OF MOLECULES OF GAS
C*** N.B. 'BUBBL' IS ONLY A ROUGH INDEX -- PROGRAMME UNDER DEVELOPMENT
      BUBBL=UN2MT**1.2*C23
      UN2MT=UN2MT+Y
C COMPUTE PARTIAL PRESSURES
  670 SN2PR=SN2MT*C26
      TN2PR=TN2MT*C28
C TISS. CO2 EXCHANGES; U=METAB.; .001 CONVERTS CC TO LITRES
      TC2MT=TC2MT+(FTCOC*(EC2CT-TC2CT)+TRQ*U)*.001
C COMPUTE PART.PRESS. FROM TOTAL CO2 AND STAND. BICARB.
      TC2PR=(TC2MT*C30-TC3MT*C36+C33)*C43
C FY STORES CHANGE IN TISS. CO2 FOR ADJUSTING TISS/. HCO3 BUFFERS
      FY=TC2PR-TC2RF
      TC2RF=TC2PR
C .4 IN LINE BELOW REPRESENTS BUFFERS OF LACTIC ACID PARTLY INSIDE
C CELLS, SO THAT THE DISPLACEMENT OF BICARBONATE IS LESS
C THAN STRICT MOLAR EQUIVALENCE
      TC3MT=TC3MT+FTCOC*.1*(VC3MT*C1-TC3MT*C13)-.4*V
      Y=(TC2PR-40.)*C3
  690 TC3CT=TC3MT*C13+Y
      IF (TC3CT) 940,940,700
  700 TPH=PHFNC(TC3CT,TC2PR)
```

MACPUF MAIN PROGRAMME
CONTINUED

```
        CALL GASES (TO2PR,TC2PR,TO2CT,TC2CT,TPH,SAT)
C AMTS OF GASES IN VENOUS POOL INC.BY ARRIVING BLOOD FROM
C TISSUES AND DECREMENTED BY BLOOD GOING TO LUNGS. SAME FOR
C BICARBONATE. CONTENTS V-2CT THEN DETERMINED
        X=C(69)*COADJ*FTCO
        VC2MT=VC2MT+FTCOC*TC2CT-FTCO*(VC2CT*C14-RC2CT*SHUNT)+X*EC2CT
        VO2MT=VO2MT+FTCOC*TO2CT-FTCO*(VO2CT*C14-RO2CT*SHUNT)+X*EO2CT
        VC3MT=VC3MT+FTCOC*.1*(TC3MT*C13-VC3MT*C1)+ADDC3
        X=TC3AJ*C10
        TC3AJ=TC3AJ-ADDC3+V-X
        TC3MT=TC3MT-FY*C(64)+X*.67
        VO2CT=VO2MT*C2
        VC2CT=VC2MT*C2
C*** S/R DELAY CAN BE OMITTED WITH LOSS OF ACCURACY ONLY
C*** WHEN USING SHORT ITERATION INTERVALS
        CALL DELAY
        VC3CT=VC3MT*C1+Y
        IF (VC3CT) 940,940,710
    710 VPH=PHFNC(VC3CT,TC2PR)
        GO TO 740
C THIS  SECTION - RARELY NEEDED - IS FOR DIFFUSION RESPIRATION
    720 FD=XVENT*C12
        AO2MT=AO2MT-FD*FIO2
        AC2MT=AC2MT-FD*FIC2
        AN2MT=AN2MT-FD*Z
        GO TO 850
C PREVENT LATER DIVISION ERRORS IF GAS EXCHANGE ZERO
    730 QA=.001
        QB=E
        GO TO 840
C NEXT LONG SECTION CONCERNS GAS EXCH.IN LUNGS.PC IS FRACTION OF
C CARD.OUTPUT PERFECTLY MIXED WITH ALVEOLAR GASES.U AND V=AMTS OF
C EACH GAS TAKEN IN PER UNIT FRACT TIME(FT)
    740 PC=FTCO*C14*PC
        X=AVENT*C12
        U=X*FIO2
        V=X*FIC2
C NEXT 3 STS.COMPUTE NEW AMTS.OF EACH GAS IN LUNGS. W IS VOLUME
C AT END OF NOMINAL 'INSPIRATION'
        AO2MT=AO2MT+U
        AC2MT=AC2MT+V
        Z=100.-FIO2-FIC2
        AN2MT=AN2MT+AVENT*C12*Z
        W=AO2MT+AC2MT+AN2MT
C NOW CALC.ALVEOLAR PARTIAL PRESSURES
        X=C11/W
        PO2=AO2MT*X
        PC2=AC2MT*X
C CHANGE ALV.GAS AMTS.IN ACCORDANCE WITH BLOOD GAS CONTENTS
C ENTERING(V-2CT) AND LEAVING(P-2CT) THE LUNGS.
C PC=FINAL NEW AMT OF TOTAL GAS AT END OF ALL
        AO2MT=AO2MT+PC*(VO2CT-PO2CT)
        AC2MT=AC2MT+PC*(VC2CT-PC2CT)
        AN2MT=AN2MT+PC*(TN2PR*.00127-EN2CT)
        PC=AO2MT+AC2MT+AN2MT
C FY BECOMES + ONLY IF MORE GAS GOES OUT THAN IN, IN WHICH CASE FY
C IS LATER BROUGHT INTO THE CALCULATION OF EFFECTIVE DEAD SPACE
        IF (PL-2.) 750,770,750
    750 IF (AVENT-20.) 770,760,760
    760 FY=(PC-W)*C34/RRATE
        GO TO 780
    770 FY=0.
    780 IF (PL) 790,800,800
    790 CALL BAGER (5,PC,X,C12,SIMLT)
C XVENT IS VOL.EXHALED IN NOM.TIME (FT) DOWN TO RESTING LUNG VOL.
C IF THIS IS NEG.THERE IS SOME DIFFUSION RESP.IN WHICH CASE GO BACK
    800 XVENT=PC*C35-VLUNG
        IF (XVENT) 720,810,810
    810 DVENT=XVENT*C25/PC
```

MACPUF MAIN PROGRAMME
CONTINUED

```
C U=O2, V=CO2 UPTAKE IN FT TIME, Y,Z,PC=GAS OUTPUTS
        Y=DVENT*AO2MT
        Z=DVENT*AC2MT
        PC=DVENT*AN2MT
C ALGEBRAIC SUMMING OF INTAKE AND OUTPUT OF O2 AND CO2
        QA=U-Y
        QB=Z-V
        IF (PL-.5) 830,830,820
  820 CALL BAGER (4,XVENT,DVENT,C12,SIMLT)
        IF (DVENT+9000.) 940,830,830
  830 IF (AVENT-E) 730,730,840
C SET NEW AMTS.OF EACH GAS, THEN CAL.PARTIAL PRESSURES
  840 AO2MT=AO2MT-Y
        AC2MT=AC2MT-Z
        AN2MT=AN2MT-PC
  850 U=C11/(AO2MT+AN2MT+AC2MT)
C TAKE ACCOUNT OF INSP/EXP DURATION RATIO
        V=C37/RRATE
        IF (V-4.) 870,870,860
  860 V=4.
  870 IF (AVENT-20.) 880,890,890
  880 V=0.
C SPEED OF CHANGE OF ALV. GAS TENSIONS(X)= FUNCT. OF TIDAL VOL.
  890 X=(TIDVL+100.)*C38
C COMPUTE END-'EXPIRATORY' PARTIAL PRESSURES
        Y=AO2MT*U
        Z=AC2MT*U
C DAMP FUNCTION USED TO PREVENT OSCILLATORY SWINGS
C OF ALVEOLAR GAS PRESSURES
        AO2PR=DAMP((Y+(PO2-Y)*V),AO2PR,X)
        AC2PR=DAMP((Z+(PC2-Z)*V),AC2PR,X)
        IF (AO2PR-E) 940,940,900
  900 IF (AC2PR-E) 940,940,910
C DETERM.EXPIRED RQ(PC)THEN ALV.GAS TENSIONS, AND EVENTUALLY
C CONTENTS OF CO2 + O2 IN PULM.CAP.BLOOD(P-2CT)
  910 IF (QA) 920,930,920
  920 PC=QB/QA
  930 X=VC3MT*C1+C3*(AC2PR-40.)
        IF (X-E) 940,950,950
  940 LL5=-1
        GO TO 1455
  950 Y=PHFNC(X,AC2PR)
        CALL GASES (AO2PR,AC2PR,FO2CT,PC2CT,Y,SAT)
C NEXT DETERMINES CEREBRAL BLOOD FLOW ADJUSTMENTS IN
C RELATION TO CARDIAC OUTPUT AND BRAIN PH(PCO2 SENSITIVE)
        Z=SQRT(COADJ)*.5
        IF (Z-1.) 970,970,960
  960 Z=1.
  970 Y=(7.4-BPH)*(BC2PR*.0184-BC3AJ*.1)
        IF (Y) 990,990,980
  980 Y=300.*Y**2
  990 IF (Y-4.4) 1010,1010,1000
 1000 Y=4.4
 1010 CBF=DAMP((Y-.12)*42.5*Z,CBF*Z,C(55))
C COMP.BRAIN GAS AMTS.BY METAB.ASSUMING RQ OF .98 AND
C ALLOWING FOR DIFFERENT AMTS.SUPPLIED IN ART.BLOOD AND
C LEAVING IN VENOUS BLOOD. CHECK FOR ARITH.ERRORS
C THEN CALC. BRAIN GAS TENSIONS FROM GUESTIMATED DISSOC. CURVES
        Y=CBF*C39
        X=C41*(BO2AD+.25)
        Z=X
        IF (BO2PR-18.) 1020,1020,1040
 1020 Z=X*(BO2PR*.11-1.)
        X=X*(19.-BO2PR)
        IF (Z) 1030,1040,1040
 1030 Z=0.
 1040 BO2MT=BO2MT+Y*(RO2CT-BO2CT)-2.*Z*(BO2AD+.1)
        IF (BO2MT) 1050,1050,1060
 1050 BO2MT=.1
```

MACPUF MAIN PROGRAMME
CONTINUED

```
     1060 BC2MT=BC2MT+Y*(RC2CT-BC2CT)+2.15*X
          BO2PR=BO2MT*1.6
          BC2PR=BC2MT*.078
          W=BC2PR-40.
          Y=BC3CT+BC3AJ+.2*W
C A SMALL PROPORTION OF ADDED BICARBONATE IS ADDED ALSO
C TO CSF, THUS AFFECTING BREATHING APPROPRIATELY
          BC3AJ=BC3AJ+((RC3CT-24.)*.3-BC3AJ)*C42
C ADJ.BICARB.TO PCO2 THEN CALC./BRAIN PH'IE.PH AT
C RECEPTOR, THEN PROCEED TO DETERMINE CONTENTS OF O2
C AND CO2 IN BLOOD LEAVING BRAIN
          X=PHFNC(2.*Y+RC3CT,2.*BC2PR+RC2PR)
          Z=((ABS(X-BPH)+E)*100.)**2+.04
          IF (Z-C17) 1080,1080,1070
     1070 Z=C17
     1080 BPH=DAMP(X,BPH,Z)
C RESTRICT RATE OF CHANGE OF BRAIN RECEPTOR PH
          Z=PHFNC(VC3MT*C1+(BC2PR-40.)*C3,BC2PR)
          CALL GASES (BO2PR,BC2PR,BO2CT,BC2CT,Z,SAT)
C NOW FOLLOW VENTILATION CALCULATIONS, STARTING WITH
C NARTI=0 WHICH IS ARTIFICIAL VENT.  COMPUTE TOTAL DEAD
C SPACE, ANAT + PHYSIOL., THEN ALV.VENT.(AVENT)
          IF (NARTI) 1090,1090,1100
     1090 DVENT=C(51)
C NAT.VENT.CONTROLS. TOTL.VENT(U AND SVENT)=SUM OF CENTRAL CO2(PH)
C CHEMORECEPTOR DRIVE(SLOPE X, INTERCEPT Z)  O2 LACK
C RECEPTOR(SLOPE Y)  CENTRAL NEUROGENIC DRIVE(PROPNL. TO
C O2 CONSUMPTION C7, + CONSTANT ETC.), AZ ETC. ARE
C FOR MANUAL ADJUSTMENTS OF VENTILATORY CONTROLS
     1100 Y=(118.-PJ)*.05
          Z=Y*.002
          X=(C(65)+Z-BPH)*1000.*Y
          IF (X) 1110,1120,1120
     1110 X=0.
     1120 W=(C(66)+Z-BPH)*150.*Y
C HIGH BRAIN PH OR LOW PCO2 ONLY INHIBITS VENT.IF LEARNT
C INTRINSIC DRIVE (CZ) IS REDUCED OR ABSENT
          IF (W) 1130,1150,1150
     1130 IF (C(67)) 1150,1150,1140
     1140 W=0.
     1150 Z=(BC2PR-120.)*.25
          IF (Z) 1160,1170,1170
     1160 Z=0.
     1170 Y=(98.-PJ)*(RC2PR-25.)*.12
          IF (Y) 1180,1190,1190
     1180 Y=0.
C BO2AD IS INDEX OF BRAIN OXYGENATION ADEQUACY
C AND LOWERS AND EVENTUALLY STOPS BREATHING IF TOO LOW
     1190 U=BO2PR-11.
          IF (U) 1210,1200,1200
     1200 U=1.
          GO TO 1220
     1210 U=0.
     1220 BO2AD=DAMP(U,BO2AD,C(63))
C PREVENT IMMEDIATE CHANGES IN SPECIFIED VENT. CAPACITY
          XRESP=DAMP(C(46),XRESP,C(68))
C COMPUTE TOTAL ADDITIVE EFFECTS OF VENT. STIMULI
          U=(C44*(X+W)+C(45)*Y+XRESP-Z)*C(47)
C RESTRICT TO MAX. VALUE, PREDICTED OR ASSUMED
          IF (U-C6) 1240,1240,1230
     1230 U=C6
C DAMP SPEED OF RESPONSE ACCORDING TO CARD.OUTPUT AND DEPTH
C OF BREATHING, INCLD. BRAIN OXYGENATION INDEX
     1240 X=(COADJ+5.)*C(62)/(TIDVL+400.)
          SVENT=BO2AD*DAMP(U,SVENT,X)
          IF (PL) 1280,1250,1250
C IF VENT. STIMULI INADEQUATE, =APNOEA
     1250 IF (SVENT-C(48)) 1260,1260,1290
     1260 IF (NARTI) 1290,1290,1280
```

MACPUF MAIN PROGRAMME
CONTINUED

```
 1280 DVENT=E
      RRATE=.0001
      GO TO 1350
C RESP.RATE CALC.FROM CONSTANT + ELASTANCE +TOTAL VENTN.+ART PO2
C ALLOWING FOR MANUAL ADJUSTMT.OF BREATHING CAP(PR)
 1290 IF (NARTI) 1320,1320,1300
 1300 DVENT=SVENT
      RRATE=(C(49)+DVENT**.7*.37)*C(50)/(PJ+40.)
      IF (RRATE-1.) 1350,1350,1310
 1310 IF (COADJ-.5) 1350,1350,1320
C CALC DYNAMIC DEAD SPACE AS SUM OF ANAT.FACTORS + THOSE
C DEPENDENT ON VENTN. AND PERFUSION, THEN CALC.ALV.VENTN.
 1320 U=AO2PR*.15
      IF (U-70.) 1340,1340,1330
 1330 U=70.
 1340 DSPAC=DAMP((C(52)+DVENT*100./RRATE**1.12+20.*DVENT/(COADJ+
     X5.)+U+FY+C(54)*(TIDVL+500.)),DSPAC,C(55))
 1350 TIDVL=DVENT*1000./RRATE
 1360 AVENT=(TIDVL-DSPAC)*RRATE*FT
C RESTRICT TIDAL VOL. TO MAXIMUM(C20), THEN IF NECESSARY GO
C BACK TO RECOMPUTE RESP. RATE, PROVIDING ARTIF.VENT. NOT IN USE
      IF (NARTI) 1380,1380,1365
 1365 X=TIDVL-C20
      IF (X) 1380,1380,1370
 1370 TIDVL=C20
      RRATE=DVENT*1000./TIDVL
      GO TO 1360
 1380 IF (AVENT) 1390,1390,1400
 1390 AVENT=E
 1400 FVENT=AVENT*C(56)
C TND,J3,ND CONCERNED WITH TIMING MARKS. PG IS INDEX OF TIME
C BRAIN HAS BEEN DEPRIVED OF OXYGEN.  IF TOO GREAT DEATH RESULTS
      TND=TND+C(57)
      IF (BO2AD-.3) 1410,1410,1420
 1410 PG=PG-(BO2AD-1.)*C(58)
      GO TO 1430
 1420 PG=PG-BO2AD*C(59)
 1430 IF (TND-60.) 1450,1440,1440
 1440 TND=TND-60.
      J3=J3+1
 1450 ND=INT(TND)
C TEST FOR DEATH, OR GIVE ERROR MESSAGE IF LL5 = -1
 1455 CALL DEATH (LL1,LL5)
      IF (LL1-2) 1457,1600,1600
C OUTPUT SUPPRESSION INSTRUCTIONS
 1457 IF (NB-1) 1470,1590,1460
 1460 IF (MORAN-NREPT) 1590,1500,1590
 1470 IF (ISPAR-2) 1500,1480,1490
 1480 IF (LL4-6) 1590,1500,1590
 1490 IF (LL4-30) 1590,1500,1590
C RESET LOOP COUNTER
 1500 LL4=0
C CHOOSE TYPE OF DISPLAY
      IF (NC-3) 1510,1515,1515
 1510 CALL BRETH
      GO TO 1590
C CONVERT ALL PRESSURES IN MM HG TO SI UNITS IF PREVIOUSLY SPECIFIED
C BEFORE OUTPUT
 1515 CALL UNITS(1,SIMLT)
      IF(NC-3) 1540,1540,1520
 1520 WRITE (KL,1530) T
 1530 FORMAT (1X,10F7.2)
      GO TO 1580
 1540 DO 1550 J=1,8
      JOKE=NE(J)
 1550 TJJ(J)=T(JOKE)
      WRITE (KL,1560) J3,ND,(TJJ(J),J=1,8)
 1560 FORMAT (1X,I3,1H,,I2,2F8.3,6F8.1)
C CONVERT ALL PRESSURE UNITS BACK TO MM HG BEFORE GOING ON
```

```
MACPUF MAIN PROGRAMME
CONTINUED

 1580 CALL UNITS(2,SIMLT)
 1590 CONTINUE
C RESET BICARBONATE ADDITION INDEX TO ZERO
      ADDC3=0.
C ENTER SR.DEADY TO ALLOW MANUAL CHANGES OF VARIABLES
 1600 CALL UNITS (1,SIMLT)
      CALL DEADY (LL1,LL2,LL5,NREPT,SIMLT)
C RESET UNITS TO MM HG
      CALL UNITS(2,SIMLT)
      NREPT=NA
 1610 IF (LL1-1) 190,190,170
      END
```

SUBROUTINE BAGER (N,CA,CB,CC,SIMLT)

```
        SUBROUTINE BAGER (N,CA,CB,CC,SIMLT)
C THIS DEALS WITH BAG REBREATHING ETC
        COMMON KT,KL,INI,NW1,NW2,JKL,ITRIG(73),NEOF,NW
        COMMON NFLAG,J3,ISPAR,NA,NB,NC,ND,NE(8)
        COMMON NARTI,MT,K2,K4,INDEX
C COMMON ARRAY USES T1,T2 ETC. IN MANY SUBROUTINES TO SAVE UNUSED LISTS
C OF NAMED VARIABLES
        COMMON FIO2,FIC2,T1(4),VLUNG,T2(5),BARPR,TEMP,T3(22),BAGO,BAGC,
      X AO2MT,AC2MT,T4(6),TIDVL,RRATE,T5(21),DSPAC,REFLV,T6(7),QB,
      X PW,FT,T7(17),AVENT,PL,T8(12),QA,T9(2),BAG
        GO TO (100,430,430,440,500,510,230), N
  100 IF (NW2.GT.19) GO TO 120
        WRITE (KT,110)
  110 FORMAT (' DO YOU WANT TO MAKE YOUR SUBJECT',/,' 1.CLOSE THE GLOTTI
      XS,    2.COLLECT EXPIRED AIR IN A BAG',/,/,' 3.REBREATHE FROM A BAG,
      X   4.SAME, WITH CO2 ABSORBER ATTACHED',/,/,' 5.RESTORE STATUS QUO -
      XBREATHING AIR, GLOTTIS OPEN, NO BAG')
        NW2=0
  120 CALL NXTWD (7,XXX,NNN,1,5)
C INDEX PL CODES BAGER CALLS FROM MAIN PROGRAMME
        PL=0.
        GO TO (410,150,140,130,170), NNN
  130 PL=PL+1.
  140 PL=PL+1.
  150 PL=PL+1.
        IF (NNN-2) 160,160,200
C*** COLLECTION OF EXPIRED AIR INTO EMPTY BAG
  160 BAG=.00001
        BAGO=.0000001
        GO TO 300
C*** RESTORE ALL TO NORMAL. BAG STAYS FILLED AS IT WAS LEFT.
  170 VLUNG=REFLV
        FIO2=20.93
        FIC2=0.03
        WRITE (KL,180)
  180 FORMAT (' *** GLOTTIS OPEN - BAG DISCONNECTED - BREATHING AIR')
  190 RETURN
C*** BAG REBREATHING OPTIONS
  200 IF (NW2.GT.19) GO TO 220
        NW2=0
        WRITE (KT,210)
  210 FORMAT (' DO YOU WANT..1. 100% O2, 2. A GAS MIXTURE, 3. TO GO ON W
      XITH PREVIOUS BAG')
  220 CALL NXTWD (7,XXX,NNNN,1,3)
C SET BTPS/STPD CORRECTION FACTORS
  230 X=BARPR/SIMLT-1.2703*TEMP
        CORR=(273.+TEMP)/(X*.3592)
        IF (N-7) 240,530,240
  240 IF (NNNN-3) 250,390,250
  250 IF (NW2.GT.19) GO TO 280
        NW2=0
  260 WRITE (KT,270)
  270 FORMAT (' GIVE INITIAL GAS VOLUME IN BAG, IN CC (BTPS)')
  280 CALL NXTWD (7,BAG,NN,300,30000)
        IF (NNNN-2) 290,310,390
  290 BAGO=BAG/CORR
  300 BAGC=.0000001
        GO TO 390
  310 IF (NW2.GT.19) GO TO 330
        NW2=0
        WRITE (KT,320)
  320 FORMAT (' SPECIFY PERCENT CO2')
  330 CALL NXTWD (7,BAGC,NNN,0,100)
        IF (NW2.GT.19) GO TO 350
        NW2=0
        WRITE (KT,340)
  340 FORMAT (' NOW PERCENT OXYGEN')
  350 CALL NXTWD (7,BAGO,NNN,0,100)
        X=BAGO+BAGC
```

```
SUBROUTINE BAGER (N,CA,CB,CC,SIMLT)
CONTINUED

        IF (X-100.) 380,380,360
  360 WRITE (KT,370)
  370 FORMAT (' RIDICULOUS - TRY AGAIN')
        GO TO 310
  380 X=BAG*.01/CORR
        BAGO=BAGO*X
        BAGC=BAGC*X
  390 X=CORR*100./BAG
        XXX=BAGO*X
        X=BAGC*X
        WRITE(KL,400) BAG,XXX,X
  400 FORMAT(' ***',F7.0,'CC BAG CONNECTED, CONTAINING',F6.1,'% O2 + ',F
     X5.1,'% CO2')
        RETURN
C*** GLOTTIS CLOSED; STORE INITIAL LUNG VOLUME FOR REFERENCE
  410 WRITE (KL,420)
  420 FORMAT (' *** GLOTTIS CLOSED UNTIL FACTOR 100 CHANGED AGAIN')
        REFLV=VLUNG
        PL=-1.
        RETURN
C SET INSPIRED GASES EQUAL TO MIXTURE IN THE BAG
  430 X=1./(BAG*CC+.00001)
        FIO2=BAGO*X
        FIC2=BAGC*X
        IF (PL.GT.2.5) FIC2=0.
        RETURN
C DSPVT IS GAS IN UPPER AIRWAY BREATHED OUT INTO BAG
  440 IF (PL.GT.1.) GO TO 450
C*** NEXT SECTION FOR BAG COLLECTION ONLY
        X=DSPAC*RRATE*FT
        BAG=BAG+CA*X
        X=X*CC
        BAGO=BAGO+CB*AO2MT+FIO2*X
        BAGC=BAGC+CB*AC2MT+FIC2*X
        RETURN
C TEST IF TIDAL VOL. GT. THAN BAG VOLUME; IF SO CODE EXIT FROM MAIN PROG.
  450 IF (BAG.GT.TIDVL) GO TO 470
        WRITE (KL,460)
  460 FORMAT(' *** TIDAL VOL. TOO BIG FOR BAG')
        CB=-10000.
        RETURN
  470 IF (PL.LT.2.5) GO TO 480
        BAG=BAG-AC2MT*.01/CC
        BAGC=0.
        GO TO 490
C THIS ST. SKIPPED IF CO2 ABSORBER IN CIRCUIT
  480 BAGC=BAGC+QB
  490 BAGO=BAGO-QA
        BAG=BAG-AVENT+CA
        RETURN
  500 VLUNG=CA*.01/CC
        RETURN
  510 WRITE (KT,520) VLUNG
  520 FORMAT (' LUNG VOLUME=',F6.0,' CC(BTPS)')
        RETURN
C DISPLAY SECTION FOR 'INSPECT' TABLE IN S/R DEADY
  530 IF (BAG.LT..001) BAG=.001
        X=X*(273.+TEMP)/(273.*BAG)
        BAGP=BAGC*X*SIMLT
        BAGPO=BAGO*X*SIMLT
        XNMT=BAG/CORR-BAGO-BAGC
        WRITE (KL,540) BAGPO,BAGP,BAGO,BAGC,XNMT,BAG
  540 FORMAT (' ***** BAG.',F7.1,F8.1,16X,F8.0,F8.0,'  *N2=',F7.0,',' *
     XBAG VOL.',F7.0,' (BTPS)')
        RETURN
        END
```

SUBROUTINE BRETH

```
      SUBROUTINE BRETH
C THIS DOES GRAPHICAL OUTPUT OF TOTAL VENT.(DVENT IN MAIN
C PROGRAMME),RESP.RATE(RRATE),ARTERIAL PCO2(RC2PR) AND
C ARTERIAL PO2(RO2PR). T1,T2 ETC. USED AS IN S/R BAGER
      INTEGER DOT(1),BLANK(1),C(1),O(1),F(1),V(1),X(1),XLINE(65)
      COMMON KT,KL,INI,NW1,NW2,JKL,ITRIG(73),NEOF,NW
      COMMON NFLAG,J3,ISPAR,NA,NB,NC,ND,NE(8)
      COMMON NARTI,MT,K2,K4,INDEX
      COMMON T1(47),RRATE,T2(2),DVENT,T3(20),RO2PR,T4,RC2PR
     X ,T5(8),BUBBL
      DATA DOT,BLANK,C,O,F,V,X/1H.,1H ,1HC,1HO,1HF,1HV,1H*/
      IOK(I)=(I-1)*(65-I)
      IFUNC(Z)=INT(Z*.5+1.1)
      KD=IFUNC(RO2PR)
      KK=IFUNC(RC2PR)
      KR=IFUNC(RRATE)
      KH=IFUNC(DVENT)
      KN=IFUNC(BUBBL)-1
      DO 100 K=1,65
  100 XLINE(K)=BLANK(1)
      XLINE(1)=DOT(1)
      IF (IOK(KD)) 110,105,105
  105 XLINE(KD)=O(1)
  110 IF (IOK(KK)) 120,115,115
  115 XLINE(KK)=C(1)
  120 IF (IOK(KR)) 130,125,125
  125 XLINE(KR)=F(1)
  130 IF (IOK(KH)) 140,135,135
  135 XLINE(KH)=V(1)
  140 IF (IOK(KN)) 150,145,145
  145 XLINE(KN)=X(1)
  150 CONTINUE
C*** ALTERNATIVE VERSION *** NEXT FOUR LINES
C**    MAX=MAXO(KD,KH,KK,KR)
C**     IF (MAX-65) 154,154,152
C*152 MAX=65
C*154 WRITE (KL,160) J3,ND,(XLINE(I),I=1,MAX)
      WRITE (KL,160) J3,ND,XLINE
  160 FORMAT (1H ,I3,1H.,I2,65A1)
      RETURN
      END
```

SUBROUTINE CLIN1(SIMLT)

```
        SUBROUTINE CLIN1(SIMLT)
C THIS SUBROUTINE PRODUCES PRESET PATIENTS
         COMMON KT,KL,INI,NW1,NW2,JKL,ITRIG(73),NEOF,NW
         COMMON NFLAG,J3,ISPAR,NA,NB,NC,ND,NE(8)
         COMMON NARTI,MT,K2,K4,INDEX
        COMMON FIO2,FIC2,CO,PD,FADM,BULLA,VLUNG,ELAST,VADM,AZ,
     X   BZ,CZ,BARPR,TEMP,TRQ,TC2MT,TVOL,HB,PCV,VBLVL,
     X   ADDC3,BC3AJ,DFG,PR,FITNS,SPACE,COMAX,SHUNT,VC,PEEP,
     X   VO2CT,PA ,RPH,VPH,FVENT,BPH,AO2CT,AC2CT,AO2MT,AC2MT,
     X   AO2PR,AC2PR,DPH,XLACT,BO2PR,BC2PR,TIDVL,RRATE,RO2CT,VC2MT,
     X   DVENT,SVENT,PC2CT,PO2CT,TO2CT,TC2CT,BO2CT,BC2CT,TPH,RC3CT,
     X   VC2CT,RO2MT,RC2MT,XRESP,AN2MT,BO2MT,BC2MT,CBF,PC,DSPAC,
     X   REFLV,RO2PR,CONSO,RC2PR,PG,PJ,TND,RC2CT,QB,PW,
     X   FT,CONOM,BUBBL,PK,TC3MT,VC3MT,TC3CT,VC3CT,TLAMT,RLACT,
     X   BC3CT,BO2AD,COADJ,EO2CT,TO2MT,TO2PR,TC2PR,VO2MT,AVENT,PL,
     X   EC2CT,TN2MT,TN2PR,FEV,SN2PR,EN2CT,UN2MT,RN2MT,X109,X110,
     X   TC3AJ,SN2MT,QA,RVADM,XDSPA,BAG,XMALE,HT,WT,AGE
      IF (NW2.GT.19) GO TO 110
      WRITE (KT,100)
  100 FORMAT (' DO YOU WANT..1.PRESET PATIENTS OR  SUBJECTS',/,' 2.TO SP
     XECIFY YOUR OWN PATIENTS  OR SUBJECTS')
      NW2=0
  110 NA=18
      FT=.16667
      NARTI=1
      ISPAR=1
      NEOF=1
      CALL NXTWD (7,XXX,NNN,1,2)
      GO TO (120,280), NNN
  120 IF (NW2.GT.19) GO TO 140
      WRITE (KT,130)
  130 FORMAT (' THE FOLLOWING PRESET PATIENTS ARE AVAILABLE ',/,' 1. NOR
     XMAL FIT SUBJECT EXERCISING AT 300 KPM/MIN',/,' 2. SAME, AT 900 KPM
     X/MIN',/,' 3. UNFIT NORMAL SUBJECT EXERCISING AT 900 KPM/MIN',/,' 4
     X. NORMAL SUBJECT, COMPRESSED TO 10 ATMOSPHERES FOR 25 MINUTES',/,'
     X 5. CHRONIC AIRWAYS OBSTRUCTION WITH VENTILATORY FAILURE',/,' 6. S
     XAME, BUT WITH ACUTE EXACERBATION, EG. ADDED BRONCHOPNEUMONIA',/,'
     X7. CHEYNE-STOKES BREATHING DUE TO BRAIN STEM DAMAGE AND HEART DISE
     XEASE',/,' ...TYPE NUMBER')
      FT=.16667
      NW2=0
  140 CALL NXTWD (7,XXX,NNN,1,7)
      GO TO (150,160,170,190,200,240,250), NNN
C**PRESET 1 - NORMAL SUBJECT EXERCISING AT 300 KPM/MIN
  150 PD=400.
      TRQ=.88
      GO TO 180
C**PRESET 2 - NORMAL SUBJECT EXERCISING AT 900 KPM/MIN
  160 PD=800.
      TRQ=.98
      GO TO 180
C**PRESET 3 - UNFIT NORMAL SUBJECT EXERCISING AT 900 KPM/MIN
  170 FITNS=35.5
      GO TO 160
  180 NA=36
      GO TO 255
C**PRESET 4 - NORMAL SUBJECT COMPRESSED FOR 25 MIN
  190 BARPR=7600.*SIMLT
      NA=30
      SN2MT=2750.
      J3=20
      GO TO 230
C**PRESET 5 - CHRONIC AIRWAYS OBSTRUCTION WITH VENTILATORY FAILURE
  200 VADM=28.
      VC=1.2
      VLUNG=5000.
  210 PR=30.
      TC3MT=480.
      BC3AJ=4.
```

```
SUBROUTINE CLIN1(SIMLT)
CONTINUED

        TC2MT=15.7
        VC2MT=2600.
        BC2MT=1000.
        ELAST=34.
  220 NA=72
  230 ISPAR=2
        GO TO 260
C**PRESET 6 - CHRONIC AIRWAYS OBSTRUCTION WITH ACUTE EXACERBATION
  240 VC=1.
        BULLA=30.
        VADM=60.
        XDSPA=30.
        AZ=50.
        VLUNG=7000.
        GO TO 210
C**PRESET 7 - CHEYNE-STOKES BREATHING DUE TO BRAIN STEM DAMAGE + HEART
C    DISEASE.
  250 CZ=0.
        AZ=160.
        BZ=50.
        CO=58.
        VADM=30.
        XRESP=0.
        AC2MT=90.
  255 FT=.0833334
  260 NB=2
        IF (NW2.GT.19) RETURN
        WRITE (KL,270)
  270 FORMAT (' TIME SCALE IS ALTERED FOR THIS SIMULATION',/,' WAIT WHIL
       XE I WORK THIS OUT!')
        RETURN
C** CLIN2 IS THE ROUTINE FOR CREATING INDIVIDUAL PATIENTS AND INSERTING
C PULM. FUCNTION TEST RESULTS
  280 CALL CLIN2
        GO TO 220
        END
```

```
      SUBROUTINE CLIN2
C THIS SUBROUTINE IS USED ONLY FOR CREATING SUBJECTS TO ORDER,
C AND FOR ALLOWING AS FAR AS POSSIBLE FOR FUNCTION TEST RESULTS
      DIMENSION T(120),ARRAY(3,10)
      COMMON KT,KL,INI,NW1,NW2,JKL,ITRIG(73),NEOF,NW
      COMMON NFLAG,J3,ISPAR,NA,NB,NC,ND,NE(8)
      COMMON NARTI,MT,K2,K4,INDEX
      COMMON FIO2,FIC2,CO,PD,FADM,BULLA,VLUNG,ELAST,VADM,AZ,
     X  BZ,CZ,BARPR,TEMP,TRQ,TC2MT,TVOL,HB,PCV,VBLVL,
     X  ADDC3,BC3AJ,DPG,PR,FITNS,SPACE,COMAX,SHUNT,VC,PEEP,
     X  VO2CT,PA ,RPH,VPH,FVENT,BPH,AO2CT,AC2CT,AO2MT,AC2MT,
     X  AO2PR,AC2PR,DPH,XLACT,BO2PR,BC2PR,TIDVL,RRATE,RO2CT,VC2MT,
     X  DVENT,SVENT,PC2CT,PO2CT,TO2CT,TC2CT,BO2CT,BC2CT,TPH,RC3CT,
     X  VC2CT,RO2MT,RC2MT,XRESP,AN2MT,BO2MT,BC2MT,CBF,PC,DSPAC,
     X  REFLV,RO2PR,CONSO,RC2PR,PG,PJ,TND,RC2CT,QB,PW,
     X  FT,CONOM,BUBBL,PK,TC3MT,VC3MT,TC3CT,VC3CT,TLAMT,RLACT,
     X  BC3CT,BO2AD,COADJ,EO2CT,TO2MT,TO2PR,TC2PR,VO2MT,AVENT,PL,
     X  EC2CT,TN2MT,TN2PR,FEV,SN2PR,EN2CT,UN2MT,RN2MT,X109,X110,
     X  TC3AJ,SN2MT,QA,RVADM,XDSPA,BAG,XMALE,HT,WT,AGE
      EQUIVALENCE (FIO2,T(1))
C ARRAY STORES NORMAL FUNCTION TESTS' RESULTS FOR FUNCTIONS
C USED LATER (FUNC1 AND FUNC2)
      DATA ARRAY/.026,.009,2.18,.047,.0075,4.583,
     X  .0452,.024,2.852,.0582,.025,4.241,.035,.025,1.932,
     X  .0363,.032,1.26,.382,.732,100.,-.125,.951,100.,
     X  .221,.683,100.,-.011,.782,100./
      FUNC1(HT,AGE,X,Y,Z)=X*HT-Y*AGE-Z
      FUNC2(HT,X,Y)=X+(HT*.01)**3*Y
C INITIALISE PREDICTED FEV,VC AND DCO IN CASE NEXT SECTION SKIPPED
      PFEV=FEV
      PVC=VC
      PDCO=20.
      IF (NW2.GT.19) GO TO 110
      WRITE (KT,100)
  100 FORMAT (' 70 KG AVERAGE MAN. DO YOU WANT TO SPECIFY SOMEONE ELSE..
     X1.YES, 2.NO')
      NW2=0
  110 CALL NXTWD (7,XXX,NNN,1,2)
      GO TO (120,280), NNN
C*** BUILD UP THE SPECIFIED SUBJECT
  120 IF (NW2.GT.19) GO TO 140
      WRITE (KT,130)
  130 FORMAT (' PLEASE SPECIFY..1.MALE, 2.FEMALE')
      NW2=0
  140 CALL NXTWD (7,XXX,NNN,1,2)
      IF (NNN.EQ.2) XMALE=0.
      IF (NW2.GT.19) GO TO 160
      WRITE (KT,150)
  150 FORMAT (' GIVE ME THE HEIGHT IN CM (183 CM=6 FT)')
      NW2=0
  160 CALL NXTWD (7,HT,NNN,95,200)
      IF (NW2.GT.19) GO TO 180
      WRITE (KT,170)
  170 FORMAT (' NOW WEIGHT IN KG')
      NW2=0
  180 CALL NXTWD (7,WT,NN,20,200)
      RAT=WT*5880./HT**1.6
      IF (XMALE.LT..5) RAT=RAT*1.064
      IF (NW2.GT.19) GO TO 200
      WRITE (KT,190)
  190 FORMAT (' AND AGE IN YEARS')
      NW2=0
  200 CALL NXTWD (7,AGE,NNN,8,100)
      K=INT(XMALE)+1
      VLUNG=FUNC1(HT,AGE,ARRAY(1,K),ARRAY(2,K),ARRAY(3,K))
      K=K+2
      X=ABS(20.-AGE)
      PDCO=(7.6*VLUNG+5.)*(100.-X)*.01
      VLUNG=VLUNG*1000.
```

```
SUBROUTINE CLIN2
CONTINUED


      IF (AGE.LT.17.) GO TO 210
      PVC=FUNC1(HT,AGE,ARRAY(1,K),ARRAY(2,K),ARRAY(3,K))
      K=K+2
      PFEV=FUNC1(HT,AGE,ARRAY(1,K),ARRAY(2,K),ARRAY(3,K))
      GO TO 220
  210 K=K+4
      PVC=FUNC2(HT,ARRAY(1,K),ARRAY(2,K))
      K=K+2
      PFEV=FUNC2(HT,ARRAY(1,K),ARRAY(2,K))
  220 CONSO=WT**.75*10.33
      X=PVC-PFEV-.1
      IF (X.LT.0.) PVC=PFEV+.1
      CONOM=CONSO*.0195
      IF (XMALE.GT..5) GO TO 230
      CONOM=CONOM*.9
      HB=13.5
      PCV=41.
  230 VBLVL=CONOM*300.+1500.
      TVOL=(WT**.6*.465)+6.
      X=TVOL*.084
      TC3MT=TC3MT*X**1.35
      TC2MT=TC2MT*X
      SN2MT=SN2MT*X
      WRITE (KT,240) PFEV,PVC,PDCO,CONSO,CONOM,RAT
  240 FORMAT (14X,'LITRES',4X,'CC/MM/MIN',4X,'CC/MIN',4X,'LITRES/MIN',5X
     X,' %IDEAL',/,1X,'PREDICTED  FEV1',4X,'VC  DIFF.CAP.  O2 CONSN.  C
     XARD.OUTPUT      WEIGHT',/,13X,F3.1,F6.1,F9.1,F12.0,F12.1,F13.0,/)
      COMAX=(210.-.65*AGE)*.0008*HT
      IF (NW2.GT.19) GO TO 260
      NW2=0
      WRITE (KT,250)
  250 FORMAT (' DO YOU WANT TO ENTER SPIROMETRY RESULTS..1,YES, 2,NO')
  260 CALL NXTWD (7,XXX,NNN,1,2)
      GO TO (280,270), NNN
  270 VC=PVC
      FEV=PFEV
      GO TO 400
C*** INCORPORATE SPIROMETRY RESULTS
  280 IF (NW2.GT.19) GO TO 310
  290 WRITE (KT,300)
  300 FORMAT (' GIVE ME THE VALUE FOR FEV1 IN LITRES')
      NW2=0
  310 CALL NXTWD (7,FEV,NNN,0,6)
      IF (FEV.GT..13) GO TO 330
      WRITE (KT,320)
  320 FORMAT (' VERY UNLIKELY - RECHECK AND')
      GO TO 290
  330 IF (NW2.GT.19) GO TO 360
  340 WRITE (KT,350)
  350 FORMAT (' NOW THE VALUE FOR VC')
      NW2=0
  360 CALL NXTWD (7,VC,NNN,0,7)
      IF (VC.GE..2) GO TO 380
      WRITE (KT,370)
  370 FORMAT (' PROBABLY A TECHNICAL ERROR - PLEASE REPEAT')
      GO TO 340
  380 IF (VC.GT.FEV) GO TO 400
      WRITE (KT,390)
  390 FORMAT (' IT CAN NEVER BE THE SAME AS, OR LESS THAN THE FEV1.',/,'
     X X LET*S HAVE BOTH AGAIN TO BE SURE')
      GO TO 290
  400 RATIO=FEV/VC
      X=RATIO*100.
      WRITE (KT,410) RATIO,X
  410 FORMAT (' THE FEV1/VC RATIO IS ',F4.2,' I.E. ',F4.0,' PER CENT')
      RAT=PFEV/FEV
      TAR=1./RAT
      XDSPA=20.*RAT**.7-20.
      IF (RATIO.GE.0.65) GO TO 460
```

```
SUBROUTINE CLIN2
CONTINUED

        WRITE (KT,420)
    420 FORMAT (' THESE VALUES INDICATE AIRWAYS OBSTRUCTION.',/)
        IF (NW2.GT.19) GO TO 440
        WRITE (KT,430)
    430 FORMAT (' IS YOUR PATIENT',/,'...1.ACUTELY BREATHLESS,  2.NOT MUCH
       X CHANGED IN LAST WEEK OR SO')
        NW2=0
    440 CALL NXTWD (7,XXX,NNN,1,2)
C** SET VALUES FOR OBSTRUCTED SUBJECT
        VLUNG=VLUNG*(.5+.43/RATIO)
        IF (NNN-1) 450,445,450
C ACUTE OBSTRUCTION ONLY
    445 ELAST=FEV+60./(FEV+1.)-11.
        VADM=2.*RAT**1.7
        IF (VADM.GT.85.) VADM=85.
        CZ=30.*RAT+70.
        IF (CZ.GT.140.) CZ=140.
        IF (FEV.LT.1.) CZ=140.*FEV
        GO TO 580
C** ADD IN CHANGES APPROPRIATE FOR CHRONIC OBSTRUCTED SUBJECTS
    450 BC3AJ=.35*RAT-.35
        ELAST=FEV+96./(FEV+4.)-11.
        X=1.2*RAT-1.2
        IF (X.LE.0.) X=0.
        X=X**.52
        IF (PFEV-FEV-2.5) 454,452,452
    452 PR=(FEV+3.)*21.
    454 TC3MT=TC3MT+TVOL*3.*X
        CZ=10.*RAT+90.
        XDSPA=XDSPA*1.2
        VADM=2.*RAT**1.1
        TC2MT=TC2MT+TVOL*.045*X
        GO TO 470
C** UNOBSTRUCTED SUBJECTS
    460 VADM=VADM*RAT**1.6
        IF (FEV.LT.1.) VADM=7.*RAT
        ELAST=FEV+72./(FEV+2.)-11.
        CZ=20.*RAT+80.
    470 IF (NW2.GT.19) GO TO 490
        WRITE (KT,480)
    480 FORMAT (' HAVE YOU MEASURED DIFFUSING CAPACITY..1.YES,  2.NO ')
        NW2=0
    490 CALL NXTWD (7,XXX,NNN,1,2)
C*** INCORPORATE DIFFUSING CAPACITY MEASUREMENTS
C REMAINING STATEMENTS ADJUST EFFECTIVE VENOUS ADMX. ACCORDING TO DIFF.
C CAPACITY ESTIMATES OR MEASUREMENTS.
        GUESS=PDCO*(1.+TAR)*.5
        IF (NNN.EQ.1) GO TO 510
        WRITE (KT,500) GUESS
    500 FORMAT (' IN THAT CASE I SHALL ASSUME THAT IT IS ',F4.1,' CC/MM HG
       X/MIN.',/,' THIS WOULD BE AN AVERAGE SORT OF FIGURE FOR YOUR SUBJEC
       XT',/)
        GO TO 580
    510 IF (NW2.GT.19) GO TO 530
        WRITE (KT,520)
    520 FORMAT (' GOOD. PLEASE GIVE ME YOUR VALUE IN CM/MM HG/MIN')
        NW2=0
    530 CALL NXTWD (7,XXX,NNN,3,100)
        X=PDCO+7.
        IF (XXX.LT.X) GO TO 550
        WRITE (KT,540) GUESS
    540 FORMAT (' THIS SEEMS LIKE NONSENSE, UNLESS THE VALUE WAS OBTAINED
       XDURING EXERCISE',/,' I AM GOING TO ASSUME IT WAS ',F4.1)
        XXX=GUESS
    550 TEST=XXX/GUESS
        IF (TEST.LT.1.4.AND.TEST.GT..6) GO TO 570
        WRITE (KT,560)
    560 FORMAT (' UNUSUAL... BUT YOU*RE THE BOSS',/)
C MAKE CHANGE WITH DIFFERENT DIFFUSING CAP. REALLY DIFFERENT
```

```
SUBROUTINE CLIN2
CONTINUED

   570 RVADM=GUESS/XXX-1.
       XDSPA=XDSPA*2./(1.+TEST)
   580 BO2MT=30.
       TO2MT=700.
       IF (ELAST.GT.75.) ELAST=75.
       RETURN
       END
```

SUBROUTINE CONST(C,NREPT,SIMLT)

```
      SUBROUTINE CONST(C,NREPT,SIMLT)
C THIS S/R COMPUTES ALL PARAMETERS CONSTANT DURING A RUN
      DIMENSION C(70)
        COMMON KT,KL,N(99)
        COMMON FIO2,FIC2,CO,PD,FADM,BULLA,VLUNG,ELAST,VADM,AZ,
     X    BZ,CZ,BARPR,TEMP,TRQ,TC2MT,TVOL,HB,PCV,VBLVL,
     X    ADDC3,BC3AJ,DPG,PR,FITNS,SPACE,COMAX,SHUNT,VC,PEEP,
     X    VO2CT,PA ,T(10),DPH,T2(3),TIDVL,RRATE,T3(24),CONSO,T4(7),FT,
     X    CONOM,T5(16),AVENT,PL,T6(3),FEV,T7(4),T8(4),QA,RVADM,
     X    XDSPA,T9(2),HT,WT
      IF (N(85).GT.1.OR.N(84).EQ.1) GO TO 111
      WRITE (KL,100)
  100 FORMAT (' (KPA)(0)',12X,'(4)',12X,'(8)',11X,'(12)',11X,'(16)',/,'
     X MINS 0',8X,'20',8X,'40',8X,'60',8X,'80',8X,'100',7X,'120')
      WRITE (KL,110)
  110 FORMAT (8H +SECS .,12(4X,1H.))
  111 X=TIDVL*RRATE
      IF ((CO.GT.340..OR.PD.GT.950..OR.SHUNT.GT..5).AND.FT.GT..04)
     X GO TO 112
      IF ((CO.GT.210..OR.PD.GT.350..OR.FIO2.LT.7..OR.CO.LT.5..OR.
     X PL.LT.0..OR.X.LT.1..OR.PR.LT.5.).AND.FT.GT..09) GO TO 114
      GO TO 120
  112 FT=.0333334
      GO TO 116
  114 FT=.0833334
  116 WRITE (KT,118)
  118 FORMAT (' ITERATION INTERVAL TOO LONG FOR THIS SITUATION.  I HAVE
     XSHORTENED IT.',/,/,' TO CHANGE BACK, USE *4,RUN CHANGE* OPTION',/)
  120 IF ((N(95).EQ.0.AND.X.LT.1.).OR.PL.LT.-.5.OR.PR.LT.1.) AVENT=.001
      IF (TEMP.GE.30.) GO TO 140
      WRITE (KT,130)
  130 FORMAT (' *SORRY - NO CAN DO - LET*S SAY 30 DEGREES')
      TEMP=30.
  140 C(1)=1000./VBLVL
      C(2)=100./VBLVL
      C(3)=.0203*HB
      C(4)=(ELAST+105.)*.01
      C(5)=2.7/(VC+.4)
      C(6)=FEV*25.+29.
      C(7)=CONSO*PD*.00081*(TEMP-26.)**1.05
      C(8)=(30.-PEEP*5./ELAST)*.0016*CONOM*(TEMP-12.2)
      C(9)=(C(7)-CONSO)*.01
      C(10)=FT*.005
      C(11)=BARPR/SIMLT-1.2703*TEMP
      C(12)=C(11)*.003592/(273.+TEMP)
      C(13)=.9/TVOL
      C(14)=SHUNT+1.
      C(15)=2./WT
      C(16)=CO*.01
      C(17)=FT*10.
      C(18)=VADM*80.
      C(19)=(PD-90.)*RVADM*.05
      IF (C(19).LT.-1.) C(19)=-1.
      C(20)=650.*VC
      IF (BULLA.GT.0.) C(20)=C(20)+SQRT(BULLA)*15.
      C(21)=(40.-PEEP)*.025
      C(22)=4.5/FT
      C(23)=20.*SIMLT/BARPR
      C(24)=CONOM*.3
      C(25)=100.*C(12)
      C(26)=7./TVOL
      C(27)=FT*.1
      C(28)=30000./(VBLVL+1000.)
      C(29)=FT*.0039*WT**.425*HT**.725
      C(30)=520./TVOL
      C(31)=2.7/TVOL
      C(32)=C(29)+.0000001
      C(33)=C(3)*308.-TVOL*.65*C(30)
      C(34)=.004/(C(12)*FT)
```

```
SUBROUTINE CONST(C,NREPT,SIMLT)
CONTINUED

      C(35)=.01/C(12)
      C(36)=7.7*C(13)
      C(37)=SPACE/FT
      C(38)=20./VLUNG
      C(39)=FT*.127
      C(40)=C(29)*(PD-25.)*1.3
      C(41)=FT*(TEMP-24.5)*1.82
      C(42)=.003*C(29)
      C(43)=1./(1.+7.7*C(3))
      X=(PD*.01)**.8*VC*.2
      C(44)=AZ*X*.0132
      C(45)=BZ*X*.008
      C(46)=CZ*.78*((C(7)*.00051)**.97+.01)
      X=.5+356./C(11)
      IF (X.GT.1.) X=1.
      C(47)=PR*.000214*(TEMP-29.)**1.5*X
      C(48)=.04*(TEMP-26.)*VC
      C(49)=9.+SQRT(ELAST*1.25)
      C(50)=(150.+PR)*.0275*(TEMP-17.)
      C(51)=RRATE*TIDVL*.001
      C(52)=VLUNG*.03-20.+BULLA
      C(53)=.8/FT
      C(54)=XDSPA*.001
      C(55)=.1/FT
      C(56)=.001/FT
      C(57)=FT*60.
      C(58)=FT*1.27
      C(59)=FT*.3
      C(60)=FT*.008
      C(61)=.22/FT
      C(62)=FT*240000./(CZ+300.)
      C(63)=FT*C(7)*.12
      C(64)=.01488*HB*(TVOL+VBLVL*.001)
      C(65)=7.324-CZ*.00005
      C(66)=C(65)-.002
      C(67)=CZ-30.
      C(68)=FT*3000./(PD+200.)
      C(69)=(FITNS-20.)*.00035
      C(70)=C(29)*1.3
      ADDC3=ADDC3/FLOAT(NREPT)
      DPH=7.4+(DPG-3.8)*.025
      IF (DPH.GT.7.58) DPH=7.58
      IF (DPG.GT.13.) DPG=13.
      RETURN
      END
```

SUBROUTINE DEADY (LL1,LL2,LL5,NREPT,SIMLT)

```
        SUBROUTINE DEADY (LL1,LL2,LL5,NREPT,SIMLT)
C THIS SR. PRINTS OUT VALUES AT THE END OF A RUN, AND ASKS FOR,
C INTERPRETS AND ACTS ON VARIOUS CHANGE OPTIONS, USING S/R NXTWD TO
C INPUT KEYBOARD INSTRUCTIONS. THEN RETURN TO MAIN PROGRAMME
        DIMENSION T(120),IANS(10),ICHAR(5)
        COMMON KT,KL,INI,NW1,NW2,JKL,ITRIG(73),NEOF,NW
        COMMON NFLAG,J3,ISPAR,NA,NB,NC,ND,NE(8)
        COMMON NARTI,MT,K2,K4,INDEX
        COMMON FIO2,FIC2,CO,PD,FADM,BULLA,VLUNG,ELAST,VADM,AZ,
      X    BZ,CZ,BARPR,TEMP,TRQ,TC2MT,TVOL,HB,PCV,VBLVL,
      X    ADDC3,BC3AJ,DPG,PR,FITNS,SPACE,COMAX,SHUNT,VC,PEEP,
      X    VO2CT,PA ,RPH,VPH,FVENT,BPH,BAGO,BAGC,AO2MT,AC2MT,
      X    AO2PR,AC2PR,DPH,XLACT,BO2PR,BC2PR,TIDVL,RRATE,RO2CT,VC2MT,
      X    DVENT,SVENT,PC2CT,PO2CT,TO2CT,TC2CT,BO2CT,BC2CT,TPH,RC3CT,
      X    VC2CT,RO2MT,RC2MT,XRESP,AN2MT,BO2MT,BC2MT,CBF,PC,DSPAC,
      X    REFLV,RO2PR,CONSO,RC2PR,PG,PJ,TND,RC2CT,QB,PW,
      X    FT,CONOM,BUBBL,TC2RF,TC3MT,VC3MT,TC3CT,VC3CT,TLAMT,RLACT,
      X    BC3CT,BO2AD,COADJ,EO2CT,TO2MT,TO2PR,TC2PR,VO2MT,AVENT,PL,
      X    EC2CT,TN2MT,TN2PR,FEV,SN2PR,EN2CT,UN2MT,RN2MT,X109,X110,
      X    TC3AJ,SN2MT,QA,RVADM,XDSPA,BAG,XMALE,HT,WT,AGE
        EQUIVALENCE (FIO2,T(1))
        DATA ICHAR/1H1,1H/,1H5,1H/,1H /
        IF(LL1-2) 360,380,300
300     WRITE (KT,310)
310     FORMAT(' ..1.BACKTRACK, 2.CONTINUE, 3.RESTART, 4.INSPECT, 5.STOP')
        NW2=0
        CALL NXTWD (7,XX,NNN,1,6)
        GO TO (330,600,600,500,1120,610), NNN
330     NW=0
        GO TO 920
360     ITRIG(73)=ITRIG(73)+1
        IF (NC-2) 370,1110,1110
370     IF (NB.EQ.1) GO TO 470
        IF (MT.LT.1) GO TO 1110
380     X=10.*2.**(ABS(8.-RPH)*3.33)
        WRITE (KL,390) RO2PR,RO2CT,PJ,RC2PR,RC2CT,RPH,X,RC3CT
390     FORMAT (/,' FINAL VALUES FOR THIS RUN WERE...',//,' ARTERIAL PO2 =
      X',F6.1,'  O2 CONT =',F6.1,', O2 SAT=',F5.0,'%',/,' ARTERIAL PCO2='
      X,F6.1,'  CO2 CONT=',F6.1,/,' ARTERIAL PH =',F5.2,'(',F4.0,'NM), AR
      XTERIAL BICARBONATE =',F5.1,/)
        WRITE (KL,400) RRATE,TIDVL,DVENT,COADJ,DSPAC,PW
400     FORMAT (' RESPIRATORY RATE =',F5.1,', TIDAL VOL.=',F6.0,' ML',/,'
      XTOTAL VENTILATION=',F6.1,' L/MIN, ACTUAL CARD.OUTPUT=',F6.1,' L/MI
      XN',/,' TOTAL DEAD SPACE=',F5.0,' CC, ACTUAL VENOUS ADMIXTURE=',F6.
      X1,' PERCENT',/)
        IF (LL1.EQ.2) GO TO 300
C ITRIG(73) CONTROLS PRINT OUT OF THE FIRST 6 FACTORS AT THE END OF RUN
        IF (ITRIG(73).GT.2) GO TO 1110
        WRITE (KT,410) (T(I),I=1,6)
410     FORMAT (' 1.INSP.O2=',F5.0,', 2.CO2=',F5.0,' PERCENT, 3.',/'NOM.CAR
      XD.OUTP.=',F5.0,'PER CENT',/,' 4.TISS.METAB.=',F5.0,' , 5.VENOUS',/'
      X ADMXT.=',F5.0,' , 6.D.SPACE+=',F6.0,' ML',/)
        IF (ITRIG(73).EQ.2) WRITE (KT,420)
420     FORMAT (' (THE FACTOR LIST ABOVE WILL NOW DISAPPEAR - REFER TO HAN
      XDBOOK)')
        GO TO 1110
430     NW=0
        CALL CLIN1(SIMLT)
        IF (NB.EQ.2) RETURN
        GO TO 470
C IF NOT NEW SUBJECT(NW=0) INSERT '1/5/' IN INPUT BUFFER TO
C RENEW THE SUBJECT FROM INITIAL VALUES, THEN RETURN TO CLIN1
440     IF (NW.GT.0) GO TO 430
        NB=1
        KYY=69-NW1
        DO 450 I=1,KYY
450     ITRIG(73-I)=ITRIG(69-I)
        DO 460 I=1,4
460     ITRIG(NW1+I-1)=ICHAR(I)
```

```
SUBROUTINE DEADY (LL1,LL2,LL5,NREPT,SIMLT)
CONTINUED

        IF (NW2.LE.19) ITRIG(NW1+3)=ICHAR(5)
        NW2=20
        GO TO 600
 470 IF (NW2.GT.19) GO TO 490
        WRITE (KT,480)
 480 FORMAT (' DO YOU WANT TO..1.CHANGE, 2.CONTINUE, 3.RESTART, 4.INSPE
    XCT, 5.STOP',/)
        NW2=0
 490 CALL NXTWD (15,XXX,NNN,1,6)
        JKL=0
        GO TO (640,630,600,500,1120,610), NNN
 500 X=T(22)+T(91)
        Y=T(16)*1000.
        WRITE (KL,510) T(72),T(74),T(49),T(78),T(62),T(63),T(33),T(60),T(4
    X1),T(42),T(76),T(39),T(40),T(41),T(42),T(54),T(53),T(45),T(46),T(5
    X7),T(58),T(66),T(67),T(36),X,T(96),T(97),T(55),T(56),T(95),Y,T(59)
    X,T(96),T(97),T(31),T(61),T(98),T(50),T(34),T(88)
 510 FORMAT ('                   P.PRESSURES          CONTENTS CC%    AMOUNTS IN C
    XC     PH      HCO3-',/,12X,3(3X,'O2',5X,'CO2',3X),/,/,' ARTERIAL ',4F8.
    X1,2F8.0,F7.3,F6.1,/,' ALV./LUNG',2F8.1,'  (SAT=',F4.0,'%'),4X,2F8.0
    X,/,' (PULM.CAP)',F7.1,3F8.1,/,' BRAIN/CSF',4F8.1,2F8.0,F7.3,F6.1,/
    X,' TISSUE/ECF',F7.1,'   (',F5.1,')',F7.1,F8.1,2F8.0,F7.3,/,' MIXED
    XVEN. (',F5.1,')  (',F5.1,')',F7.1,F8.1,2F8.0,F7.3,F6.1)
        IF (PL.GE.1.) CALL BAGER (7,X,Y,PPH,SIMLT)
        WRITE (KL,520) RLACT
 520 FORMAT (' PLASMA LACTATE CONC.=',F4.1,' MMOL/L')
        IF (LL1.EQ.2.OR.LL5.LT.0) GO TO 300
        RR=DSPAC/(TIDVL+.000001)
        X=QA/FT
        Y=QB/FT
        WRITE (KL,530) X,Y,PC
 530 FORMAT (/,' O2 UPTAKE= ',F6.0,'  CO2 OUTPUT= ',F6.0,' CC/MIN(STPD)
    X EXPIRED R.Q.=',F5.2)
        WRITE (KL,540) DVENT,FVENT,RRATE,PW
 540 FORMAT (' TOT.VENT.=',F5.1,'  ALV.VENT(BTPS)=',F4.1,' R.RATE=',F4.
    X1,'  VEN.ADMX.=',F4.1)
        IF (DVENT.LT..2) GO TO 560
        WRITE (KL,550) DSPAC,TIDVL,RR
 550 FORMAT (' DEAD SPACE(BTPS)=',F5.0,'  TIDAL VOL.=',F5.0,' D.SP./TID
    X.VL.RATIO=',F4.2)
 560 IF (COADJ.GT..1) WRITE (KL,570) COADJ,CBF
 570 FORMAT (' CARDIAC OUTPUT=',F5.1,'    CEREBRAL BLOOD FLOW=',F4.0,' M
    XL/100G/MIN')
        IF (BUBBL.GT.0.) WRITE (KL,580) BUBBL
 580 FORMAT (' NITROGEN SUPERSATURATION INDEX=',F6.0)
        IF (PL.LT.0.) CALL BAGER (6,X,Y,PPH,SIMLT)
        WRITE (KL,590)
 590 FORMAT (/)
        IF (LL1-2) 470,300,300
 600 MT=0
        LL1=3
        RETURN
 610 WRITE (KL,620) T
 620 FORMAT (1X,10F7.2)
        IF (LL1-2) 470,300,300
 630 IF (NB.EQ.1) NB=0
        NREPT=NA
        RETURN
 640 IF (NW2.GT.19) GO TO 660
        WRITE (KT,650)
 650 FORMAT (' 1.CHANGE VALUES, 2.NAT/ART VENT, 3.STORE/BKTRK, 4.RUN CH
    XANGE, 5.PRESETS')
        NW2=0
 660 CALL NXTWD (3,XXX,NNN,1,5)
        IF (NNN.NE.5) NW=0
        GO TO (930,820,920,670,440), NNN
 670 IF (NW2.GT.19) GO TO 690
        WRITE (KT,680)
 680 FORMAT (' TYPE NO.OF SECONDS FOR RUN(1800 MAX.)')
```

```
SUBROUTINE DEADY (LL1,LL2,LL5,NREPT,SIMLT)
CONTINUED

    690 CALL NXTWD (7,XT,NNN,2,1800)
        IF (NW2.GT.19) GO TO 710
        WRITE (KT,700)
    700 FORMAT (' TYPE INTERVAL BETWEEN COMPUTATIONS IN SECS.(10 MAX.)')
    710 CALL NXTWD (12,XXX,NNN,1,10)
        FT=XXX/60.+.000001
        NA=INT(XT/XXX)
        IF (NW2.GT.19) GO TO 730
        WRITE (KT,720)
    720 FORMAT (' DO YOU WANT 1.ALL, 2.EVERY 6TH, OR 3.EVERY 30TH VALUE PR
       XINTED')
    730 CALL NXTWD (11,XXX,ISPAR,1,3)
        IF (NW2.GT.19) GO TO 750
        WRITE (KT,740)
C THIS USE OF NXTWD ALLOWS A STRING OF 1 TO 8 NUMBERS TO
C BE FED INTO ARRAY(NE)
    740 FORMAT (' DO YOU WANT..1.GRAPHS + TEXT, 2.GRAPHS ONLY, 3.SELECTED
       XVALUES')
    750 CALL NXTWD (5,XXX,NC,1,4)
        MT=1
        GO TO (470,810,760,470), NC
    760 IF (NW2.GT.19) GO TO 780
        WRITE (KT,770)
    770 FORMAT (' TYPE UP TO 8 NOS. - 69 IS STANDARD')
        NW2=0
    780 NEOF=8
        NL=0
        JKL=1
    790 CALL NXTWD (6,XXX,NNN,1,120)
        NW2=NW2+1
        NL=NL+1
        IF (JKL.EQ.0) GO TO 800
        IF (NEOF.EQ.0) GO TO 470
        NE(NL)=NNN
        GO TO 790
    800 NE(NL)=NNN
    810 MT=0
        GO TO 470
    820 IF (NW2.GT.19) GO TO 840
        WRITE (KT,830)
    830 FORMAT (' 1.GIVE ARTIFICIAL, 2.RETURN TO NATURAL VENTILATION')
    840 CALL NXTWD (7,XXX,NARTI,1,2)
        NARTI=NARTI-1
        IF (NARTI) 850,850,841
    841 PEEP=0.
        WRITE (KL,842)
    842 FORMAT (' *** NATURAL VENTILATION')
        GO TO 470
    850 IF (NW2.GT.19) GO TO 870
        WRITE (KT,880)
    860 FORMAT (' GIVE TIDAL VOLUME IN ML')
    870 CALL NXTWD (7,RRATE,NNN,0,200)
        IF (RRATE.LE..001) RRATE=.001
        IF (NW2.GT.19) GO TO 890
        WRITE (KT,860)
    880 FORMAT (' NOW VENTILATION RATE IN CYCLES/MIN')
    890 CALL NXTWD (8,TIDVL,NNN,0,5000)
        IF (TIDVL.LE..001) TIDVL=.001
        NW=0
        IF (NW2.GT.19) GO TO 910
        WRITE (KT,900)
    900 FORMAT (' POSITIVE END EXPIRATORY PRESSURE - TYPE EITHER *O*',/,'
       XOR NUMBER OF CM WATER (UP TO 15)')
    910 CALL NXTWD (16,PEEP,NNN,0,15)
        WRITE (KL,912) RRATE,TIDVL,PEEP
    912 FORMAT (' *** ART.VENT. AT',F4.0,'/MIN.,',F6.0,'ML TID.VOL., AND',
       XF4.0,'CM PEEP')
        GO TO 470
    920 CALL DUMP (LL1)
```

```
SUBROUTINE DEADY (LL1,LL2,LL5,NREPT,SIMLT)
CONTINUED


      NB=0
      GO TO 470
  930 IF (NW2.GT.19) GO TO 950
      WRITE (KT,940)
  940 FORMAT (' TYPE NUMBER OF FACTORS (1-30) TO CHANGE, OR 100 FOR BAG
     XEXPTS., ETC.')
      NW2=0
  950 NEOF=10
      NL=0
      KYY=-1
      JKL=1
  960 CALL NXTWD (9,XXX,NNN,1,120)
      IF (NNN.EQ.100) GO TO 1100
      KYY=KYY+1
      NW2=NW2+1
      NL=NL+1
      IF (JKL.EQ.0) GO TO 980
      IF (NEOF.EQ.0) GO TO 990
      IANS(NL)=NNN
      IF (NNN.GT.30) WRITE (KT,970) NNN
  970 FORMAT (' POINTLESS -- FACTOR',I4,' WILL BE CHANGED BACK AGAIN DUR
     XING THE NEXT RUN')
      GO TO 960
  980 IANS(NL)=NNN
      KYY=KYY+1
  990 IF (NW2.GT.19) GO TO 1000
      NW2=0
 1000 DO 1040 IJ=1,KYY
      I=IANS(IJ)
      IF (NW2.GT.19) GO TO 1020
      WRITE (KT,1010) I,T(I)
 1010 FORMAT (' FACTOR ',I3,' (CURRENT VALUE=',F7.1,'), SPECIFY NEW VALU
     XE')
 1020 CALL NXTWD (10,XXX,NNN,-500,16000)
      WRITE (KT,1030) I,XXX,T(I)
 1030 FORMAT (' FACTOR ',I3,' =',F7.1,' (PREVIOUSLY =',F7.1,')')
      T(I)=XXX
      IF (T(I).EQ..0) T(I)=.00000001
 1040 CONTINUE
 1050 NW=0
      REFLV=VLUNG
      GO TO 470
 1100 CALL BAGER (1,X,Y,PPH,SIMLT)
      GO TO 1050
C CHECK FOR VARIOUS SYMPTOMS
 1110 IF (NB.EQ.2) CALL DUMP (LL1)
      CALL SYMPT (SIMLT)
      GO TO 470
 1120 WRITE (KT,1130)
C*** LOCAL ARRANGEMENTS
 1130 FORMAT (' THANK YOU FOR YOUR INTEREST. PLEASE LET ',
     X'YOUR TUTOR',
     X/,' HAVE ANY COMMENTS, SUGGESTIONS OR CRITICISMS')
      STOP
      END
```

SUBROUTINE DEATH (LL1,LL5)

```
      SUBROUTINE DEATH (LL1,LL5)
C THIS SUBROUTINE CHECKS FOR 1.ERRORS, 2.DEATH, 3.INTOLERABLE ACIDOSIS
      DIMENSION MM(6)
      COMMON KT,KL,NTAB(99),T(95)
      EQUIVALENCE (PD,T(4)),(TPH,T(59)),(PG,T(75)),(BUBBL,T(83))
      DATA MM/60,87,88,95,41,42/
      IF (LL5) 90,140,140
C*** ERRORS DIAGNOSIS
   90 DO 100 I=1,6
      LL5=MM(I)
      IF(T(LL5)-.001) 110,100,100
  100 CONTINUE
      LL5=0
  110 WRITE (KT,120) LL5
  120 FORMAT (' *** FACTOR ',I2,' HAS GONE NEGATIVE - TIME INTERVAL PROB
     XABLY TOO LONG')
      LL1=3
      GO TO 360
C*** CHECK FOR LETHAL CONDITIONS
  140 LL1=1
      IF (PG) 145,150,150
  145 PG=0.
  150 IF (PG-7.) 160,160,190
  160 IF (TPH-6.63) 210,210,170
  170 IF (TPH-7.8) 180,180,230
  180 IF (BUBBL-280.) 300,300,240
  190 WRITE (KL,200)
  200 FORMAT (/,' ANOXAEMIA HAS BEEN SEVERE AND IRRECOVERABLE')
      GO TO 270
  210 WRITE (KL,220)
  220 FORMAT (/,' TISSUE PH HAS FALLEN TO A LETHALLY LOW LEVEL')
      GO TO 270
  230 WRITE (KL,260)
      GO TO 270
  240 WRITE (KL,250)
  250 FORMAT (/,' THE BRAIN IS IRRECOVERABLY FULL OF GAS BUBBLES')
  260 FORMAT (/,' TISSUE PH HAS RISEN TO A LETHALLY HIGH LEVEL')
  270 WRITE (KT,280)
  280 FORMAT (/,' YOUR PATIENT HAS DIED')
  290 LL1=2
      GO TO 360
C*** CHECK FOR INTOLERABLE ACIDOSIS DURING EXERCISE
  300 IF(PD-290.) 360,310,310
  310 IF(TPH-7.1) 320,320,360
  320 WRITE (KL,350)
  350 FORMAT (' ....I CAN*T GO ON....')
  360 RETURN
      END
```

SUBROUTINE DELAY

```
      SUBROUTINE DELAY
      COMMON KT,KL,INI,NW1,NW2,JKL,ITRIG(73),NEOF,NW
      COMMON NFLAG,J3,ISPAR,NA,NB,NC,ND,NE(8)
      COMMON NARTI,MT,K2,K4,INDEX
      COMMON T1(30),VO2CT,T2(29),VC2CT,T3(19),FT,T4(4),VC3MT,T5(6),
     X COADJ,T6(3),TC2PR,T7(23),TDLAY(40)
C DELAY LINE FOR CIRCULATION OF GASES ETC
      NFT=IFIX(13.2*SQRT(COADJ*FT))
      IF (NFT-10) 110,110,100
  100 NFT=10
  110 M=INDEX+NFT-1
      DO 140 I=INDEX,M
      N=I
      IF (N-10) 130,130,120
  120 N=N-10
  130 TDLAY(N)=VO2CT
      TDLAY(N+10)=VC2CT
      TDLAY(N+20)=VC3MT
  140 TDLAY(N+30)=TC2PR
      N=INDEX+NFT
      IF (N-10) 160,160,150
  150 N=N-10
  160 VO2CT=TDLAY(N)
      VC2CT=TDLAY(N+10)
      VC3MT=TDLAY(N+20)
      TC2PR=TDLAY(N+30)
      INDEX=N
      RETURN
      END
```

SUBROUTINE DUMP (LL1)

```
      SUBROUTINE DUMP (LL1)
C THIS S/R ALLOWS STORAGE AND BACKTRACKING
      COMMON KT,KL,INI,NW1,NW2,JKL,ITRIG(73),NEOF,NW
      COMMON NTAB(20),T(160)
      COMMON NDUMP(20),TDUMP(160)
      IF (LL1.GT.9) GO TO 140
      IF (NTAB(5).EQ.2) GO TO 120
      IF (LL1.GT.1) GO TO 170
      IF (NW2.GT.19) GO TO 110
      WRITE (KT,100)
  100 FORMAT (' DO YOU WANT TO 1.STORE PRESENT STATE, 2.BACKTRACK TO LAS
     XT STORED STATE')
  110 CALL NXTWD (14,XXX,NNN,1,2)
      GO TO (120,170), NNN
  120 WRITE (KL,130)
  130 FORMAT (' STORED AT THIS POINT ************')
  140 DO 150 I=2,20
  150 NDUMP(I)=NTAB(I)
      DO 160 I=1,160
  160 TDUMP(I)=T(I)
      RETURN
  170 WRITE (KL,180)
  180 FORMAT (' *********** BACKTRACK TO LAST STORE')
      DO 190 I=2,20
  190 NTAB(I)=NDUMP(I)
      DO 200 I=1,160
  200 T(I)=TDUMP(I)
      LL1=1
      RETURN
      END
```

SUBROUTINE GASES (PO2,PC2,O2CON,C2CON,PH,SAT)

```
      SUBROUTINE GASES (PO2,PC2,O2CON,C2CON,PH,SAT)
C THIS SR TAKES ANY VALUES OF PO2,PCO2,AND PH AND WORKS
C OUT O2 CONTENT AND CO2 CONTENT(AND SAT.OF O2) AND
C RETURNS RESULTS TO CALLING ROUTINE. MATHS IS THAT OF
C KELMAN WHO HAS PUBLISHED THESE COMPUTER ROUTINES
C TEMPERATURE,HAEMOGLOBIN AND PCV ALSO ALLOWED FOR
C .....REFER TO KELMAN'S PAPERS FOR DETAILS
      COMMON NTAB(101)
      COMMON Y1(13),TEMP,Y2(3),HB,PCV,Y3(23),DPH
C ABOVE CONTAINS ALL NECESSARY VARIABLES WHICH,TO SAVE SPACE,
C ARE REFERRED BY ARRAY NUMBERS RATHER THAN IDENT.LETTERS.
C SEE MAIN PROGRAMME FOR NAMES OF VARIABLES IN ARRAY Y()
      DATA A1, A2, A3, A4, A5, A6, A7/-8.532229E3, 2.121401E3,
     X    -6.707399E1, 9.359609E5, -3.134626E4, 2.396167E3, -6.710441E1/
      X=PO2*10.**(.4*(PH-DPH)+.024*(37.-TEMP)+.026057669*(ALOG(40./
     XPC2)))
      IF (X-.01) 100,110,110
100   X=.01
110   IF (X-10.) 120,130,130
120   SAT=(.003683+.000584*X)*X
      GO TO 140
130   SAT=(X*(X*(X*(X+A3)+A2)+A1))/(X*(X*(X*(X+A7)+A6)+A5)+A4)
140   O2CON=HB*SAT*1.34+.003*PO2
      P=7.4-PH
      PK=6.086+P*.042+(38.-TEMP)*(.00472+.00139*P)
      T=37.-TEMP
      SOL=.0307+(.00057+.00002*T)*T
      DOX=.590+(.2913-.0844*P)*P
      DR=.664+(.2275-.0938*P)*P
      T=DOX+(DR-DOX)*(1.-SAT)
      CP=SOL*PC2*(1.+10.**(PH-PK))
      CC=T*CP
      H=PCV*.01
      C2CON=(CC*H+(1.-H)*CP)*2.22
      RETURN
      END
```

SUBROUTINE GSINV (PO2,PC2,O2CON,C2CON,PH,SAT)


```
      SUBROUTINE GSINV (PO2,PC2,O2CON,C2CON,PH,SAT)
C THIS SR REVERSES GASES AND BY AN OPTIMISED PROCESS OF
C SUCCESSIVE APPROXIMATION USES O2 AND CO2 CONTENTS TO
C COMPUTE THE RESPECTIVE PARTIAL PRESSURES
      COMMON NTAB(101)
      COMMON Y1(13),TEMP,Y2(3),HB,PCV,Y3(23),DPH,Y4(40),PK
      DATA ERR,FACT/.01,1./
C FLAGS ICH1/3 SIGNIFY STATES IN APPROXIMATION OF PO2,
C ICH2/4= SIMILARLY FOR PCO2
C ICH1=0 MEANS PO2 IS WELL ENOUGH APPROXIMATED WITH ABS.ACCURACY
C 'ERR' IN O2CON
C ICH1=1 MEANS A BRACKETING PROCEDURE TO ESTABLISH BOUNDS ON THE
C PO2 VALUE IS IN PROGRESS
C ICH3=1 A BRACKET HAS BEEN ESTABLISHED AND A LINEAR INTERPOLATION
C MADE FOR NEXT ESTIMATE OF PO2
C ICH3=0 NO BRACKET AT THIS TIME
C SET MAGNITUDE INITIAL STEP LENGTHS FOR BRACKETING PROCEDURE TO FIND
C BOUNDS WITHIN WHICH PO2 AND PCO2 MUST LIE
C SET INITIAL FLAG VALUES AS IF CURRENT VALUES FOR PO2 AND PCO2
C WERE AS INTERPOLATED AT A BRACKET
      D1Z=2.
      D2Z=2.
      ICH1=1
      ICH2=1
      ICH3=1
      ICH4=1
C START SEARCH FROM CURRENT ESTIMATES OF PO2 AND PCO2
  100 CALL GASES(PO2,PC2,X,Y,PH,SAT)
C XX2/YY2 STORE DISCREPANCY BETWEEN KNOWN CONTENTS AND VALUES
C COMPUTED USING CURRENT GUESSES OF PRESSURES
      XX2=X-O2CON
      YY2=Y-C2CON
C AVOID ERROR IN SIGN FUNCTION BELOW
      IF(XX2) 120,110,120
  110 XX2=.001
  120 IF(YY2) 140,130,140
  130 YY2=.001
C XP2/YP2 STORE PRESSURE ESTIMATES CORRESPONDING TO DISCREPANCIES
C XX2/YY2. THESE ARE ALL USED IN INTERPOLATION PROCEDURE BELOW.
C FORM NEW SEARCH VECTORS D1/D2, AFTER BRACKETING AND
C INTERPOLATION, ACCORDING TO SIGN OF DISCREPANCIES XX2/YY2.
C RESET ICH3/ICH4 TO ZERO
  140 XP2=PO2
      YP2=PC2
      IF(ICH3-1)160,150,160
  150 ICH3=0
      D1=SIGN(D1Z,-XX2)
  160 IF(ICH4-1)210,170,210
  170 ICH4=0
      D2=SIGN(D2Z,-YY2)
C TEST FOR CONVERGENCE OF CALCULATED AND GIVEN CONTENTS.  SET FLAGS
C ICH1/ICH2 TO ZERO IF CONTENTS APPROXIMATED WELL ENOUGH
      IF(ABS(XX2)-ERR) 180,180,190
  180 ICH1=0
  190 IF(ABS(YY2)-ERR) 200,200,210
  200 ICH2=0
C FINISH IF BOTH CONTENTS APPROXIMATED WELL ENOUGH
      IF(ICH1+ICH2)450,450,210
C COMPUTE TRIAL INCREMENT DS FOR PO2 ENFORCING A LIMIT OF
C -PO2*.75 IF IT IS NEGATIVE. (STOP NEGATIVE TRIAL
C VALUES AND SMOOTH APPROACH TO A SOLUTION).
  210 DS=D1*ICH1
      X=PO2+DS-PO2*.25
      IF (X) 220,230,230
  220 DS=-PO2*.75
  230 PO2=PO2+DS
C COMPUTE TRIAL INCREMENT OF PCO2 AS FOR PO2 ABOVE
      DS=D2*ICH2
      X=PC2+DS-PC2*.25
```

```
SUBROUTINE GSINV (PO2,PC2,O2CON,C2CON,PH,SAT)
CONTINUED

        IF (X) 240,250,250
  240 DS=-PC2*.75
  250 PC2=PC2+DS
C ENFORCE LOWER BOUND ON PO2/PCO2
        IF(PO2-.1) 260,270,270
  260 PO2=.1
  270 IF(PC2-.1)280,290,290
  280 PC2=.1
C COMPUTE CONTENTS WITH TRIAL INCREMENTS MADE TO PO2/PCO2
  290 CALL GASES(PO2,PC2,X,Y,PH,SAT)
C SAVE LAST BUT ONE PAIRS OF VALUES PO2/O2CON DISCREPANCY IN
C XX1/XP1, SIMILARLY FOR PC2/C2CON DISCREPANCY IN YY1/YP1.
C THEN PLACE LATEST PAIRS OF VALUES IN XX2/XP2, YY2/YP2 AS BEFORE
        XX1=XX2
        XX2=X-O2CON
        XP1=XP2
        XP2=PO2
        YY1=YY2
        YY2=Y-C2CON
        YP1=YP2
        YP2=PC2
C FIRST LOOK AT DISCREPANCY IN O2CON (ICH1=0). IF WITHIN LIMIT
C 'ERR' ACCEPT VALUES OF PO2 AND LOOK AT C2CON
        IF(ABS(XX2)-ERR) 300,300,310
  300 ICH1=0
        GOTO 360
C IF O2CON DISCREPANCY STILL TOO HIGH TEST WHETHER TRIAL PO2 HAS
C OVERSHOT THE CORRECT SOLUTION
  310 ICH1=1
        IF(XX2*D1) 320,360,350
C IF NOT OVERSHOT, SOLUTION LIES FURTHER ALONG DIRECTION OF TRIAL
C INCREMENT.  COMPUTE A NEW TRIAL INCREMENT BASED ON LAST 2 PAIRS
C OF CONTENTS/PRESSURES VALUES. FACTOR 'FACT' WAS USED IN
C IN OPTIMISING THE ALGORITHM IN PRACTICE
  320 IF(XP2-XP1) 340,330,340
  330 D1=SIGN(D1Z,-XX2)
        GO TO 360
  340 D1=(XP2-XP1)*ABS(XX2)/(FACT*ABS(XX2-XX1))
        GO TO 360
C IF OVERSHOT, (I.E. BRACKET FOUND ON PO2) LINEARLY INTERPOLATE
C USING LAST 2 PAIRS OF PRESSURES/CONTENTS VALUES TO GET NEW TRIAL
C VALUE FOR PO2. SET ICH3=1 TO INDICATE BRACKETED INTERPOLATED
C VALUE FOR NEW SEARCH TO BE INITIATED AT STATEMENT 100. REDUCE
C INITIAL SEARCH VECTOR TO AID CONVERGENCE
  350 ICH3=1
        PO2=XP1+(XP2-XP1)*ABS(XX1)/(ABS(XX2)+ABS(XX1))
        D1Z=D1Z/2.
C NOW REPEAT ABOVE PROCEDURE FOR DISCREPANCY IN C2CON
  360 IF(ABS(YY2)-ERR) 370,370,380
  370 ICH2=0
        GO TO 430
  380 ICH2=1
        IF(YY2*D2) 390,430,420
C KEEP GOING
  390 IF(YP2-YP1) 410,400,410
  400 D2=SIGN(D2Z,-YY2)
        GO TO 430
  410 D2=(YP2-YP1)*ABS(YY2)/(FACT*ABS(YY2-YY1))
        GO TO 430
C BRACKET FOUND
  420 ICH4=1
        PC2=YP1+(YP2-YP1)*ABS(YY1)/(ABS(YY1)+ABS(YY2))
        D2Z=D2Z/2.
C FINISH IF BOTH O2CON AND C2CON WELL ENOUGH APPROXIMATED.  IF EITHER
C PO2 OR PCO2 SEARCH IS AT A BRACKET ESTABLISH NEW SEARCH AT
C STATEMENT 100.  ELSE, IF BOTH ARE CONTINUING ALONG PREVIOUS
C DIRECTIONS OF SEARCH PROCEED FROM STATEMENT 210
  430 IF(ICH1+ICH2) 450,450,440
  440 IF(ICH3+ICH4-1) 210,100,100
  450 RETURN
        END
```

SUBROUTINE MINIT (LL1,LL3,LL4,NREPT,SIMLT)

```
      SUBROUTINE MINIT (LL1,LL3,LL4,NREPT,SIMLT)
C INITIALIZE ALL VALUES AND INDICES FOR A NEW SUBJECT
      DIMENSION REFER(120)
        COMMON KT,KL,INI,NW1,NW2,JKL,ITRIG(73),NEOF,NW
        COMMON NFLAG,J3,ISPAR,NA,NB,NC,ND,NE(8)
        COMMON NARTI,MT,K2,K4,INDEX
        COMMON T(120),TDLAY(40)
C CONSTANTS FOR INTIALIZING A NEW SUBJECT
      DATA REFER/20.93,.03,2*100.,2*.0,3000.,5.,3.,100.,
     X 2*100.,760.,37.,,8,13.38,12.,14.8,45.,3000.,,
     X 0.,0.,3.8,100.,33.,,4,35.,0.,5.,0.,
     X 14.56,1.,7.4,7.37,4.26,7.33,2*0.,348.1,143.3,
     X 101.9,39.75,7.40,0.,28.89,52.8,461.9,12.82,19.54,1540.,
     X 2*5.92,47.25,19.66,14.47,51.4,10.05,56.62,7.37,23.82,
     X 51.33,195.44,473.5,10.99,1987.,18.06,677.,51.94,.80,129.2,
     X 3000.,94.18,240.,39.9,0.,97.13,-10.,47.35,33.29,2.36,
     X .166667,4.6,0.,45.43,318.,71.55,2*25.48,34.63,.99,
     X 22.7,1.,5.01,19.54,178.4,40.13,45.43,437.,710.8,0.,
     X 47.35,76.07,571.1,4.,564.,,73,0.,7.26,1.,1.,
     X -.03,967.,41.61,3*0.,,1.,178.,70.,40./
      WRITE(KL,100)
  100 FORMAT (//,' --- NEW SUBJECT ----',/)
      IF (LL1.LT.10) GO TO 200
      T(81)=.166667
      CALL QUERY (LL3)
      NW2=0
      CALL NXTWD (7,XXX,LL3,0,2)
C ITRIG(73) CONTROLS PRINT OUT OF THE FIRST 6 FACTORS AT THE END OF RUN
C OTHER INDICES MOSTLY CONCERNED WITH INTERACTIVE DIALOGUE(S/R NXTWD)
      IF (LL3) 120,150,120
  120 IF (LL3-2) 140,130,140
  130 ITRIG(73)=-5
  140 CALL QUERY (LL3)
      GO TO 160
  150 NC=3
  160 IF (NW2.GT.19) GO TO 170
      WRITE (KT,102)
  102 FORMAT(' TO USE S.I. UNITS(KPA) TYPE 1, FOR MM HG TYPE 2',/)
      NW2=0
  170 CALL NXTWD (7,XXX,NNN,1,2)
      SIMLT=1.
      IF(NNN.EQ.1) SIMLT=.1332
  200 NW=1
      NARTI=1
      J3=0
      MT=1
      K2=0
      K4=0
      IF (NC-3) 250,220,250
  220 IF (LL1-10) 260,230,260
  230 CALL QUERY (18)
  260 WRITE (KL,270) NE
  270 FORMAT (10H MINS       ,7(1H,,I3,1H),3X),1H(,I3,1H))
  250 INDEX=1
      NREPT=1
      X=T(81)
      DO 320 I=1,120
  320 T(I)=REFER(I)
      DO 330 I=1,10
      TDLAY(I)=T(31)
      TDLAY(I+10)=T(61)
      TDLAY(I+20)=T(86)
  330 TDLAY(I+30)=T(97)
      T(13)=T(13)*SIMLT
      IF (LL1.LT.10) GO TO 240
      CALL DUMP (LL1)
      LL1=1
  240 T(81)=X
      T(77)=-X*60.
      LL4=-1
      RETURN
      END
```

SUBROUTINE NXTWD (LL3,XXX,NNN,IMIN,IMAX)

```
      SUBROUTINE NXTWD (LL3,XXX,NNN,IMIN,IMAX)
C THIS S/R AND FUNCTIONS VALUE AND V1 ALLOW NUMBERS TO BE ENTERED IN
C FREE FORMAT AND RETRIEVED IN STANDARD REAL OR INTEGER FORM, OR FED
C INTO ARRAYS IF NEEDED OR, IF *Q* IS TYPED, REFERENCE IS MADE TO
C S/R QUERY TO EXPLAIN THE MEANING OF THE QUESTION. OTHERWISE
C THIS SR.AND FUNCTIONS ARE SELF EXPLANATORY
      DIMENSION ICHAR(18),ITEM(20)
      COMMON KT,KL,INI,NW1,NW2,JKL,ITRIG(73),NEOF
      DATA ICHAR/1H ,1H1,1H2,1H3,1H4,1H5,1H6,1H7,1H8,1H9,1H0,
     X          1H.,1H-,1H/,1HB,1HF,1HU,1HQ/
      XMIN=IMIN
      XMAX=IMAX
100   DO 110 J=1,20
      ITEM(J)=1
110   CONTINUE
      IF (NW2.GE.1) GO TO 200
      NREF=NEOF
      DO 120 J=1,72
120   ITRIG(J)=ICHAR(1)
      IL=1
      WRITE (KT,130)
130   FORMAT (1X,'?')
      READ (INI,140) (ITRIG(IM),IM=1,72)
140   FORMAT (72A1)
150   IF (ITRIG(1).NE.ICHAR(1).AND.ITRIG(1).NE.ICHAR(14)) GO TO 190
160   WRITE (KT,170)
170   FORMAT (' A NUMBER MUST BE ENTERED')
      GO TO 240
180   CALL QUERY (LL3)
      GO TO 240
190   IF (ITRIG(IL).EQ.ICHAR(18)) GO TO 180
      NW1=IL
200   L=0
      DO 280 IL=NW1,72
      DO 210 J=1,14
      IF (ITRIG(IL).EQ.ICHAR(J)) GO TO 260
210   CONTINUE
      IF ((ITRIG(IL).EQ.ICHAR(15).OR.ITRIG(IL).EQ.ICHAR(16)).AND.ITRIG(I
     XL+1).EQ.ICHAR(17)) GO TO 340
220   WRITE (KT,230)
230   FORMAT (' ONLY NUMBERS ARE ACCEPTABLE')
240   WRITE (KT,250)
250   FORMAT (' PLEASE TRY AGAIN')
      NW2=0
      NEOF=NREF
      GO TO 100
260   IF (J.NE.1.AND.J.NE.14) GO TO 270
      IF (L) 280,280,290
270   L=L+1
      IF (L.EQ.20) GO TO 360
      ITEM(L)=J
      IF (J.EQ.1) GO TO 290
280   CONTINUE
      IL=72
      IF (NW2.GT.19) GO TO 160
290   NW1=IL+1
C DETECT SLASH / DELIMITER
      IF (J.EQ.14) GO TO 330
      IF (J.EQ.1.AND.NEOF.LE.1) NW2=0
      IF (J.EQ.1.AND.ITRIG(NW1).EQ.ICHAR(1).AND.
     X NW2.GT.19) GO TO 380
300   IF (NW1.GE.72) GO TO 320
      XXX=VALUE(ITEM)
      IF (XXX.LT.XMIN.OR.XXX.GT.XMAX) GO TO 360
      NNN=INT(XXX)
310   NEOF=NEOF-1
      RETURN
320   NEOF=1
      NW2=0
```

```
SUBROUTINE NXTWD (LL3,XXX,NNN,IMIN,IMAX)
CONTINUED

        GO TO 310
  330 NW2=20
        JKL=0
        NEOF=1
        GO TO 300
  340 WRITE (KT,350)
  350 FORMAT (' DON*T USE RUDE WORDS')
        GO TO 220
  360 WRITE (KT,370)
  370 FORMAT (' I*M AFRAID YOUR NUMBER IS NO GOOD')
        GO TO 240
  380 JKL=0
        NW2=0
        GO TO 300
        END
```

REAL FUNCTION VALUE(ITEM)

```
      REAL FUNCTION VALUE(ITEM)
      INTEGER ITEM(20)
      VALUE=0.
      I=1
      VALUE=V1(ITEM,I)
      IF ((ITEM(I).EQ.1).OR.(I.GE.20)) RETURN
      I=I+1
      VALUE=VALUE*(10.**V1(ITEM,I))
      RETURN
      END
```

REAL FUNCTION V1(ITEM,I)

```
      REAL FUNCTION V1(ITEM,I)
      DIMENSION DIGIT(13)
      INTEGER ITEM(20)
      DATA DIGIT/0.,1.,2.,3.,4.,5.,6.,7.,8.,9.,0.,0.,-1./
      S=1.
      V1=0.
      P=0.
      NDOT=0
  100 IF ((ITEM(I).EQ.1).OR.(I.GE.20)) GO TO 150
      IF (ITEM(I).EQ.12) GO TO 120
      IF (ITEM(I).EQ.13) GO TO 130
      IF (NDOT.EQ.1) GO TO 110
      IZ=ITEM(I)
      V1=(V1*10.+DIGIT(IZ))
      GO TO 140
  110 P=P+1.
      IZ=ITEM(I)
      V1=(V1+(DIGIT(IZ)/(10.**P)))
      GO TO 140
  120 NDOT=NDOT+1
      GO TO 140
  130 IZ=ITEM(I)
      S=DIGIT(IZ)
  140 I=I+1
      GO TO 100
  150 V1=V1*S
      RETURN
      END
```

SUBROUTINE QUERY (LL3)


```
        SUBROUTINE QUERY (LL3)
C THIS DOES EXPLANATIONS OF QUESTIONS, AND IS ALSO USED WHEN
C CALLING UP MODEL. LL3 IS ALSO 1ST ARG. OF S/R NXTWD, AND DETERMINES
C OUTPUT TEXT FOR START, AND QUERY CALLS.
        COMMON KT,KL,INI
        GO TO (170,140,260,320,280,300,320,320,360,380,200,340,320,220,240
     X,400,100,120), LL3
  100 WRITE (KT,110)
C*** LOCAL ARRANGEMENTS
  110 FORMAT (' TO PROCEED TYPE 1 THEN PRESS CAR/RET KEY,',/
     X,' TO GET BRIEF DESCRIPTION AND INSTRUCTIONS TYPE 2 + C/R',/)
        GO TO 420
  120 WRITE (KT,130)
  130 FORMAT (' *UNLESS CHANGED LATER, COLUMNS REFER AS FOLLOWS...FACTOR
     X NUMBERS BELOW',/,10X,'EXP.RQ   ART.PH   TOT-VENT-ALV      HCO3  ALV.
     XPO2   PO2-ART-PCO2',/)
        GO TO 420
  140 WRITE (KT,150)
  150 FORMAT (/,' MACPUF IS A MODEL OF THE HUMAN RESPIRATORY SYSTEM DESI
     XGNED AT MCMASTER',/,' UNIVERSITY MEDICAL SCHOOL, CANADA AND ST.BAR
     XTHOLOMEWS HOSPITAL',/,' MEDICAL COLLEGE, ENGLAND, BY DR.C.J.DICKIN
     XSON, DR.E.J.M.CAMPBELL,',/,' DR.A.S.REBUCK, DR.N.L.JONES, DR.D.ING
     XRAM AND DR.K.AHMED.',/,' HE WAS CREATED TO STUDY GAS TRANSPORT AND
     X EXCHANGE.',/,' HE CONTAINS SIMULATED LUNGS, CIRCULATING BLOOD AND
     X',/,' TISSUES. INITIALLY HE BREATHES AT A RATE AND DEPTH DETERMINE
     XD',/,' BY KNOWN INFLUENCES UPON VENTILATION.',/)
        WRITE (KT,160)
  160 FORMAT (' ONCE INTO A STANDARD RUN OF 3 MINUTES (CHANGEABLE)',/,'
     XTHE DISPLAY UNIT PLOTS A VERTICAL GRAPH OF VENTILATION, RATE OF',/
     X,' BREATHING, ART.PCO2 + PO2(SYMBOLS V,F,C + O RESPECTIVELY).',//,
     X' AFTER EACH RUN YOU CAN CHANGE ANYTHING (EG. INSPIRED OXYGEN %)',
     X/,' THEN RUN ANOTHER 3 MINS AND WATCH RESULTS.')
  170 WRITE (KT,180)
C*** LOCAL ARRANGEMENTS
  180 FORMAT (/,' IF ANYTHING GOES WRONG NOTE WHAT YOU DID AND INFORM ',
     X'YOUR TUTOR.',/,1X,'A PRIZE OF $1',
     X' WILL BE GIVEN TO ANYONE CONVINCINGLY SHOWING IMPOSSIBLE',/,' BEH
     XAVIOUR OF THE MODEL IN A POSSIBLE CLINICAL SITUATION....ANY TIME Y
     XOU',/,' CAN*T UNDERSTAND AN INSTRUCTION TYPE Q(QUERY) AND PRESS *C
     X/R*.',//,' OK, LET*S GO ...')
        WRITE (KT,190)
  190 FORMAT (/,' SYMBOLS--- VV= TOT.VENT., FF=FREQ.BR., CC= ART.PCO2,'
     X,' OO= ART.PO2',/,'               **= N2 SUPERSAT.INDEX,IF PRESENT',/)
        GO TO 420
  200 WRITE (KT,210)
  210 FORMAT (' IF EVERY 6TH VALUE PRINTED COMPUTATION WILL STILL TAKE P
     XLACE',/,' AS SPECIFIED IN PREVIOUS REQUESTS..SIMILARLY FOR *30TH*'
     X)
        GO TO 420
  220 WRITE (KT,230)
  230 FORMAT (' THIS ALLOWS YOU TO STORE THE PRESENT STATE OF YOUR SUBJE
     XCT AND TO',/,' RECREATE HIM AGAIN THROUGH USE OF THIS SAME OPTION,
     X BY BACKTRACKING')
        GO TO 420
  240 WRITE (KT,250)
  250 FORMAT (' 1 IS OBVIOUS, 2 STARTS ANOTHER RUN OF STANDARD 3 MIN',/,
     X' 3 STARTS AGAIN WITH A NEW SUBJECT, 4 PRINTS A TABLE OF MOST',/,'
     X USEFUL VALUES, 5 STOPS THE PROGRAMME')
        GO TO 420
  260 WRITE (KT,270)
  270 FORMAT (' 1 IS OBVIOUS, 2 WILL RETURN TO NATURAL VENTILATION IF',/
     X,' ARTIFICIAL HAS BEEN USED AND ALLOWS YOU TO STOP VENTILATION OR
     XTO GIVE',/,' GRADED ARTIFICIAL VENTILATION, 3 ALLOWS YOU TO STORE
     XTHE',/,' PRESENT STATE BY A DUMP INSTRUCTION, AND ALSO BRING THIS
     XSTATE BACK',/,' AGAIN BY A BACKTRACK INSTRUCTION, 4 ALLOWS YOU TO'
     X,/,' ALTER LENGTH OF RUN AND ALSO GET SELECTED VALUES PRINTED TO O
     XRDER',/,' 5 GIVES PRESET PATIENTS AND INSERTION OF FUNCTION TESTS'
     X)
        GO TO 420
```

```
SUBROUTINE QUERY (LL3)
CONTINUED

  280 WRITE (KT,290)
  290 FORMAT (' 1 GIVES THE GRAPH FORMAT YOU HAVE SEEN,',/,' 2 SUPPRESSE
     XS TEXT AND VALUES AND LEAVES JUST GRAPHS,',/,' 3 WILL ALLOW COLUMN
     XS OF UP TO 8 SELECTED VARIABLES TO BE PRINTED',/,' INSTEAD.')
      GO TO 420
  300 WRITE (KT,310)
  310 FORMAT (' THIS IS THE SPECIAL TYPE OF OUTPUT. REFER TO THE ',/,' H
     XANDBOOK FOR INTERPRETATIVE CODE. *69* WILL GIVE THE FOLLOWING',/,'
     X IN COLUMNS  1.TIME, 2. EXP.R.Q., 3.ART.PH, 4.TOT.VENTLN.',/,' 5.A
     XLV.VENTLN., 6.ART.BICARB., 7.ALV.PO2 8.ART.PO2, 9.ART.PCO2',/,' OT
     XHER VARIABLES CAN BE OBTAINED BY TYPING IN A DIFFERENT NUMBER',/,'
     X OR STRING OF NUMBERS...REFER TO HANDBOOK')
      GO TO 420
  320 WRITE (KT,330)
  330 FORMAT (' IF YOU CAN*T UNDERSTAND THIS, GIVE UP!')
      GO TO 420
  340 WRITE (KT,350)
  350 FORMAT (' NORMAL IS 10, BUT FOR BIG METAB.RATES,CARDIAC OUTPUTS OR
     X VENTILATIONS,',/,' A SMALLER ITERATION INTERVAL,EG.5 SECS.WOULD B
     XE BETTER')
      GO TO 420
  360 WRITE (KT,370)
C*** LOCAL ARRANGEMENTS
  370 FORMAT (' TYPE EACH FACTOR NO. YOU WANT TO ALTER AS A STRING OF NU
     XMBERS',/,' SEPARATED BY BLANKS..CAR/RET AT END.',/,' TYPING 100 AL
     XLOWS YOU TO DO SPECIAL EXPERIMENTS, E.G. CLOSE',/,' GLOTTIS, EXPIR
     XE INTO OR REBREATHE FROM A BAG')
      GO TO 420
  380 WRITE (KT,390)
C*** LOCAL ARRANGEMENTS
  390 FORMAT (' TYPE IN THE VALUE IN USUAL UNITS, E.G. TO ALTER FACTOR 1
     X FROM',/,' ITS PRESENT VALUE TO 10(PERCENT OXYGEN) TYPE *10*',/,'
     XAND PRESS C/R KEY')
      GO TO 420
  400 WRITE (KT,410)
  410 FORMAT (' POSITIVE END EXPIRED PRESSURE TENDS TO REDUCE CARDIAC OU
     XTPUT',/,' BUT CAN IMPROVE OXYGEN UPTAKE UNDER SOME CONDITIONS')
  420 RETURN
      END
```

SUBROUTINE SYMPT(SIMLT)

```
      SUBROUTINE SYMPT(SIMLT)
C THIS S/R SPECIFIES VARIOUS SYMPTOMS UNDER APPROPR. CONDITIONS
      COMMON KT,KL,INI,NW1,NW2,JKL,ITRIG(73),NEOF,NW
      COMMON NFLAG,J3,ISPAR,NA,NB,NC,ND,NE(8)
      COMMON NARTI,MT,K2,K4,INDEX
      COMMON T1(12),BARPR,T2(4),HB,T3(26),BO2PR,BC2PR,T4,RRATE,RO2CT,
     X T5,DVENT,SVENT,T6(6),TPH,T7(15),PG,T8(5),FT,CONOM,BUBBL,T9(19),
     X TN2PR
C K1-K4 CONCERNED WITH IMPROVEMENT SYMPTOMS (LOGIC IS COMPLEX)
      X=1./SIMLT
  100 K1=0
      K3=0
      IF (TN2PR*X-6000.) 110,110,130
  110 IF (12.5-BO2PR*X) 120,120,130
  120 IF (BC2PR*X-91.) 150,150,130
  130 WRITE (KT,140)
  140 FORMAT (/,' YOUR PATIENT IS UNROUSABLE')
      K1=1
      GO TO 428
  150 IF (BO2PR*X-13.9) 160,160,180
  160 WRITE (KT,170)
  170 FORMAT (/,5X,'MY EYES ARE GOING DIM')
      K1=1
  180 IF (BUBBL-160.) 210,210,190
  190 WRITE (KT,200)
  200 FORMAT (/,5X,'I HAVE AWFUL PAINS IN MY LEGS')
      K1=1
      GO TO 240
  210 IF (BUBBL-101.) 240,240,220
  220 WRITE (KT,230)
  230 FORMAT (/,5X,'MY SKIN IS ITCHING')
      K3=1
  240 IF (TN2PR*X-4300.) 250,250,260
  250 IF (BC2PR*X-80.) 280,280,260
  260 WRITE (KT,270)
  270 FORMAT (/,5X,'I AM FEELING DROWSY')
      K3=1
  280 IF (NARTI) 390,390,290
  290 IF (RRATE-46.) 330,330,300
  300 WRITE (KT,310)
  310 FORMAT (/,5X,'THIS....IS....IMPOSSIB... ...')
  320 K1=1
      GO TO 390
  330 IF (RRATE-35.) 360,360,340
  340 WRITE (KT,350)
  350 FORMAT (/,5X,'I AM VERY SHORT OF BREATH')
      GO TO 320
  360 IF (RRATE-27.) 390,390,370
  370 WRITE (KT,380)
  380 FORMAT (/,5X,'I AM RATHER SHORT OF BREATH')
      K3=1
  390 IF (TPH-7.59) 420,420,400
  400 WRITE (KT,410)
  410 FORMAT (/,5X,'I AM GETTING TINGLING AND CRAMPS IN MY HANDS')
      K3=1
  420 IF (TPH-7.13) 424,424,428
  424 WRITE (KT,426)
  426 FORMAT (/,5X,'I DON*T FEEL WELL AT ALL')
      K3=1
  428 IF (TPH-7.08) 430,450,450
  430 WRITE (KT,440)
  440 FORMAT (/,' YOUR PATIENT IS TWITCHING')
      K1=1
  450 IF (NARTI) 460,460,490
  460 X=SVENT*.9-DVENT
      IF (X) 490,490,470
  470 WRITE (KT,480)
  480 FORMAT (/,' YOUR PATIENT IS FIGHTING THE VENTILATOR')
      K3=1
```

```
SUBROUTINE SYMPT(SIMLT)
CONTINUED

  490 X=1.3*HB-RO2CT
      IF (X-7.) 520,500,500
  500 WRITE (KT,510)
  510 FORMAT (/,' YOUR PATIENT IS VERY BLUE')
      K1=1
      GO TO 550
  520 IF (X-5.) 550,530,530
  530 WRITE (KT,540)
  540 FORMAT (/,' YOUR PATIENT IS BLUE')
      K3=1
  550 IF (K1-K3) 570,570,560
  560 K3=1
  570 K5=K1+K3
      IF (K2-K5) 600,600,580
  580 WRITE (KT,590)
  590 FORMAT (/,5X,'GOD BLESS YOU DOCTOR. I FEEL REALLY WELL AGAIN',/,5X
     X,'IT*S LIKE A MIRACLE',/)
      GO TO 660
  600 IF (K2-K1) 630,630,610
  610 WRITE (KT,620)
  620 FORMAT (/,5X,'I FEEL BETTER BUT NOT RIGHT YET.',/,5X,'CAN*T YOU DO
     X SOMETHING ELSE FOR ME?',/)
      GO TO 660
  630 IF (K4-K3) 660,660,640
  640 WRITE (KT,650)
  650 FORMAT (/,5X,'THAT*S BETTER DOCTOR ..... ',/,5X,'BUT ARE YOU GOING
     X TO DO ANY OTHER NASTY THINGS TO ME?',/)
  660 K2=K1
      K4=K3
      IF (NB.NE.2) GO TO 670
C ALTER NO. OF ITERATIONS AFTER CLIN1 AND 2 SUBJECTS IN STEADY STATE
      NA=30
      IF (FT.LT..1) NA=18
      NB=0
  670 RETURN
      END
```

```
SUBROUTINE UNITS(N,SIMLT)


      SUBROUTINE UNITS(N,SIMLT)
C TRANSFORM PRESSURE VARIABLES TO S.I. UNITS, IF NECESSARY
C SIMLT HAS VALUE OF 1 FOR MM HG, .1332 FOR SI(KPA)
      COMMON NTAB(101),T(105)
      DIMENSION NSI(10)
C NSI CONTAINS FACTOR NUMBERS OF ALL P.PRESS. VARIABLES FOR
C SI CONVERSION BEFORE OUTPUT DISPLAY
      DATA NSI/41,42,45,46,72,74,96,97,103,105/
      X=SIMLT
      IF(N-2) 10,5,10
    5 X=1./X
   10 DO 20 I=1,10
      J=NSI(I)
   20 T(J)=T(J)*X
      RETURN
      END
```

Appendix V

TECHNICAL DETAILS; STORAGE SPACE; SEGMENT INTER-
CONNECTIONS AND OVERLAYS; EXECUTION TIME;
COPYRIGHT; COST

The technical details in this section may be of no interest to the general
reader, to the physiologist or clinician wanting to use the model, apart from
the final section on the cost of operating MacPuf on various systems. However, the details are given here to help him or a programmer with no knowledge of the physiology involved to be able with least trouble to load and run
MacPuf.

Fortran was chosen because it is the most widely available high-level
language, and a Fortran compiler is available on almost every computer
except the very smallest. The merits of the Basic language have been urged
upon me by many people, but at this late stage it would be a major undertaking to convert the model, and its speed of operation would be unacceptably
slow. In any case many computers have no Basic interpreter, and Basic
compilers are in their infancy. High level simulation languages are not widely
available and would have been more difficult to work with.

The programme of Appendix IV, i.e. the whole programme of the model,
contains approximately 1760 Fortran statements, about 90% of which are
executable. However, much of this material is concerned with interaction
between an operator and the model (see Table II). The main-line programme
contains about 360 statements (excluding store instructions), subroutine
GASES contains 27 and subroutine DELAY contains 28. Between them these
segments perform all the computations needed during a run. Those who
wanted to fit the programme into the smallest possible computer, and were
not concerned with user interaction and symptom generation, could set up
the main-line programme and these two subroutines, feed the data of subroutine MINIT into the common store from cards (to initialise a new intact
subject), read in changes in parameters if necessary using subroutine CONST,
and run the iterative DO loop of the main programme to examine their chosen
problem. If subroutine BAGER is included, the scope of experiments simul-
able includes glottis closure, bag collection and rebreathing experiments.
Inclusion of CLIN2 allows the creation of patients to order, by allowing
specifications of body dimensions, sex and age, and by specifying the results
of respiratory function tests. Subroutine SYMPT is entirely dispensable and
its omission results only in the disappearance of symptoms. Subroutine
DUMP is also only relevant for interactive use, allowing the recreation of

Table II   Principal functions of Programme segments

Name	Number of Fortran statements (excluding comments)	PDP11 module size (decimal words)	Functions
BLANK COMMON		505	Store of variables
MAIN	361	3201	Introduction; iterate main programme for all computations except dissociation curves and delay line
BAGER	120	1189	Perform all manoeuvres and computations associated with glottis closure, collection or rebreathing procedures using bags; display
BRETH	33	614	Graphical display of ventilation, frequency, and artificial gas tensions
CLIN1	91	659	Create preset patients
CLIN2	201	2134	Create patients specified by age, size, sex, and pulmonary function test results
CONST	98	1154	Initialise all parameters before each set of main programme iterations
DEADY	270	2942	Provide operator interaction for changing parameters, time scale, and display
DEATH	44	362	Test each programme iteration for lethal or illegal conditions
DELAY	28	158	Insert delays in venous line for gas contents, bicarbonate, etc.
DUMP	28	239	Copy current values of all COMMON variables into store; or retrieve previously stored values and copy back into store
GASES	27	353	Compute gas contents from partial pressures, pH, etc.
GSINV	83	684	Compute partial pressures from contents, by reversing S/R GASES
MINIT	69	600	Initialise all values for a normal average young adult; on first call dump same into storage (TDUMP)
NXTWD	78	559	Read in operator's instructions as numbers, blanks or slashes. Using real functions VALUE and V1 convert same to free format
VALUE	10	70	
V1	28	185	
QUERY	100	1980	Print initial text; explain meaning of questions in interactive dialogue
SYMPT	102	850	Test relevant values for symptom occurrence at end of each run, and print same
UNITS	12	74	Interconvert SI and mmHg units before and after display routines
LIBRARY		4954	

previously stored states. CLIN1 is rather in the same category, since it is concerned with the generation of preset patients whose parameter changes could equally well be read in from cards. Subroutine BRETH is concerned with graphical output during iterative repetition of the main programme loop. The largest subroutine (DEADY) is the focal point of user interaction, by which changes in parameters can be made and by which end-of-run values can be displayed. Subroutine DEATH tests for lethal conditions and potential arithmetical errors. Subroutine NXTWD and its associated function subprogrammes VALUE and V1 are mainly used in the interactive dialogue of subroutine DEADY.

The main functions of each individual part of the programme are summarised in Table II, which also indicates the length of each segment in terms of the number of Fortran statements and the approximate module size for a PDP11, in decimal words.

Storage space

The COMMON store of the model contains 120 basic parameters and computed variables in array 'T'. Another 40 are stored in array TDLAY, which holds the values for the venous return delay line. If storage of variables is a problem (which is likely only on an extremely small computer) TDLAY could be omitted, and subroutine DELAY also omitted. This makes surprisingly little difference to the operation of the programme, though the speed of transit of gases becomes unduly fast, and inaccurate phase relationships occur during rapid changes, especially at short iteration intervals. Subroutine DUMP allows the current state of the model to be stored in its entirety, in array TDUMP. On a 'STORE' instruction, array T and array TDLAY are copied into TDUMP; on a 'BACKTRACK' instruction TDUMP is copied back into T and TDLAY. Subroutine DUMP and array TDUMP could be omitted, with their interactive dialogue in subroutine DEADY, with no effect on the model save for the loss of this storage/retrieval facility.

Interactive dialogue is centred on subroutine DEADY, and subroutine NXTWD and its associated function subprogrammes VALUE and V1 perform all reading in of an operator's instructions. These routines allow free format reading, but use standard Fortran format statements throughout. For example, typing 20, 20., or 020.000 sets the integer argument NNN and the floating point argument XXX to the value 20. Entry of 'QUERY' or 'Q' calls subroutine QUERY, which could be omitted to save space. Since subroutine QUERY contains many text strings, it occupies a lot of storage in the compiled programme. CLIN1 and CLIN2, especially the latter, make MacPuf much more useful to a clinician, but do not affect the main computational process. Subroutine BAGER and all the calls to it in the main programme and from subroutine DEADY could likewise be omitted, with loss of the special facilities it contains, but without otherwise affecting the programme.

Segment interconnexions and overlays

An experienced programmer wanting to pack MacPuf into a small computer must devise a suitable form of overlay consistent with core available and any limitations of the Fortran compiler and linker structure. A larger machine will, of course, allow the programme to be run without the need for any segmenting. It can simply be fed in, edited to insert, if necessary, correct logical numbers for input and output devices, and the model will at once be fully operational. The overlay facilities available on different machines vary so greatly that it is not possible to make a general statement regarding the best way to organise the programme. I have seen MacPuf working well on a PDP12 machine with 16K of core but the programmer had to split the main-line programme to get it in. This raised a few problems with local variables in array 'C' which are computed outside the main programme loop in subroutine CONST (see Appendix IV). These could readily be inserted into a subroutine assigning new values before each run into a COMMON ARRAY or into an argument list.

Probably the best place for splitting the main programme loop is either just before or just after the venous blood pool exchanges, i.e. either at or just after statement 700 or after statement 710. It might be better still to take gas transport starting between statements 380 and 390 and ending just after statement 950 and put all this into a subroutine called from the main-line programme DO loop. Care would be needed anyway to retain the values of local variables as subroutine arguments or as a labelled common store.

The programme can be loaded without overlaying on a PDP11 computer with 28K of core. It has also been built to run as an overlaid programme within 16K of core. To achieve this subroutine DEADY was modified to avoid calls to subroutine BAGER, CLIN1, etc., and renamed DEADZ. A new routine DEADY was written to perform the calls to these routines and communicate with DEADZ to perform all other functions of the original DEADY. In this way the large routine DEADZ could be placed in a common overlay region with CLIN1, CLIN2, SYMPT, BAGER, etc. and the total programme could be fitted into 16K. The best overlay structure was as shown in Figure AV.1.

Execution time

On a dedicated PDP11/10 in overlaid form the programme took about 2 s to compute each iteration (simulating 2 to 10 s). On the PDP12 with floating point processor, again in overlaid form, it took about $\frac{1}{2}$ s to compute each iteration. The totally core resident version on the PDP11/10 does not run appreciably faster than the overlaid version since the speed of the output device and operator response time are usually the limiting factors. The overlay structure is designed to minimise disc transfers during the main loop of the programme—most overlaying occurs during user interaction at the end of a run. At the other end of the scale the programme runs on a PDP11/45 with floating point processor at a rate of between $\frac{1}{10}$ and $\frac{1}{30}$ s per iteration

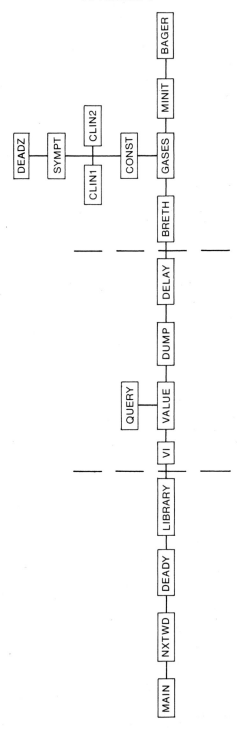

Figure AV.1   Suggested overlay structure suitable for limited core size

depending on the Fortran compiler in use. On the PDP12 version, therefore, respiratory computations can run about 20 times as fast as real time in a clinical situation, and on the PDP11/45 about 200 times as fast. The output device is usually the limiting factor. Speed of execution on time-sharing systems depends on the size, speed and other-user load and it is difficult to generalise. However, a class using MacPuf on 8 separate terminals supported on an HP 3000 time-sharing system noted no delay at all, and all 30 character/second printers were operating at full speed throughout.

Copyright

As in the case of other self-teaching simulations programmes that my colleagues and I have developed at McMaster University, University College Hospital and St. Bartholomew's Hospital Medical Colleges we have not, fortunately, been so hard pressed for financial support that we have had to restrict availability of the software to those who can help recoup the development costs, which have so far been met by our research and education budgets. We are very pleased this is so and hope it may remain so, especially so that duplication of effort in many schools can be avoided. My colleagues and I therefore make no claim to copyright of the programme itself nor of the manual examples in Appendix VII, though the remainder of the book is, of course, copyright. We trust that other users will do us the courtesy of retaining the acknowledgements of authorship and sponsorship which are incorporated in the text of the programme, in subroutine QUERY, and which are displayed when a user first makes acquaintance with the model.

Cost

The cost of operating computers depends so much on local circumstances that it is difficult to generalise. In ordinary usage on a commercial time-sharing system MacPuf on average runs up a *computation* time (i.e. CPU) bill of about $5 per hour. (The British pound seems to be sliding so fast that current costing in dollars seems more helpful!) A student, going slower, would use less, e.g. $2–3 per hour; an experienced user might use $15 CPU time per hour for extensive work. In addition there would, of course, be rental charges and telephone charges. A commercial time-sharing service in London (England) currently (1976) offered a package deal including:

1. rent of a Teletype or similar terminal and coupler
2. unlimited low-priority connect-time
3. limited file storage (enough for MacPuf and 2 or 3 other large programmes)
4. 20 minutes CPU time per month

for a basic charge of $350 per month, i.e. about $4000 per annum. This amount of CPU time would be easily enough for regular demonstrations and limited clinical use; it would need to be supplemented by extra CPU time for the widespread use of a large class.

The situation is transformed if MacPuf is only one computer resource amongst many. If there are 10 similar teaching or clinical 'packages', for example, the running cost would probably be only twice as much as for MacPuf alone, per year. For example, if reasonable student and faculty use was already taking up, say, $6000 p.a., it would probably be possible by spending another $6000 p.a. to maintain and effectively use 10 large instructional programmes on a commercial system.

Any department with a small dedicated computer can obviously run MacPuf at virtually no extra cost at all other than a small amount of once-and-for-all programmer's time interfacing the model with his system.

Appendix VI

LIST OF FORTRAN SYMBOLIC NAMES

Floating point variables

The standard method of construction of most of the Fortran symbolic names for variables in the programme was described in Chapter 4. Summarising, the first letter specifies a compartment:

A—Alveolar; B—Brain; E—Effluent arterial blood flowing to tissues; P—Pulmonary capillary (idealised); R—Arterial; S—Slow tissue store (for nitrogen); T—Tissue; U—Bubbles in tissues (if present); V—Venous

The second two letters specify the nature of the material or measurement, e.g.:

O2—Oxygen; C2—Carbon dioxide; C3—Bicarbonate; N2—Nitrogen

The final two letters specify the type of measurement, e.g.:

MT—Amount of something in cc STPD (gas) or mmol (bicarbonate); CT—Content of something, in cc STPD/100 ml (gas) or mmol/litre (bicarbonate); PR—Partial pressure, in mmHg (torr); PH—pH (second 2 letters omitted—e.g. brain pH is represented by 'BPH')

Thus arterial blood carbon dioxide content is represented by RC2CT, and AN2MT represents the amount of nitrogen in the alveolar compartment.

Non–standard floating point variables in main programme

Other floating point, i.e. non-integer, variables are mostly chosen to have some mnemonic value. A complete list of these non-standard, non-integer symbols appears below, in alphabetical order:

ADDC3 Manually changeable variable specifying number of mmol bicarbonate to be added to the body: initialised at 0, and returned to zero after use

AGE Age in years

AVENT Alveolar ventilation, in cc/iteration interval (BTPS)

AZ Percentage normal response of ventilation to altered H^+ and PCO_2 stimuli

BAG	Volume of a bag, if used, in cc BTPS
BAGC	Volume of CO_2 in the bag, in cc STPD
BAGO	Volume of O_2 in the bag, in cc STPD
BARPR	Barometric pressure, mmHg or KPa
BO2AD	Index of brain oxygenation adequacy (normally = 1.0)
BULLA	Symbolic name for added dead space—normal value = 0 cc (BTPS)
BZ	Percentage normal response of ventilation to hypoxia
C	Array storing precalculated run parameters (see subroutine CONST)
CBF	Cerebral blood flow, in ml/100g/min
CO	Cardiac function, as percentage normal average for the subject
COADJ	Effective cardiac output, from nominal cardiac output and adjustments, l/min
COMAX	Maximum cardiac output, in l/min
CONOM	Nominal resting cardiac output, l/min
CONSO	Tissue oxygen consumption, nominal resting value, cc/min STPD
CZ	Percentage normal response of ventilation to increased metabolic requirements and to intrinsic neurogenic drive
DSPAC	Dead space, in cc BTPS
DVENT	Total ventilation, l/min (BTPS)
ELAST	Elastance, cm H_2O/l
FADM	Fixed venous admixture, i.e. complete right-to-left shunt, as percentage of cardiac output
FEV	Forced expired volume in 1 second
FIC2	Inspired carbon dioxide percentage
FIO2	Inspired oxygen percentage
FT	Fractional time interval, in min (normal 0.16667, = 10 s)
FTCO	Local variable incorporating effective cardiac output and fractional time
FTCOC	Same but including an allowance for wasted tissue perfusion, related to fitness
FVENT	Alveolar ventilation, in l/min
FY	Local variable describing (1) tissue buffering with changing PCO_2, and (2) extra dead space under certain conditions (Chapter 11)
HB	Haemoglobin, in g/100 ml
HT	Height, in cm
PC	Respiratory exchange ratio during last iteration interval (also used as a local variable)
PC2	Local variable, arterial or end inspiratory PCO_2, mmHg
PCV	Packed cell volume, percentage
PD	Metabolic rate as percentage normal resting value
PEEP	Positive end-expiratory pressure (cm H_2O)
PG	Index affected by severity and time of brain oxygen inadequacy, to determine death and syptoms
PJ	Arterial oxygen saturation, percentage
PL	Index determining operative mode during bag collection, re-

	breathing and tracheal obstruction experiments (see subroutine BAGER)
PO2	Local variable, arterial or end-inspiratory alveolar PO_2, mmHg
PR	Percentage normal coupling of ventilatory drives to resultant ventilation
PW	Effective operative venous admixture effect (percentage cardiac output), taking all factors into account
QA	Net oxygen uptake per unit time interval, cc STPD
QB	Net carbon dioxide output per unit time interval, cc STPD
REFER	120-element DATA array for initialisation of new subjects (see subroutine MINIT)
REFLV	Reference volume of the lungs, used to return lung volume after prolonged tracheal obstruction
RRATE	Respiratory rate, in breaths/min
RVADM	Extra shunt effect brought in for emphysematous patients when specified (normally $=0$)
SAT	Local saturation returned to main programme from subroutine GASES
SHUNT	Right-to-left shunt, as a ratio of the unshunted flow
SIMLT	Multiplier for S.I. unit/mmHg conversion
SPACE	Inspiratory/expiratory duration ratio (normally 0.4)
SVENT	Total effective drive to ventilation, taking most variables into account, l/min
T	120-member array containing COMMON variables and parameters
TC2RF	Reference value for detecting changes in tissue PCO_2
TDLAY	40-member array storing tissue CO_2 content and pressure, pH and bicarbonate for the venous delay line
TDUMP	160-member array storing similar sets of values for use in backtracking
TEMP	Body temperature, in °C
TIDVL	Tidal volume, cc BTPS
TJJ	Eight-member array storing a string of variables to be output in columns
TND	Counter in seconds
TRQ	Tissue respiratory quotient
TVENT	Total stimulus to ventilation, in l/min
TVOL	Effective tissue fluid volume, as litres of extracellular fluid
U	Local variable—used in several places
V	Local variable—used in several places
VADM	Nominal value for dynamic venous admixture, varying with lung oxygenation, etc. (percentage)
VBLVL	Venous blood volume, in ml
VC	Vital capacity, in litres
VLUNG	Volume of the lung, in cc BTPS
W	Local variable—used in several places
WT	Weight, in kg
X	Local variable—used in several places
X109–X110	Spare variables not in present use

XDSPA	Extra dead space specified by altered function tests for specified subjects (cc BTPS)
XMALE	Index specifying male (1) or female (0)
XVENT	Local variable describing volume ventilated out in one iteration interval (cc BTPS)
Y	Local variable—used in several places
Z	Local variable—used in several places

Integer factors and variables

The list that follows is in alphabetical order:

I	Local integer variable
INDEX	Keeps a log of the position of the 'pointer' in the venous delay line in subroutine DELAY
INI	Logical number of the input unit. In interactive use this will always be the console Teletype or equivalent; otherwise could be a card-reader
ISPAR	Index specifying suppression of 5 out of 6 lines of output (2), 29 out of 30 lines (3) or no suppression (1)
ITRIG	72-element array representing 72 spaces across a line of the keyboard typewriter, each element being a single alphanumeric character. Reading of instructions is transferred into this array as blanks, numbers or separators
ITRIG(73)	The 73rd element of this (same) array is used to control printing of current values of the first 6 parameters after each run. If less than 2, the table is printed; otherwise printing is suppressed
J	Local integer variable
J3	Time in minutes since creation of a new subject
JKL	Index governing input of sequences of numbers separated by blanks. Normal value = 1; zero ends sequence of numbers (see subroutines DEADY and NXTWD)
K2	Index specifying previous occurrence of severe symptoms (= 1); or absence of same (= 0) (for comparison with K1)
K4	Index specifying previous occurrence of minor symptoms (= 1); or absence of same (= 0) (for comparison with K3)
KL	Logical number of unit displaying output most suitable for a lineprinter if available (cf. KT). If output is all to be directed to a Teletype or equivalent, KT and KL should be the same
KT	Logical number of output most suitable for operator interaction. If all output is to be directed to a Teletype or equivalent, KT should have the same logical number as KL
LL1	1st entry to MINIT inserts normal values into DUMP store (LL1 = 10). After new subject set up, LL1 = 1. LL1 = 2 calls for a new subject after 'DEATH'; LL1 = 3 calls for the same, after arithmetic errors.
LL2	Spare index not in present use.

LL3 — Index controlling output from subroutine QUERY displaying text when setting up the model: normal = 2; abbreviated introduction = 1; research application without introduction or graphs (= 0). Subsequently codes explanations from subroutine QUERY in response to typing 'Q'

LL4 — Counter (1 to 6) for suppression of 5 out of 6 lines of output, when specified by index ISPAR

LL5 — Normal acceptable values (= 0). Impossible values make this index = −1 and lead to same situation as simulated 'DEATH'

MORAN — Local integer variable controlling main programme loop

MT — Prints final computed values after each run (= 1); or not (= 0)

N — Local integer variable

NA — Specifies number of iterations of main programme loop until next halt (default = 18)

NARTI — Specifies natural ventilation (1), or artificial ventilation (0)

NB — Specifies suppression of main programme output display during creation of preset or specially created patients, using CLIN1 or CLIN2 subroutine (= 2); or no such suppression, as in normal use (= 1). If NB = 0 graph scales are printed

NC — Type of output: standard (1); graphs only (2); selected values (3); all values (4)

ND — Time in seconds

NDUMP — 20-element array holding COMMON integer values from NFLAG to INDEX, used during 'BACKTRACK' by means of subroutine DUMP

NE — Eight-element array holding the factor numbers of 8 variables whose values can be displayed by the 'SELECTED VALUES' option. Default values for NE(8) are: 69 33 51 35 60 41 72 and 74. These numbers correspond to expired R.Q.; arterial pH; total ventilation; alveolar ventilation; arterial bicarbonate; alveolar PO_2; arterial PO_2; and arterial PCO_2. Changeable by user interaction from subroutine DEADY

NEOF — Specifies maximum number of integer or floating point numbers that the next call to subroutine NXTWD can accommodate. Normal (= 1): set to zero after call completed

NFLAG — Normal use (1). If 'BACKTRACK' after 'DEATH' is requested, NFLAG = 0, which prevents the creation of a new subject by subroutine MINIT

NO — 20-element array held for reference in a DATA statement, and used for initialising COMMON integer values from NFLAG to INDEX

NREPT — Specifies number of repetitions of main programme loop. During setting up of a new subject, NW = 1; thereafter is set equal to index NA at end of each run

NTAB — 20-element array equivalent to COMMON integer values from NFLAG to INDEX

NW — Index specifying that a new subject has been created and not so far changed (1); or that changes have already been made (0)

NW1   Maintains a pointer of a 72-character line of input instruc-
           tions, taking them in sequence from left to right. Initialised
           before every READ at unity
NW2   Initialised at zero before the first call to NXTWD. If greater
           than zero further calls to NXTWD take instructions from
           array ITRIG rather than from the keyboard. If greater than
           19, all text questions are suppressed

Appendix VII

OPERATING HANDBOOK (abbreviated)

The operating handbook for the model, including a block diagram and full operating instructions, is available at nominal cost from the Software Supervisor, Computation Services Unit, McMaster University Medical Center, Main Street West, Hamilton, Ontario, Canada. The illustrations that follow are examples taken from the handbook which give some idea of the range of experimental simulation possible.

The last item in Appendix VII is the list of changeable parameters or factors (30 in all) which are listed in the handbook and which can be changed by operator interaction. Their usual values and units are also shown. In addition, the factor numbers for most of the important variables in different compartments are listed and the final section indicates the meaning and cause of various errors which can arise during operation of the model, and the remedy suggested to circumvent or prevent them. The whole of this section (the only indispensable part of the handbook) appears as comment cards at the end of the complete Fortran programme when this is supplied as a card deck on a magnetic tape by McMaster University Medical Center.

```
SYMBOLS-- VV= TOT.VENT.,, FF=FREQ.BR.,, CC= ART.PCO2, OO= ART.PO2
       **= N2 SUPERSAT.INDEX,IF PRESENT

TO USE S.I. UNITS(KPA) TYPE 1, FOR MM HG TYPE 2

?_2
(KPA)(O)              (4)            (8)          (12)          (16)
 MINS 0       20        40        60        80      100        120
+SECS .     .     .     .     .     .     .     .     .     .     .
  0. 0.  V  F                C                            O

FINAL VALUES FOR THIS RUN WERE...

ARTERIAL PO2 =  94.2  O2 CONT =  19.5, O2 SAT=  97.%
ARTERIAL PCO2=  39.9  CO2 CONT=  47.3
ARTERIAL PH = 7.40( 40.NM), ARTERIAL BICARBONATE = 23.8

RESPIRATORY RATE = 12.8, TIDAL VOL.=  462. ML
TOTAL VENTILATION=   5.9 L/MIN, ACTUAL CARD.OUTPUT=    5.0 L/MIN
TOTAL DEAD SPACE= 129. CC, ACTUAL VENOUS ADMIXTURE=    2.4 PERCENT

1.INSP.O2=  21., 2.CO2=   0. PERCENT, 3.NOM.CARD.OUTP.= 100.PER CENT
4.TISS.METAB.= 100. , 5.VENOUS ADMXT.=   0. ,  6.D.SPACE+=   0. ML

DO YOU WANT TO..1.CHANGE, 2.CONTINUE, 3.RESTART, 4.INSPECT, 5.STOP

?_2
(KPA)(O)              (4)            (8)          (12)          (16)
 MINS 0       20        40        60        80      100        120
+SECS .     .     .     .     .     .     .     .     .     .     .
  0.10.  V  F                C                            O
  0.20.  V  F                C                            O
  0.30.  V  F                C                            O
  0.40.  V  F                C                            O
   {      {  {               {                            {
   {      {  {               {                            {
  2.50.  V  F                C                            O
  3. 0.  V  F                C                            O

FINAL VALUES FOR THIS RUN WERE...

ARTERIAL PO2 =  94.2  O2 CONT =  19.5, O2 SAT=  97.%
ARTERIAL PCO2=  39.9  CO2 CONT=  47.3
ARTERIAL PH = 7.40( 40.NM), ARTERIAL BICARBONATE = 23.8

RESPIRATORY RATE = 12.8, TIDAL VOL.=  462. ML
TOTAL VENTILATION=   5.9 L/MIN, ACTUAL CARD.OUTPUT=    5.0 L/MIN
TOTAL DEAD SPACE= 129. CC, ACTUAL VENOUS ADMIXTURE=    2.4 PERCENT

1.INSP.O2=  21., 2.CO2=   0. PERCENT, 3.NOM.CARD.OUTP.= 100.PER CENT
4.TISS.METAB.= 100. , 5.VENOUS ADMXT.=   0. ,  6.D.SPACE+=   0. ML

(THE FACTOR LIST ABOVE WILL NOW DISAPPEAR - REFER TO HANDBOOK)
DO YOU WANT TO..1.CHANGE, 2.CONTINUE, 3.RESTART, 4.INSPECT, 5.STOP

?_1
1.CHANGE VALUES, 2.NAT/ART VENT, 3.STORE/BKTRK, 4.RUN CHANGE, 5.PRESETS
?_Q
1 IS OBVIOUS, 2 WILL RETURN TO NATURAL VENTILATION IF
ARTIFICIAL HAS BEEN USED AND ALLOWS YOU TO STOP VENTILATION OR TO GIVE
GRADED ARTIFICIAL VENTILATION, 3 ALLOWS YOU TO STORE THE
PRESENT STATE BY A DUMP INSTRUCTION, AND ALSO BRING THIS STATE BACK
AGAIN BY A BACKTRACK INSTRUCTION, 4 ALLOWS YOU TO
ALTER LENGTH OF RUN AND ALSO GET SELECTED VALUES PRINTED TO ORDER
5 GIVES PRESET PATIENTS AND INSERTION OF FUNCTION TESTS
PLEASE TRY AGAIN
```

Figure VII.1   Shows the output of the model when first called up, and the effect of an instruction to CONTINUE. After a graph of 3 minutes' simulated time, during which ventilation (V), frequency of breathing (F), arterial PCO_2 (C) and arterial PO_2 (O) do not change the steady state values are again printed. At the bottom of the page the effect of typing 'Q' (query) is shown

```
DO YOU WANT TO..1.CHANGE, 2.CONTINUE, 3.RESTART, 4.INSPECT, 5.STOP

?_(1)
1.CHANGE VALUES, 2.NAT/ART VENT, 3.STORE/BKTRK, 4.RUN CHANGE, 5.PRESETS
?_(2)
1.GIVE ARTIFICIAL, 2.RETURN TO NATURAL VENTILATION
?_(1)
NOW VENTILATION RATE IN CYCLES/MIN
?_(14)
GIVE TIDAL VOLUME IN ML
?_(300)
POSITIVE END EXPIRATORY PRESSURE — TYPE EITHER *0*
OR NUMBER OF CM WATER (UP TO 15)
?_(0)
*** ART.VENT. AT 14./MIN., 300.ML TID.VOL., AND  0.CM PEEP
DO YOU WANT TO..1.CHANGE, 2.CONTINUE, 3.RESTART, 4.INSPECT, 5.STOP

?_(2)
(KPA)(0)              (4)              (8)            (12)              (16)
  MINS 0       20       40        60       80        100        120
 +SECS .    .    .    .    .    .    .    .    .    .    .    .    .
    0.10. V      F           C                        O
    0.20. V      F           C                        O
    0.30. V      F           C                     O
    0.40. V      F            C                  O
    0.50. V      F            C                O
    1. 0. V      F            C              O
    1.10. V      F            C            O
    1.20. V      F            C         O
    1.30. V      F            C         O
    1.40. V      F            C       O
    1.50. V      F            C      O
    2. 0. V      F            C      O
    2.10. V      F             C     O
    2.20. V      F             C     O
    2.30. V      F             C   O
    2.40. V      F             C   O
    2.50. V      F             C   O
    3. 0. V      F             C   O

FINAL VALUES FOR THIS RUN WERE...

ARTERIAL PO2 =   74.0  O2 CONT =  18.9, O2 SAT=  94.%
ARTERIAL PCO2=   45.0  CO2 CONT=  49.6
ARTERIAL PH = 7.36( 43.NM), ARTERIAL BICARBONATE = 24.7

RESPIRATORY RATE = 14.0, TIDAL VOL.= 300. ML
TOTAL VENTILATION=   4.2 L/MIN, ACTUAL CARD.OUTPUT=   5.2 L/MIN
TOTAL DEAD SPACE= 108. CC, ACTUAL VENOUS ADMIXTURE=   3.1 PERCENT


* YOUR PATIENT IS FIGHTING THE VENTILATOR
  DO YOU WANT TO..1.CHANGE, 2.CONTINUE, 3.RESTART, 4.INSPECT, 5.STOP

  ?_(1)
  1.CHANGE VALUES, 2.NAT/ART VENT, 3.STORE/BKTRK, 4.RUN CHANGE, 5.PRESETS
  ?_(3)
  DO YOU WANT TO 1.STORE PRESENT STATE, 2.BACKTRACK TO LAST STORED STATE
  ?_(1)
  STORED AT THIS POINT ************
  DO YOU WANT TO..1.CHANGE, 2.CONTINUE, 3.RESTART, 4.INSPECT, 5.STOP
```

Figure VII.2 Use of the ARTIFICIAL VENTILATION option at a total ventilation which is inadequate to maintain normal gas tensions. Note the fall of PO_2 (symbol O) and the rise of PCO_2 (C) over the 3 minutes of the run. Notice also the patient's 'symptom' (*) at the end of the run. At the bottom is an instruction to store the existing present state

```
DO YOU WANT TO..1.CHANGE, 2.CONTINUE, 3.RESTART, 4.INSPECT, 5.STOP

?.(1)
1.CHANGE VALUES, 2.NAT/ART VENT, 3.STORE/BKTRK, 4.RUN CHANGE, 5.PRESETS
?.(1)
TYPE NUMBER OF FACTORS (1-30) TO CHANGE, OR 100 FOR BAG EXPTS., ETC.
?.(1)
FACTOR   1 (CURRENT VALUE=   20.9), SPECIFY NEW VALUE
?.(100)
FACTOR   1 =  100.0 (PREVIOUSLY =   20.9)
DO YOU WANT TO..1.CHANGE, 2.CONTINUE, 3.RESTART, 4.INSPECT, 5.STOP

?.(1)
1.CHANGE VALUES, 2.NAT/ART VENT, 3.STORE/BKTRK, 4.RUN CHANGE, 5.PRESETS
?.(2)
1.GIVE ARTIFICIAL, 2.RETURN TO NATURAL VENTILATION
?.(2)
*** NATURAL VENTILATION
DO YOU WANT TO..1.CHANGE, 2.CONTINUE, 3.RESTART, 4.INSPECT, 5.STOP

?.(2)
(KPA)(0)              (4)           (8)           (12)          (16)
MINS 0        20       40       60       80       100       120
+SECS .    .    .    .    .    .    .    .    .    .    .    .    .
  3.10.    V F              C               O
  3.20.    V F              C                           O
  3.30.  V   F            C
  3.40.  V   F            C
  3.50.  V   F            C
  4. 0.  V   F             C
  4.10.  V   F              C
  4.20.  V   F              C
  4.30.  V   F              C
  4.40.  V   F              C
  4.50.  V   F              C
  5. 0.  V   F              C
  5.10.  V   F              C
  5.20.  V   F              C
  5.30.  V   F              C
  5.40.  V   F              C
  5.50.  V   F              C
  6. 0.  V   F              C

FINAL VALUES FOR THIS RUN WERE...

ARTERIAL PO2 = 604.8  O2 CONT =   21.6, O2 SAT= 100.%
ARTERIAL PCO2=  44.7  CO2 CONT=  48.9
ARTERIAL PH = 7.36( 44.NM), ARTERIAL BICARBONATE = 24.4

RESPIRATORY RATE = 12.5, TIDAL VOL.=  454. ML
TOTAL VENTILATION=   5.7 L/MIN, ACTUAL CARD.OUTPUT=   4.5 L/MIN
TOTAL DEAD SPACE= 181. CC, ACTUAL VENOUS ADMIXTURE=   1.7 PERCENT
```

*   THAT*S BETTER DOCTOR .....
       BUT ARE YOU GOING TO DO ANY OTHER NASTY THINGS TO ME?

```
DO YOU WANT TO..1.CHANGE, 2.CONTINUE, 3.RESTART, 4.INSPECT, 5.STOP
```

Figure VII.3 Continues from the previous figure and shows the manoeuvres necessary to change the value of Factor 1 (inspired oxygen percentage) from the current value of 20.9 to a new value of 100(%). At the same time as this was done the artificial ventilation was removed and natural ventilation was restored. The graph illustrates a rapid return of breathing to normal. The arterial PO_2 rapidly goes off scale owing to the high percentage of oxygen inspired and the PCO_2 is slightly above resting values because of the removal of the minor stimulus from hypoxia. Note also the symptom of improvement!

```
DO YOU WANT TO..1.CHANGE, 2.CONTINUE, 3.RESTART, 4.INSPECT, 5.STOP

? 1
1.CHANGE VALUES, 2.NAT/ART VENT, 3.STORE/BKTRK, 4.RUN CHANGE, 5.PRESETS
? 4
TYPE NO.OF SECONDS FOR RUN(1800 MAX.)
? 30
TYPE INTERVAL BETWEEN COMPUTATIONS IN SECS.(10 MAX.)
? 3
DO YOU WANT 1.ALL, 2.EVERY 6TH, OR 3.EVERY 30TH VALUE PRINTED
? 1
DO YOU WANT..1.GRAPHS + TEXT, 2.GRAPHS ONLY, 3.SELECTED VALUES
? 2
DO YOU WANT TO..1.CHANGE, 2.CONTINUE, 3.RESTART, 4.INSPECT, 5.STOP

? 2
    6. 3. V   F                    C
    6. 6. V   F                    C
    6. 9. V   F                C
    6.12. V   F                C
    6.15. V   F                    C
    6.18. V   F                    C
    6.21. V   F                C
    6.24. V   F                    C
    6.27. V   F                    C
    6.30. V   F                    C
DO YOU WANT TO..1.CHANGE, 2.CONTINUE, 3.RESTART, 4.INSPECT, 5.STOP

? 4
                P.PRESSURES       CONTENTS CC%     AMOUNTS IN CC     PH     HCO3-
                 O2      CO2       O2     CO2        O2      CO2

ARTERIAL       618.7    44.7     21.7    48.9       217.    484.    7.360   24.4
ALV./LUNG      653.8    44.6   (SAT=100.%)          2268.   160.
(PULM.CAP)     653.8    44.6     21.8    48.7
BRAIN/CSF       44.1    53.5     15.0    54.9        28.    686.    7.320   22.7
TISSUE/ECF      48.0  ( 50.3)    16.0    52.6       213.  13583.    7.337
MIXED VEN.  ( 48.0)  ( 50.3)    16.1    52.5       482.   1576.    7.338   26.1
PLASMA LACTATE CONC.= 0.9 MMOL/L

O2 UPTAKE=    309.   CO2 OUTPUT=    176. CC/MIN(STPD) EXPIRED R.Q.= 0.57
TOT.VENT.=   5.8   ALV.VENT(BTPS)= 3.5 R.RATE=12.5   VEN.ADMX.= 1.7
DEAD SPACE(BTPS)= 183.    TIDAL VOL.= 461. D.SP./TID.VL.RATIO=0.40
CARDIAC OUTPUT=   4.5    CEREBRAL BLOOD FLOW= 74. ML/100G/MIN


DO YOU WANT TO..1.CHANGE, 2.CONTINUE, 3.RESTART, 4.INSPECT, 5.STOP

? _
```

Figure VII.4   Illustration of alteration in the type of run by the RUN CHANGE option. Note that the total length of the run, the interval between computations (iteration interval) and the type of output were determined by the operator answering a series of simple questions. At the end of the run the INSPECT option was called for and a table of current values printed

```
DO YOU WANT TO..1.CHANGE, 2.CONTINUE, 3.RESTART, 4.INSPECT, 5.STOP

?.①
1.CHANGE VALUES, 2.NAT/ART VENT, 3.STORE/BKTRK, 4.RUN CHANGE, 5.PRESETS
?.④
TYPE NO.OF SECONDS FOR RUN(1800 MAX.)
?.⑫⓪
TYPE INTERVAL BETWEEN COMPUTATIONS IN SECS.(10 MAX.)
?.④
DO YOU WANT 1.ALL, 2.EVERY 6TH, OR 3.EVERY 30TH VALUE PRINTED
?.②
DO YOU WANT..1.GRAPHS + TEXT, 2.GRAPHS ONLY, 3.SELECTED VALUES
?.③
TYPE UP TO 8 NOS. - 69 IS STANDARD
?.⑨⑥ 97 95 16 45 46 47 48⓪
DO YOU WANT TO..1.CHANGE, 2.CONTINUE, 3.RESTART, 4.INSPECT, 5.STOP

?.⑧
I*M AFRAID YOUR NUMBER IS NO GOOD
PLEASE TRY AGAIN
?.②
  0.24    40.140   45.199    178.4    13.4    28.1    52.7   451.2    39.9
  0.48    40.061   45.197    178.0    13.4    28.0    52.8   456.8    39.9
  1.12    40.036   45.274    177.9    13.4    28.2    52.8   458.9    39.8
  1.36    40.032   45.309    177.9    13.4    28.3    52.8   460.7    39.8
  2. 0    40.029   45.322    177.9    13.4    28.4    52.9   462.2    39.7




--- MACPUF -- VERSION 76.4 --- 1 NOVEMBER 1976 ---



--- NEW SUBJECT ---

TO PROCEED TYPE 1 THEN PRESS CAR/RET KEY,
TO GET BRIEF DESCRIPTION AND INSTRUCTIONS TYPE 2 + C/R

?.⓪
TO USE S.I. UNITS(KPA) TYPE 1, FOR MM HG TYPE 2

?.②
*UNLESS CHANGED LATER, COLUMNS REFER AS FOLLOWS...FACTOR NUMBERS BELOW
          EXP.RQ   ART.PH   TOT-VENT-ALV    HCO3    ALV.PO2    PO2-ART-PCO2

MINS    ( 69)    ( 33)    ( 51)    ( 35)    ( 60)    ( 41)    ( 72)    ( 74)
  0. 0    0.801    7.399     5.9      4.3     23.8    101.9     94.2     39.9
DO YOU WANT TO..1.CHANGE, 2.CONTINUE, 3.RESTART, 4.INSPECT, 5.STOP
```

Figure VII.5 An example of the 'research mode' option allowing columns of selected values to be printed by the computer instead of graphs. The eight numbers typed consecutively code for variables in the COMMON store and '96, 97, 95, 16', etc. in practice refer to tissue PO_2, tissue PCO_2, tissue O_2 stores, tissue CO_2 stores, brain PO_2, brain PCO_2, tidal volume and respiratory rate. In the lower part of the illustration the model is called up directly in standard 'research mode' by entering zero instead of options 1 or 2 in response to the initial question. This then gives a series of eight columns showing expired RQ (factor 69), arterial pH (33), total ventilation (51), alveolar ventilation (35), arterial bicarbonate concentration (60), alveolar PO_2 (41), arterial PO_2 (72), and arterial PCO_2 (74)

```
DO YOU WANT TO..1.CHANGE, 2.CONTINUE, 3.RESTART, 4.INSPECT, 5.STOP

?.1
1.CHANGE VALUES, 2.NAT/ART VENT, 3.STORE/BKTRK, 4.RUN CHANGE, 5.PRESETS
?.1
TYPE NUMBER OF FACTORS (1-30) TO CHANGE, OR 100 FOR BAG EXPTS., ETC.
?.100
DO YOU WANT TO MAKE YOUR SUBJECT
1.CLOSE THE GLOTTIS,    2.COLLECT EXPIRED AIR IN A BAG,
3.REBREATHE FROM A BAG,    4.SAME, WITH CO2 ABSORBER ATTACHED,
5.RESTORE STATUS QUO - BREATHING AIR, GLOTTIS OPEN, NO BAG
?.3
DO YOU WANT..1. 100% O2, 2. A GAS MIXTURE, 3. TO GO ON WITH PREVIOUS BAG
?.2
GIVE INITIAL GAS VOLUME IN BAG, IN CC (BTPS)
?.550
SPECIFY PERCENT CO2
?.6.5
NOW PERCENT OXYGEN
?.70
***   550.CC BAG CONNECTED, CONTAINING  70.0% O2 +   6.5% CO2
DO YOU WANT TO..1.CHANGE, 2.CONTINUE, 3.RESTART, 4.INSPECT, 5.STOP

?.2/4
 1. 5.  V   F               C                              O
 1.10.  V   F               C                                    O
 1.15.  V   F                    C                                    O
 1.20.  V   F                    C
             P.PRESSURES     CONTENTS CC%    AMOUNTS IN CC   PH    HCO3-
             O2      CO2      O2      CO2     O2      CO2

ARTERIAL     132.0    45.8    19.9    52.1    199.    509.    7.379   25.0
ALV./LUNG    145.8    47.7 (SAT= 99.%)        500.    165.
(PULM.CAP)   145.8    47.7    20.0    52.3
BRAIN/CSF     30.1    53.2    10.5    56.9     19.    682.    7.324   22.7
TISSUE/ECF    40.3  ( 45.5)   14.5    51.6    180.  13398.    7.370
MIXED VEN. ( 40.3) ( 45.5)    14.6    51.3    438.   1540.    7.373   25.6
***** BAG.   142.3    44.6                     82.     26.   *N2=    278.
* BAG VOL.   466. (BTPS)
PLASMA LACTATE CONC.= 1.0 MMOL/L

O2 UPTAKE=    155.  CO2 OUTPUT=    -23. CC/MIN(STPD) EXPIRED R.Q.=-0.15
TOT.VENT.=   5.5  ALV.VENT(BTPS)= 3.8 R.RATE=12.6  VEN.ADMX.= 1.6
DEAD SPACE(BTPS)= 135.   TIDAL VOL.= 432. D.SP./TID.VL.RATIO=0.31
CARDIAC OUTPUT=   4.9   CEREBRAL BLOOD FLOW= 57. ML/100G/MIN


DO YOU WANT TO..1.CHANGE, 2.CONTINUE, 3.RESTART, 4.INSPECT, 5.STOP

?.1
1.CHANGE VALUES, 2.NAT/ART VENT, 3.STORE/BKTRK, 4.RUN CHANGE, 5.PRESETS
?.5
DO YOU WANT..1.PRESET PATIENTS OR  SUBJECTS
2.TO SPECIFY YOUR OWN PATIENTS  OR SUBJECTS
?.1
THE FOLLOWING PRESET PATIENTS ARE AVAILABLE
1. NORMAL FIT SUBJECT EXERCISING AT 300 KPM/MIN
2. SAME, AT 900 KPM/MIN
3. UNFIT NORMAL SUBJECT EXERCISING AT 900 KPM/MIN
4. NORMAL SUBJECT, COMPRESSED TO 10 ATMOSPHERES FOR 25 MINUTES
5. CHRONIC AIRWAYS OBSTRUCTION WITH VENTILATORY FAILURE
6. SAME, BUT WITH ACUTE EXACERBATION, EG. ADDED BRONCHOPNEUMONIA
7. CHEYNE-STOKES BREATHING DUE TO BRAIN STEM DAMAGE AND HEART DISEEASE
...TYPE NUMBER
```

Figure VII.6 Illustrates the use of a BAG REBREATHING option in which a 550 cc bag filled with 6.5% CO_2 in 70% oxygen was connected to the mouth and rebreathed for 20 seconds, after which an INSPECT table displayed the volume, partial pressures and amounts of individual gases in the bag. The lower part of Figure VII.6 indicates the calling up of one of the preset subjects

```
DO YOU WANT TO..1.CHANGE, 2.CONTINUE, 3.RESTART, 4.INSPECT, 5.STOP

?(1)
1.CHANGE VALUES, 2.NAT/ART VENT, 3.STORE/BKTRK, 4.RUN CHANGE, 5.PRESETS
?(1)
TYPE NUMBER OF FACTORS (1-30) TO CHANGE, OR 100 FOR BAG EXPTS., ETC.
?(1 2)
FACTOR    1 (CURRENT VALUE=   20.9), SPECIFY NEW VALUE
?(0)
FACTOR    1 =     0.0 (PREVIOUSLY =   20.9)
FACTOR    2 (CURRENT VALUE=    0.0), SPECIFY NEW VALUE
?(5)
FACTOR    2 =     5.0 (PREVIOUSLY =    0.0)
DO YOU WANT TO..1.CHANGE, 2.CONTINUE, 3.RESTART, 4.INSPECT, 5.STOP

?(2)
(KPA)(0)               (4)             (8)          (12)           (16)
 MINS 0        20         40         60        80         100        120
+SECS .     .      .      .      .      .      .      .      .      .      .
ITERATION INTERVAL TOO LONG FOR THIS SITUATION.  I HAVE SHORTENED IT.
TO CHANGE BACK, USE *4.RUN CHANGE* OPTION

   0. 5.  V  F           C                       O
   0.10.  V  F           C               O
   0.15.  V  F            C         O
   0.20.    V  F         C     O
   0.25.       VF        CO


DO YOU WANT TO..1.CHANGE, 2.CONTINUE, 3.RESTART, 4.INSPECT, 5.STOP

?(1/1/1 2/0/5/2)
FACTOR    1 =     0.0 (PREVIOUSLY =   20.9)
FACTOR    2 =     5.0 (PREVIOUSLY =    0.0)
(KPA)(0)               (4)             (8)          (12)           (16)
 MINS 0        20         40         60        80         100        120
+SECS .     .      .      .      .      .      .      .      .      .      .
ITERATION INTERVAL TOO LONG FOR THIS SITUATION.  I HAVE SHORTENED IT.
TO CHANGE BACK, USE *4.RUN CHANGE* OPTION

   0. 5.  V  F           C                       O
   0.10.  V  F           C               O
   0.15.  V  F            C         O
   0.20.    V  F         C     O
   0.25.       VF        CO
```

Figure VII.7 Illustrates the use of the 'slash/separator' to speed up operation of the model. In the dialogue above factors 1 and 2 are successively changed to 0 and 5% respectively, after which the model is then started running. The illustration below indicates that the text can be suppressed and all the desired changes economically specified by a string of numerical instructions separated by slashes

```
                                                            APPROX.
                                                      NORMAL VALUE

 1.INSPIRED O2, %                                            20.93
 2.INSPIRED CO2, %                                            0.03
 3.CARDIAC PUMP PERFORMANCE, AS  %NORMAL (= 5 L/MIN NORMALLY) 100
 4.METABOLIC RATE, AS  %NORMAL RESTING VALUE,↑ TO SIM. EXERCISE 100
 5.EXTRA ANAT. RIGHT-TO-LEFT SHUNT, AS  %CARDIAC OUTPUT         0
 6.EXTRA DEAD SPACE, IN CC BTPS, ABOVE NORMAL VALUE            0
 7.LUNG VOLUME, CC BTPS  (END-EXPIRATION)                   3000
 8.LUNG ELASTANCE, CC H2O/LITRE  (AN INCREASE MAKES BREATHING   5
   FASTER, AND STIFFER LUNGS REDUCE ILL EFFECTS OF 'PEEP')
 9.VENOUS ADMIXTURE EFFECT AS  %CARDIAC OUTPUT                 3
   (SHUNT EFFECT OF FACTOR 9 MODIFIED BY ALV.PO2.  FACTOR 5
   SPECIFIES FIXED INDEPENDENT SHUNT - EG. CONGEN.HEART DISEASE)
10.VENTILATORY RESPONSE TO CO2 OR H+ AS  %AVERAGE NORMAL     100
11.VENTILATORY RESPONSE TO FALLING PO2, AS  %AVERAGE NORMAL  100
12.'CENTRAL NEUROGENIC (LEARNT) RESPIRATORY DRIVE' AS  %NORMAL 100
   (RISES IN PROPORTION TO %METABOLIC RATE AND O2 CONSUMPTION)
13.BAROMETRIC PRESSURE, MM HG (OR KPA -DEPENDS ON INIT.SETTING) 760
14.BODY TEMPERATURE, DEGREES CENTIGRADE                       37
15.TISSUE RESP.QUOTIENT (CO2 OUTPUT/O2 UPTAKE)               0.8
16.TISSUE CO2 STORES, LITRES STPD                            13
17.TISSUE ECF DISTRIBUTION VOLUME, LITRES                    12
18.HAEMOGLOBIN, G/100 ML BLOOD                             14.8
19.PACKED CELL VOLUME,                                       45
20.VENOUS BLOOD VOLUME, ML                                 3000
21.ADDITION OF BICARBONATE OR ACID, MMOL STANDARD BICARBONATE.  0
   (ADDITION SPECIFIED IS MADE GRADUALLY OVER SUCCEEDING RUN,
   THEN VALUE OF FACTOR 21 IS RETURNED TO ZERO.  IF A NEGATIVE
   VALUE IS ENTERED, THAT NUMBER OF MMOL STRONG ACID ARE
   ADDED INSTEAD)
22.BRAIN BICARBONATE, MMOL/L, DEVIATION FROM NORMAL VALUE (+/-)  0
   (ALLOWS SIMULATION OF CHRONIC ACID/BASE DISTURBANCES.
   BRAIN HCO3 WILL SLOWLY CHANGE ANYWAY; BUT YOU CAN SPEED UP
   EQUILIBRATION A LOT BY CHANGING THIS FACTOR APPROPRIATELY)
23.2,3-DIPHOSPHOGLYCERATE CONC. IN RED CELLS, MMOL/L        3.8
24.'BREATHING CAPACITY',  %NORMAL AVERAGE VALUE             100
   (ACTS ON SUMMATED EFFECTS OF FACTORS 10,11, AND 12 ABOVE,
   AND GOVERNS COUPLING OF VENTILATORY STIMULI TO RESPONSE).
25.STATE OF PHYSICAL FITNESS...THRESHOLD FOR SWITCH TO ANAEROBIC 33
   METABOLISM. >33 LOWERS THE THRESHOLD, THEREBY SIMULATING
   UNFITNESS.  <33 SIMULATES INCREASED FITNESS. (ARB.UNITS,
   MM HG, MIXED VENOUS PO2.  RANGE 30-37)
26.INSPIRATORY/TOTAL BREATH DURATION RATIO                  0.4
   (I.E. VALUE OF 0.4 MEANS INSPIRATION OCCUPIES 40% OF THE
   TIME TAKEN FOR ONE COMPLETE RESPIRATORY CYCLE)
27.MAXIMUM CARDIAC OUTPUT, L/MIN                             35
28.LEFT-TO-RIGHT SHUNT, AS RATIO OF CARDIAC OUTPUT -          0
   (E.G. A VALUE OF 2.0 SPECIFIES A 2/1 SHUNT)
29.VITAL CAPACITY, LITRES BTPS                                5
   (MAXIMUM TIDAL VOLUME IS LIMITED TO 60%  OF THIS VALUE)
30.POSITIVE END-EXPIRATORY PRESSURE, CM H2O                   0
```

Figure VII.8 List of changeable parameters or factors (numbered 1 to 30). (The first six are printed in abbreviated form when 'MacPuf' is first called up.)

```
                                                    APPROX.
                                             NORMAL VALUE

LUNGS************************************* ALVEOLAR/LUNG ***************
     O2- AMOUNT, CC STPD (39)                            345
          P.PRESSURE, MM HG (41)                         100
          CONTENT IN IDEALISED PULM.CAP.BLOOD, CC/DL (54)  20
     CO2- AMOUNT, CC STPD (40)                           145
          P.PRESSURE, MM HG (42)                          40
          CONTENT IN IDEALISED PULM.CAP.BLOOD, CC/DL (53)  47
     N2- AMOUNT, CC STPD (65)                           2000
ARTERIES********************************* ARTERIAL BLOOD POOL ********
     O2- AMOUNT, CC STPD (62)                            200
          P.PRESSURE, MM HG (72)                          92
          CONTENT, CC/100 ML (49)                         20
          CONTENT OF BLOOD LEAVING ART.POOL (94)          20
          SATURATION,    MAXIMUM (76)                     97
     CO2- AMOUNT, CC STPD (63)                           500
          P.PRESSURE, MM HG (74)                          40
          CONTENT, CC/100 ML (78)                         50
          CONTENT OF BLOOD LEAVING POOL (101)             50
     N2- P.PRESSURE, MM HG (108)                         570
          CONTENT OF BLOOD LEAVING POOL, CC/100 ML (106)  0.8
HCO3- CONTENT, MMOL/L (60)                                25
LACTATE- CONCENTRATION, MMOL/L (90)                      1.0
PH-  (33)                                                7.4
BRAIN************************************* BRAIN **********************
     O2- AMOUNT, CC STPD (66)                             22
          P.PRESSURE, MM HG, OF BLOOD LEAVING BRAIN (45)  33
          CONTENT, CC/100 ML, OF BLOOD LEAVING BRAIN (57) 13
     CO2- AMOUNT, CC STPD (67)                           650
          P.PRESSURE, MM HG, OF BLOOD LEAVING BRAIN (46)  55
          CONTENT, CC/100 ML, OF BLOOD LEAVING BRAIN (58) 56
HCO3- CONTENT, MMOL/L, OF BLOOD LEAVING BRAIN (22)        22
          (BUT NOTE THAT EFFECTIVE BRAIN HCO3 IS ALGEBRAIC
          SUM OF FACTOR 22 AND FACTOR 92 - FORMER=ADAPTATION)
PH- AT PUTATIVE CENTRAL CHEMORECEPTOR SITE (36)          7.35
FLOW- OF BLOOD, ML/100 G. BRAIN PER MINUTE (68)           55
TISSUES********************************* LUMPED TISSUE POOL *********
     O2- AMOUNT, CC STPD (95)                            175
          P.PRESSURE, MM HG (96)                          40
          CONTENT, CC/100 ML, OF BLOOD LEAVING TISSUES (55) 15
     CO2- AMOUNT, CC STPD (16)                         15000
          P.PRESSURE, MM HG (97) (TIME SHIFTED...APPROX. VALUE) 47
          CONTENT, CC/100 ML, OF BLOOD LEAVING TISSUES (66) 55
     N2- AMOUNT IN FAST-EQUILIBRATING COMPARTMENT, CC STPD (102)  60
          AMOUNT IN SLOWLY-EQUILIBRATING COMPARTMENT, CC STPD(112) 900
          AMOUNT HELD ABOVE NORMAL MAX.SATURATION, CC STPD (107)   0
          ARBITRARY INDEX OF RISK OF DECOMPRESSION SYMPTOMS (83)   0
          (MAXIMUM SAFE VALUE UP TO 100)
          P.PRESSURE, MM HG, IN FAST-EQUILIBRATING STORE (103)   570
          P.PRESSURE, MM HG, IN SLOWLY-EQUILIBRATING STORE (105) 570
HCO3- CONTENT, MMOL/L, OF BLOOD LEAVING TISSUES (87)      26
LACTATE- TOTAL AMOUNT IN BODY, MMOL (89)                  35

     PH- OF BLOOD LEAVING TISSUES (59)                   7.38
```

[continued

```
        LIST OF COMPUTED VARIABLES (CONTINUED)

VEINS************************************* VENOUS BLOOD POOL **********
    02- AMOUNT, CC STPD, IN WHOLE POOL (98)                         440
        P.PRESSURE, MM HG (96) (TIME SHIFTED...APPROX. VALUE)        40
        (MIXED VENOUS BLOOD P.PRESSURES BOTH OF O2 AND CO2 ARE
        NOT COMPUTED, TO ECONOMISE ON COMPUTING TIME. APPROX.
        TISSUE VALUES ARE USED INSTEAD, HENCE THE TIME SHIFT.
        BUT THE CONTENTS OF THE GASES IN MIXED VENOUS BLOOD
        ARE CORRECT, AND HAVE BEEN CORRECTLY DELAYED IN
        TRANSIT THROUGH THE VENOUS BLOOD POOL)
        CONTENT, CC/100 ML, OF BLOOD IN PULMONARY ARTERY (31)        15
    CO2- AMOUNT, CC STPD, IN VENOUS BLOOD POOL (50)                1600
        P.PRESSURE, MM HG (97) - SEE NOTE ABOVE FOR O2               47
        CONTENT, CC/100 ML, OF BLOOD IN PULMONARY ARTERY (61)        55
    HCO3- CONTENT, MMOL/L, OF MIXED VENOUS BLOOD (88)                27
      PH- OF MIXED VENOUS BLOOD (34)                               7.38
BAG*************************** BAG FOR COLLECTION OR REBREATHING ***
    VOL.- CC BTPS (116)              (ALL THESE REMAIN)              0
    O2- AMOUNT, CC STPD (37)         (UNCHANGED WHILE BAG)           0
    CO2- AMOUNT, CC STPD (38)        (IS DISCONNECTED)               0
OTHERS************************************** MISC. OTHER VALUES *********
CARDIAC OUTPUT-ACTUAL EFFECTIVE CARDIAC OUTPUT, L/MIN (93)          4.8
DEAD SPACE -    TOTAL EFFECTIVE PHYSIOLOGICAL, CC BTPS (70)         130
RESPIRATORY EXCHANGE RATIO  (69)  (CO2 OUTPUT IN LAST ITERATION     0.8
                    INTERVAL, DIVIDED BY O2 CONSUMPTION.  A NORMAL
                    VALUE SHOWS THAT THERE IS A STEADY STATE)
RESP. RATE    - CYCLES/MINUTE (48)                                  14
TIDAL VOL.    - CC BTPS (47)                                        450
VEN.ADMIXT.   - TOTAL EFFECTIVE ADMIXT., AS   %CARDIAC OUTPUT (80)   3
VENTILATION
      TOTAL   - LITRES/MIN, BTPS (51)                               6.5
    ALVEOLAR  - LITRES/MIN, BTPS (35)                               4.2
```

Figure VII.9   List of computed variables. The number in brackets after each is the corresponding factor number, allowing any of these factions to be displayed in columns by using the 'run change' option. (The 'normal values are given in mmHg, but an initial call for S.I. units will give all in KPA.)

FACTOR NEGATIVE	MEANING OF ERROR	PROBABLE CAUSE	SUGGESTED REMEDY
0	TIDAL VOL.TOO LARGE FOR BAG	BAG TOO SMALL	USE LARGER BAG OR SHORTEN RUN
OR...PUL.CAP.BLOOD	HCO3 FELL TOO FAST TO ALLOW EQUILIBRATION	SUDDEN FALL IN ALVEOLAR PCO2 (E.G. SUDDEN HYPERVENTILATION)	CHANGE CO2 OR VENTILATION MORE SLOWLY. IF THIS IS IMPOSSIBLE, SHORTEN TIME INTERVAL AND AND RERUN
41	ALVEOLAR O2 LESS THAN 0	SUDDEN FALL IN ALV.PO2	CHANGE O2 MORE SLOWLY OR SHORTEN TIME INTERVAL
42	ALVEOLAR CO2 LESS THAN 0	SUDDEN FALL IN ALV. PCO2	CHANGE CO2 OR VENTILATION OR ADD HCO3 MORE SLOWLY OR SHORTEN TIME INTERVAL
60	ART. HCO3 LESS THAN 0	SUDDEN FALL IN ALV.PCO2 OR TOO MUCH ACID GIVEN OR MADE TOO QUICKLY	SHORTEN TIME INTERVAL CONSIDERABLY AND RERUN AND/OR GIVE ACID MORE SLOWLY
87	TISSUE HCO3 LESS THAN 0	VERY RAPID ADDN. OF ACID OR TOO RAPID GEN. OF LACTIC ACIDOSIS	ADD ACID MORE SLOWLY OR RERUN AT MUCH SHORTER TIME INTERVAL
88	VENOUS HCO3 LESS THAN 0	TOO RAPID ADDN. OF ACID	ADD ACID MORE SLOWLY
95	TISSUE OXYGEN LESS THAN 0	NOT ENOUGH TIME FOR ANAEROBIC MET. TO GET GOING	SHORTEN TIME INTERVAL AND RERUN

Figure VII.10   Error messages

Index

Date D